ORAL MANIFESTATIONS OF INHERITED DISORDERS

Heddie O. Sedano, D.D.S., Dr. Odont.

Associate Professor, Department of Oral Pathology, University of Minnesota School of Dentistry; Graduate Faculty; Director of Oral Pathology Clinic, University of Minnesota School of Dentistry

John J. Sauk, Jr., D.D.S., M.S.

Associate Professor, Department of Human and Oral Genetics and Oral Pathology, University of Minnesota School of Dentistry

Robert J. Gorlin, D.D.S., M.S.

Professor and Chairman, Department of Oral Pathology, University of Minnesota School of Dentistry; Professor of Pathology, Dermatology, Pediatrics, Obstetrics and Gynecology, Otolaryngology, University of Minnesota School of Medicine

BUTTERWORTHS
Boston London

The Butterworth Group

UNITED STATES
Butterworth (Publishers) Inc.
19 Cummings Park
Woburn, MA 01801

ENGLAND
Butterworth & Co. (Publishers) Ltd.
88 Kingsway
London WC2B 6AB

AUSTRALIA
Butterworth Pty Ltd
586 Pacific Highway
Chatswood, NSW 2067

CANADA
Butterworth & Co. (Canada) Ltd.
2265 Midland Avenue
Scarborough, Ontario M1P 4S1

NEW ZEALAND
Butterworths of New Zealand Ltd.
26–28 Waring Taylor Street
Wellington 1

SOUTH AFRICA
Butterworth & Co. (South Africa) (Pty) Ltd.
152–154 Gale Street, Durban

Printed in the United States of America.

Library of Congress Cataloging in Publication Data

Sedano, Heddie O.
Oral manifestations of inherited disorders.

Bibliography: p.
Includes index.
1. Oral manifestations of general diseases. 2. Medical genetics.
I. Sauk, John J., joint author.
II. Gorlin, Robert J., joint author.
III. Title. [DNLM: 1. Hereditary diseases. 2. Oral manifestations.

WU290 S447o]
RC815.S455 616'.042 77-8363
ISBN 0-409-95050-5

Contents

Preface

During the last ten years the pathology of inherited disorders has been explored to such an extent that today a veritable plethora of possible clinical combinations have been covered in many excellent works. The presence of orodental anomalies in systemic inherited disorders is so frequent as to include the great majority of known genetic syndromes. It was, therefore, not an easy task to assemble this book.

The number of conditions that still are of debatable inheritance is such that the decision-making process "to include or not to include" became very arduous. Therefore, a number of syndromes with obvious oral manifestations were included even if their inheritance pattern is yet to be clarified. Many conditions were purposely excluded because the degree of oral involvement is minimal (or even of doubtful association with a given syndrome). Sporadic case reports are often seen in the literature presenting both oral anomalies and indications of an inheritance pattern in patients who cannot be classified within any known syndrome. It was the consensus of the authors to exclude those disorders not yet properly classified.

This book emphasizes inherited systemic disorders presenting oral manifestations which have been reported as an integral part of the disorder. Chapter 2 has been devoted to some inherited conditions affecting only calcified dental tissues, for the purpose of differential diagnosis. Classification of the conditions described in chapters 3–7 has by no means been attempted. It is almost impossible to classify such a large group of disorders in any single manner. We have decided to divide them based upon the affected orodental structures as follows:

Systemic inherited disorders with dental involvement.

Systemic inherited disorders with oral and/or perioral soft tissue involvement.

Systemic inherited disorders with involvement of jaw bones.

Systemic inherited disorders associated with facial clefting.

Systemic inherited disorders with involvement of multiple oral structures.

The basic criterion for incorporating a condition in a particular group was that only those oral structures which are constantly or characteristically affected in a given condition were used. Those oral structures which are sporadically reported as the site of anomalies in the same condition were disregarded as a parameter.

When an anomaly occurs as a consequence of a primary defect, the site of such an anomaly was also not considered for the purpose of division. For example, the crowding of teeth in Apert syndrome was considered to be secondary to maxillary hypoplasia; therefore, it was disregarded and the Apert syndrome was included with disorders associated with jaw bone involvement. Within each subdivision the different disorders were arranged alphabetically.

We hope that the effort of amalgamating these conditions in a text will be of benefit to those professionals interested not only in malformation syndromes but also in the oral manifestations of inherited disorders. Finally, the goal of this book is to provide a basis for proper genetic counseling.

We would like to gratefully acknowledge the National Institutes of Health for financial aid in grant DE-01770. Part of this work was accomplished during a sabbatical leave of absence granted to one of us (H.O.S.) by the regents of the University of Minnesota, to whom we are indebted. The completion of this book would not have been possible without the expert and patient help of LeRoy B. Christenson and the staff of Audio-Visual Media Resources, School of Dentistry, University of Minnesota, who produced the photographic material. Our thanks also go to John Molstad for his accurate graphs and drawings. Finally, we wish to express our profound thanks to Oliv A. Flück and Virginia Hansen for typing and retyping as well as for their precise and careful proofreading of the manuscript.

ORAL MANIFESTATIONS OF INHERITED DISORDERS

CHAPTER 1

Genetic Counseling and Oral Examination

1.1 Genetic Counseling

A distinctive pattern of signs and symptoms constitutes a syndrome. Knowledge of the pattern may enable the clinician to make a diagnosis. Changes and variations occur within a single syndrome, but when understood as part of the malformation processes, they actually enhance the clinical description by adding further diagnostic criteria. Labeling a disorder not only satisfies the diagnostician, but diminishes the anxiety of patients and their relatives.

Having an unknown or extremely rare disorder or one "that no one ever heard of" is distressing. Even more dangerous, however, is incorrect diagnosis. For example, we have seen a young teenager with the Melnick-Needles syndrome, an essentially benign disorder, who was told she had osteogenesis imperfecta. Considerable time and psychological support were required to correct this clinical error in judgment.

Counseling patients with inherited disorders is sometimes rewarding, but often the proband will leave the office and forget the possible consequences to which their progeny may be subject. Some forget they ever received counseling, while many others will recall that counseling was given but will not have understood the information. It is imperative, therefore, that the counselor speak at the patients' level of comprehension. It is advisable that he/she have the counselees repeat in their own words what has been discussed. Counseling can be provided by a geneticist, a physician, or a dentist. The only key requirement is that the counselor be knowledgeable concerning the disorder about which he/she is being consulted and about its inheritance pattern. The counselor should seek advice in all doubtful cases.

It is important not only that the patients and their relatives understand the chances of having similarly affected children but that they comprehend fully the prognosis for the disorder. The counselor must remember that learning that one is the carrier of a heritable disorder often awakens a marked feeling of guilt which eventually may be transferred to and shared by the nearest relatives. It is advisable that the counselor, if possible, be thoroughly familiar with the patient and that he/she fully understand the psychological complications that the diagnosis of a severe inherited condition may produce. At the risk of boring some readers, a brief review of single gene inheritance patterns is undertaken here.

Autosomal Dominant Inheritance. For an affected parent the risk of having an affected offspring is 50% in each pregnancy. One must remember that this is merely an estimate of probability. In a small family with two children for example, none, one, or both may be affected. Males and females are equally affected. The condition is therefore carried vertically from one generation to the next. Failure of the condition to be expressed at all in an individual inheriting the gene is referred to as lack of penetrance. An isolated example of a condition known to be autosomal dominant may represent a new mutation or a misrepresentation of paternity or, rarely, maternity. Autosomal dominant disorders often vary in severity among the individuals affected (variable expressivity).

Autosomal Recessive Inheritance. The parents of children with autosomal recessive disorders characteristically are phenotypically normal. They are recognized as carriers of the gene (heterozygotes) after the birth of an affected offspring. For parents who have had one affected offspring, the risk of recurrence is 25% in each pregnancy. If the gene is rare, a history of parental consanguinity is frequently present. Male and female offspring are affected in approximately equal proportion. For known heterozygote parents, the probability of having a homozygote normal offspring is 25%; the risk of having a heterozygote carrier offspring is 50% and, as mentioned above, the risk of having a homozygote affected offspring is 25% in every pregnancy.

X-linked Inheritance. Females can be either heterozygous or homozygous for a given mutant gene, because they have two X-chromosomes. Therefore, in the female, X-linked conditions can be either recessive or dominant. When a mutant gene in the X-chromosome is present in the male, it will always be expressed clinically, regardless of the dominant or recessive behavior of the same mutant gene in the female, because males are hemizygous for the X-chromosome.

Females may manifest X-linked recessive disorders in modified form, for they are heterozygous since one X-chromosome is randomly "turned off" (heteropyknotic). This is known as the Lyon hypothesis. The X chromosome in the male is transmitted to none of his sons and to all of his daughters. Therefore there is absence of male-to-male (father-to-son) transmission. There are a few conditions that have X-linked inheritance which are lethal in the male. The female is able to survive possibly due to the action of the normal allelic gene in one of the X-chromosomes. A female carrier of an X-linked recessive trait has a 50% risk of having an affected son and a 50% risk of having a carrier daughter in each pregnancy. For an affected mother with a dominant X-linked condition, the risk of having a male or female affected offspring is 50% in each pregnancy.

Genetic Heterogeneity. The term indicates that a disorder has more than one inheritance pattern, as well as differences in the degree of clinical manifestations for each inherited form.

Polygenic Inheritance. The term defines those conditions which are inherited through the participation of several genes with little environmental influence. Such conditions generally present a greater variability in clinical expression than disorders due to a single gene.

Multifactorial Conditions. The term is used to refer to a phenotype that is the result of a combination of genetic factors and environmental influences.

Codominance. The term is used to refer to those conditions in which both allelic genes are manifested in the heterozygote state. The most well known example is the AB blood group.

Consanguinity. The term that literally means related by blood is used to refer to individuals who have at least one common ancestor. Figure 1.1 illustrates the most frequent patterns of consanguinity observed in genetic counseling.

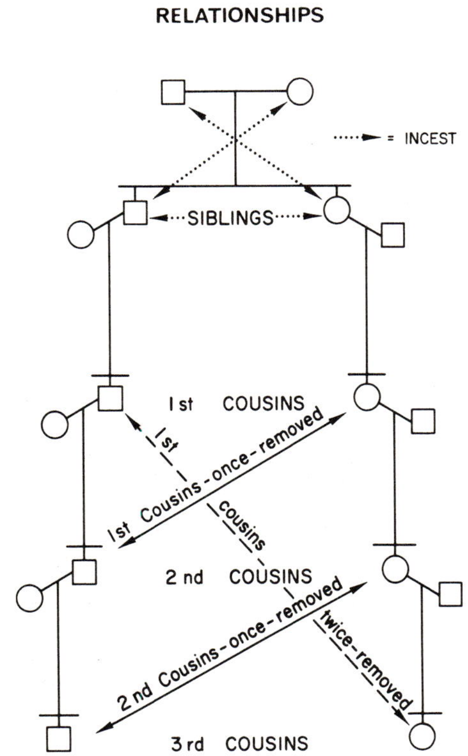

Fig. 1.1. Chart of relationships.

1.2 Physical Examination of the Oral Cavity

Many heritable syndromes have distinctive oral manifestations which aid the diagnostician; therefore, a brief review of the normal oral configuration and some of the frequent variations from normal will be undertaken here. Two indispensable aids are needed in order to perform an accurate oral examination: an intraoral mirror and good illumination. Manifestations of inherited disorders may occur in any area of the oral cavity; a systematic approach to clinical inspection is recommended. It is our preference to start by inspecting the lips, then the right buccal mucosa, palate, left buccal mucosa, tongue, floor of mouth, and fauces. Following these, the gingiva and teeth are inspected, starting from the maxillary right molar area to the left maxillary molar area, then from the mandibular left molar area to the right mandibular molar area.

The mouth is classically divided into two parts: the vestibule and the oral cavity proper. The vestibule is bounded by the teeth and gingiva on the one side and by the buccal and labial mucosae on the other. The roof and floor of this area are known as the vestibular sulci. Within the sulcus, frenulas are normally seen in the anterior maxilla and mandible, extending from the lip to the gingival mucosa (Fig. 1.2). Lateral frenulas extend from the buccal mucosa to the gingiva, generally bilaterally, at the level of both mandibular and maxillary premolars. Abnormally thick frenulas are seen in the orofacial digital I syndrome. The vestibular sulcus is entirely absent in the anterior mandibular and maxillary areas in the Ellis-van Creveld syndrome.

Lip and Buccal Mucosae. The labial and buccal mucosae are generally shiny with a pale pink color; the mucous membranes are kept moist by the constant salivary flow. Various conditions are associated with diminished or absent excretion of saliva. This can be demonstrated easily by simply touching the buccal mucosa with a finger tip. Normally the finger will run smoothly over the surface. If there is dryness of the mouth (xerostomia), the finger will adhere to the mucosal surface.

Whitening of the oral soft tissues, generally known as leukoplakia, is also associated with some inherited disorders. Other white conditions are frequently found, such as linea alba (Fig. 1.3), a bilateral white line lo-

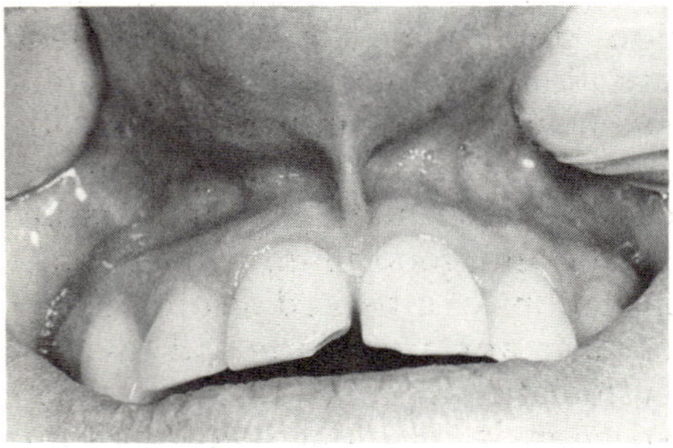

Fig. 1.2. Vestibular sulcus and labial frenulum.

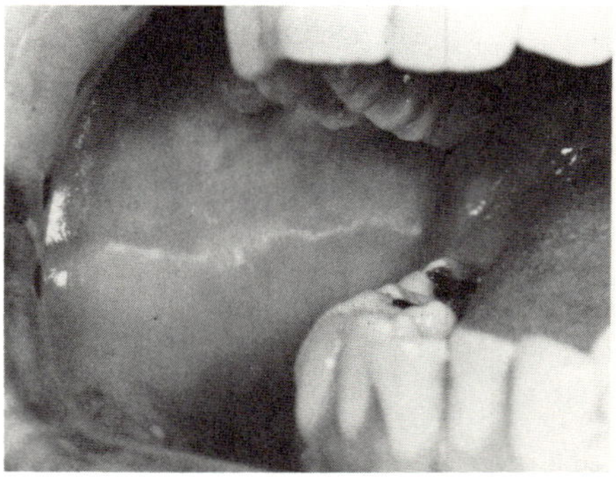

Fig. 1.3. Linea alba.

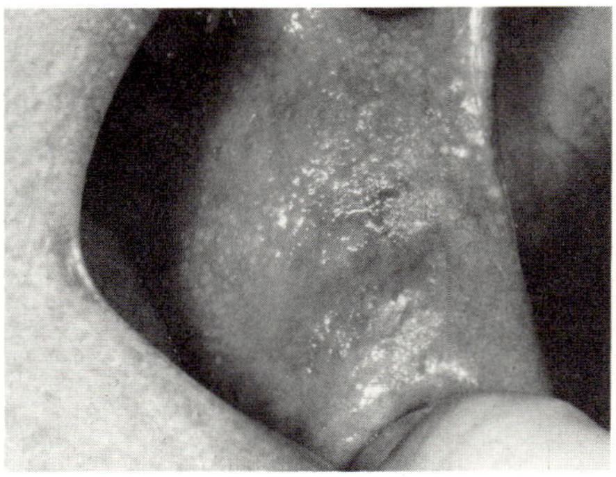

Fig. 1.4. Morsicatio buccarum.

cated on the buccal mucosa that follows the plane of occlusion. Some patients, and especially mentally retarded individuals, have the habit of chewing their labial or buccal mucosa or both (morsicatio buccarum). The tissues appear as if macerated, with an irregular white coating (Fig. 1.4). On the buccal mucosa at the level of the maxillary first molars is a triangular papilla that protects the opening of the Stensen duct (main excretory duct of the parotid gland). Both labial and buccal mucosae contain numerous minor salivary glands that occasionally may produce a pebbly appearance (Fig. 1.5). In around 80% of

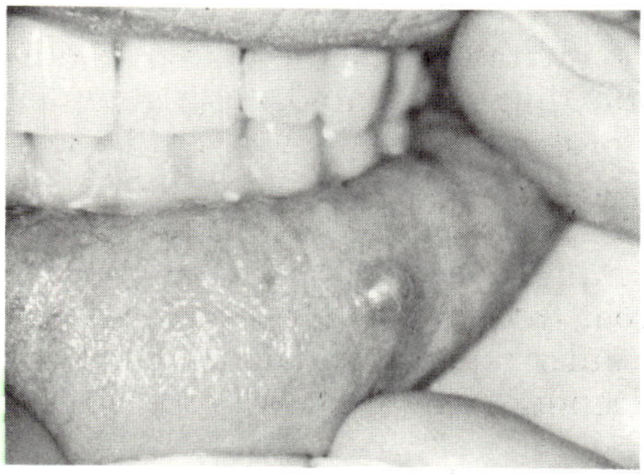

Fig. 1.5. Pebbly appearance of lower lip. Also note small protuberance which represents a mucocele (cystic retention of saliva).

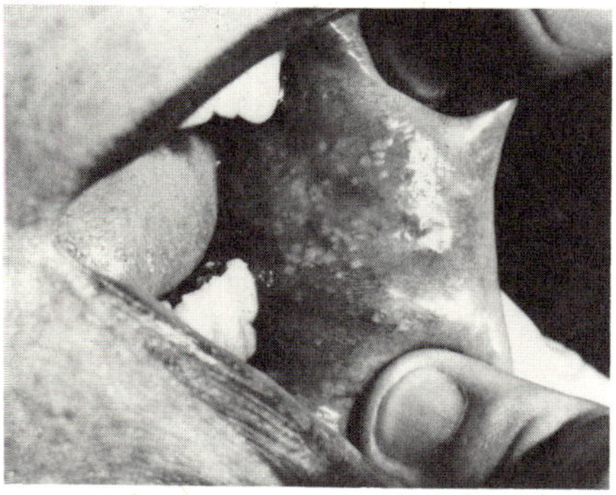

Fig. 1.6. Fordyce granules.

the population, ectopic sebaceous glands can be found both in the buccal and labial mucosae. These glands vary in shape and number, but they always present a yellowish color (Fig. 1.6). The red external margin of the lips, ie, the transition zone between skin and mucous membrane is known as the vermilion border.

Palate. The hard palate is slightly paler than the rest of the oral mucosa since it is covered by a layer of keratin. Normally, ridges called palatal rugae are seen in the anterior portion radiating from a central larger ridge, the incisive papilla (Fig. 1.7). The shape and distribution of these rugae are peculiar to each individual. In the palatal midline, running in an anteroposterior direction from the incisive papilla to the junction with the soft palate, the palatine raphe can be seen as a slightly elevated ridge. The center of the hard palate is the site, in some individuals, of a bony protuberance of variable degree and shape, known as torus palatinus (Fig. 1.8). This bony exostosis is generally only seen after puberty.

Salivary glands are also located in the posterior one-third of the hard

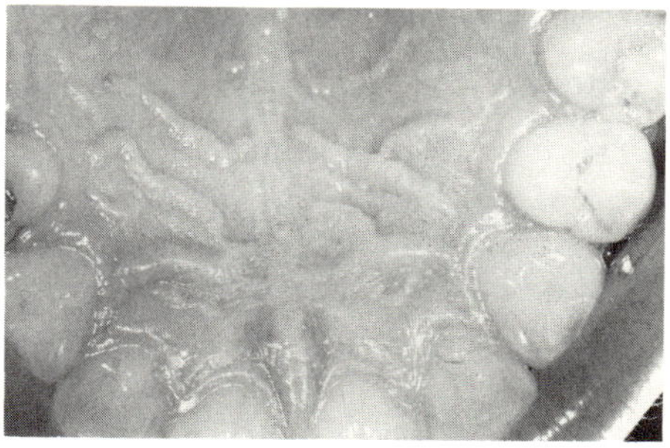

Fig. 1.7. Normal palate showing incisive papilla, palatal rugae, and palatine raphe.

palate, bilaterally and off the midline. Often the literature reads that a patient has a "high-arched palate"; generally this observation is based upon a merely visual appreciation. Accurate determination of palatal height and width can be obtained by special devices. Normal mean values for different ages have been determined by Shapiro and his colleagues.[1]

The soft palate is generally redder than the hard palate and extends toward the fauces. Laterally it fuses with the pharyngeal wall, giving rise on each side to the palatoglossal folds. The uvula is a conoid extension of soft tissue located in the midline of the free border of the soft palate.

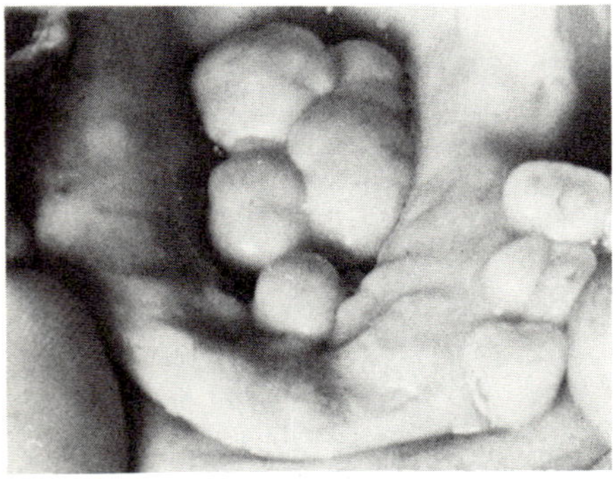

Fig. 1.8. Torus palatinus, multilobulated variety.

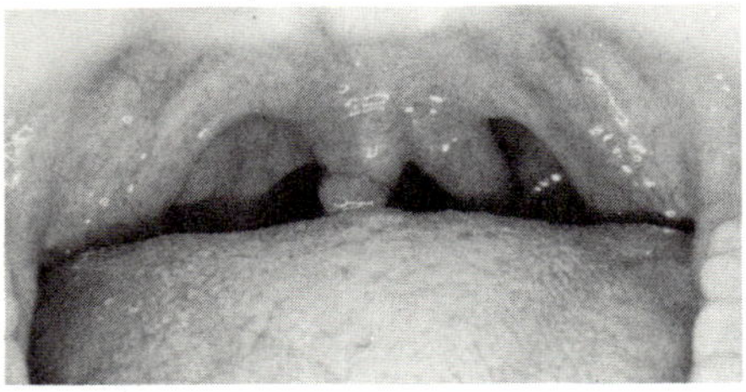

Fig. 1.9. Bifid uvula.

Submucous cleft can be detected easily by manual palpation of the palate. Bifid uvula occurs in around 1 in 100 people, and it is considered a minor form of cleft palate (Fig. 1.9). Numerous minor salivary glands are also found in the soft palatal mucosa.

Tongue. The dorsum of the tongue is divided into two sections by the sulcus terminalis and the lingual V (Fig. 1.10). The V is formed by eight to twelve vallate or circumvallate papillae, which are round and flat. At the apex of the V is the foramen cecum, a depression that represents the site of embryonal origin of the thyroid gland. Rarely, remnants of the thyroid can be found in that location (lingual thyroid) as a rounded protuberant mass (Fig. 1.11). In such a case, thyroid scanning is indicated. The posterior part of the tongue or lymphoid area is occupied by the lingual tonsils, characterized by an irregular nodular surface with cryptic openings. The anterior portion of the

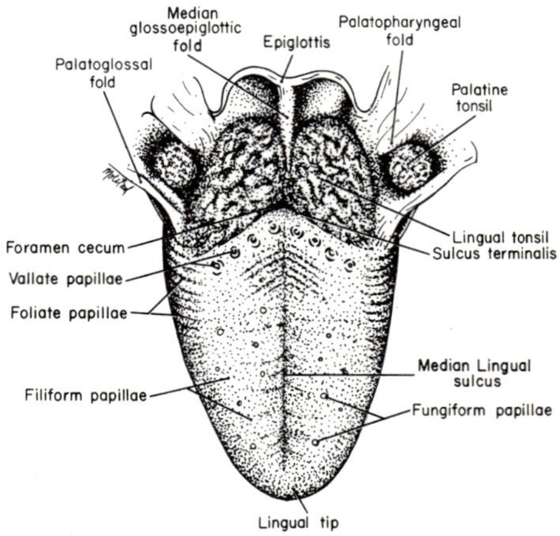

Fig. 1.10. Dorsum of the tongue.

[1]Shapiro BL, et al., Measurement of normal and reportedly malformed palatal vaults. I. Normal adult measurements. *J Dent Res* 42:1039, 1963.

lingual dorsum is occupied by numerous papillae, giving this area a rough, white appearance.

The filiform papillae on this portion are numerous; they are thin, white elongations of the corium and are covered by keratin. In the vicinity of the lingual V they also have a V-arrangement, but closer to the lingual tip they acquire a horizontal disposition. Among the filiform papillae, round, bright red structures can be seen, especially on the sides and tip of the tongue; they are the fungiform papillae. Foliate papillae can be seen on the lateral border of the tongue, but they are generally rudimentary in humans. The center of the lingual dorsum is occupied by a fissure of variable depth.

Variations are observed in the clinical picture of the tongue that are considered within normal limits; only three will be mentioned here.

Geographic tongue is characterized by areas of depapillation alternating with areas of increased keratinization, giving the tongue, as the name implies, a map-like configuration (Fig. 1.12). This phenomenon tends to change shape from day to day. There is strong evidence to support a multifactorial etiology.

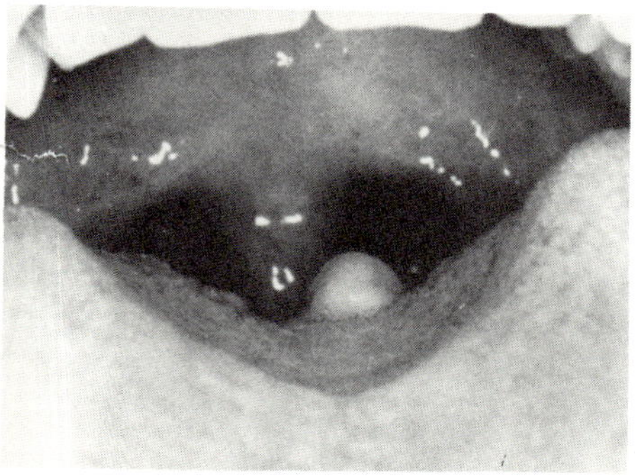

Fig. 1.11. Lingual thyroid.

Fissured tongue, also known as *scrotal tongue,* is characterized by marked intercrossing fissures of the dorsum of the tongue (Fig. 1.13). Fissured tongue is also most likely of multifactorial etiology and is frequently associated with geographic tongue.

Median rhomboid glossitis is a condition seen as an exophitic or flat rhomboidal area of variable size, which is deprived of papillae and located in the midline of the posterior third of the dorsal surface of the

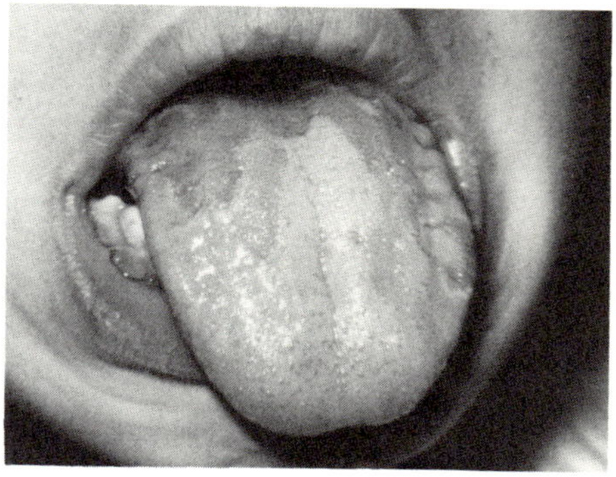

Fig. 1.12. Geographic tongue.

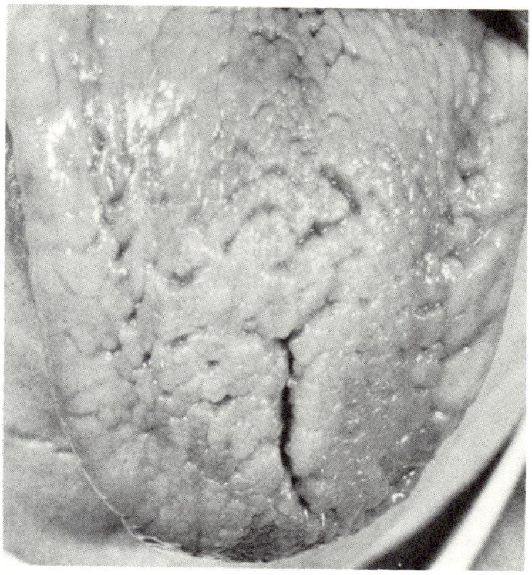

Fig. 1.13. Fissured tongue.

tongue (Fig. 1.14). The largest dimension of the rhomboid follows the anteroposterior direction. The condition represents remnants of the tuberculum impar that during embryonal development were not fully covered by the lateral lingual tubercles.

The ventral surface of the tongue is shiny, smooth, and reddish. Tongue varicosities are seen in this area, especially in older individuals (Fig. 1.15). The ventral surface is continuous with the oral floor. The lingual frenulum is located in the midline of the oral floor, extending as a bridge from the mandibular gingiva to the ventral surface of the tongue. Abnormal attachment of the frenulum produces tongue-tie (ankyloglossia) with resultant reduced ability to protrude the tongue (Fig. 1.16).

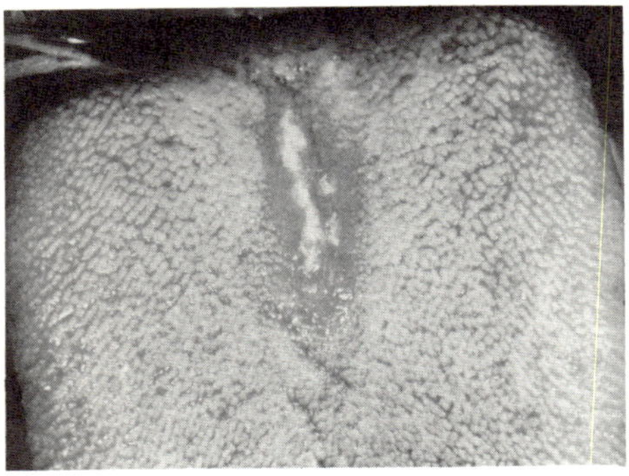

Fig. 1.14. Median rhomboid glossitis.

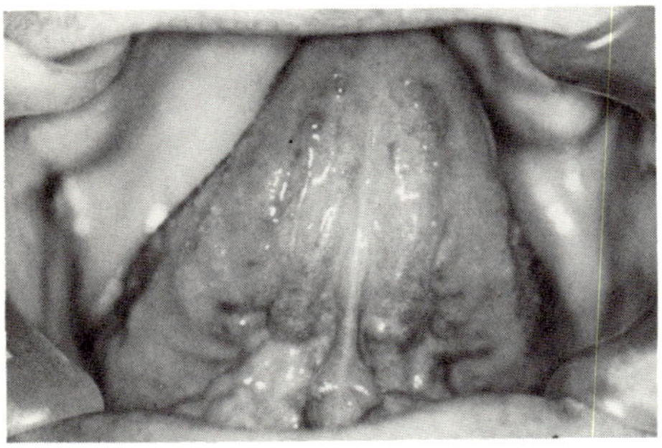

Fig. 1.15. Tongue varicosities.

Oral Floor. The floor of the mouth on each side of the midline on the one side is essentially a continuation of the ventral lingual mucosa and on the other side it is reflected onto the gingiva. In the midline and at each side of the lingual frenulum, the openings of both submandibular and sublingual glands can be seen as elevated, conical, crater-like structures, known as the sublingual caruncles. The sublingual glands located on each side of the midline produce elevations of the floor of the mouth, the sublingual folds (Fig. 1.17).

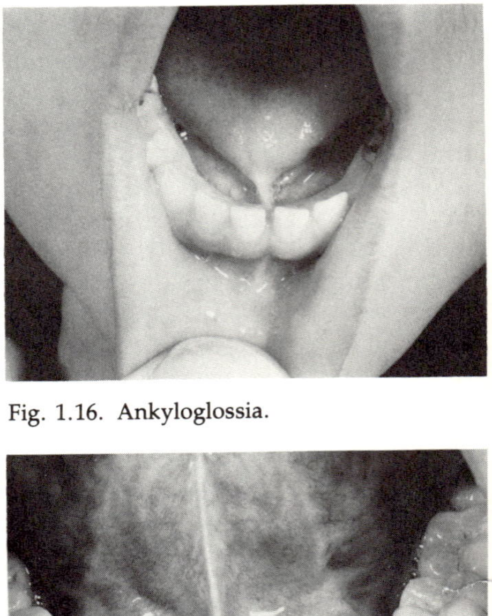

Fig. 1.16. Ankyloglossia.

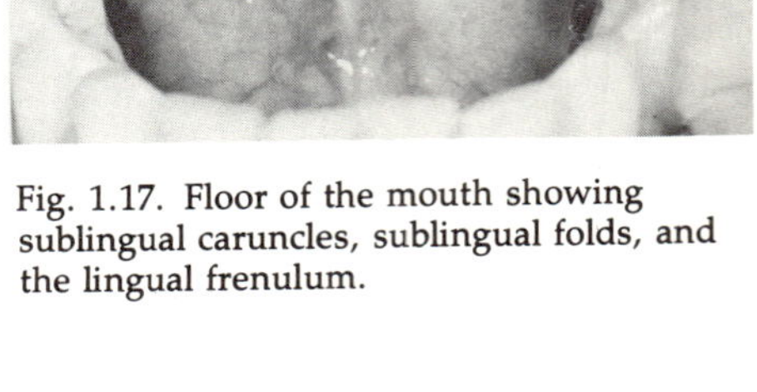

Fig. 1.17. Floor of the mouth showing sublingual caruncles, sublingual folds, and the lingual frenulum.

Gingiva. The gingiva is divided into free marginal gingiva and attached gingiva by the free marginal groove (Fig. 1.18). The free gingiva has an undulating contour; the triangular projections between the teeth are called interdental papillae. The marginal end of the gingiva folds over the tooth surface, and actual attachment of the gingiva to the tooth only takes place below the gingival border. The gingival sulcus, or crevice, is therefore created between tooth and mucosa; its depth varies from 0.1 to 0.3 cm. The attached gingiva extends from the free gingival groove to the beginning of the alveolar crest and is continuous with the alveolar mucosa. Vestibular and lingual gingiva are essentially identical in clinical appearance, presenting a whiter color due to surface keratinization which is absent in the alveolar mucosa.

The geniohyoid processes can be seen bilaterally at each side of the mandibular midline on the lingual attached gingiva. Torus mandibularis, inherited in an autosomal dominant manner, is a bony protuberance of variable shape and size, generally bilateral, located beneath the lingual attached gingiva at the level of the premolar teeth (Fig. 1.19). Multiple bony exostoses are rarely present at the level of the maxillary molars (Fig. 1.20).

Teeth. Humans are characterized by having a double dentition. The primary, temporary, deciduous, or pediatric dentition is composed of twenty teeth, 10 in each arch. The deciduous dentition correlates with the smaller bone size and facial di-

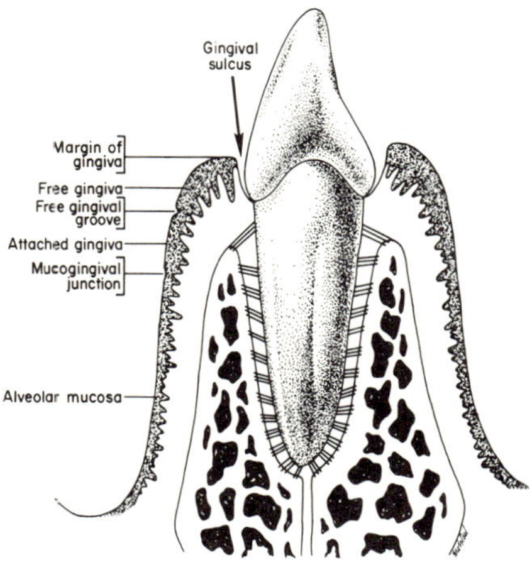

Fig. 1.18. Diagram showing tooth and surrounding structures.

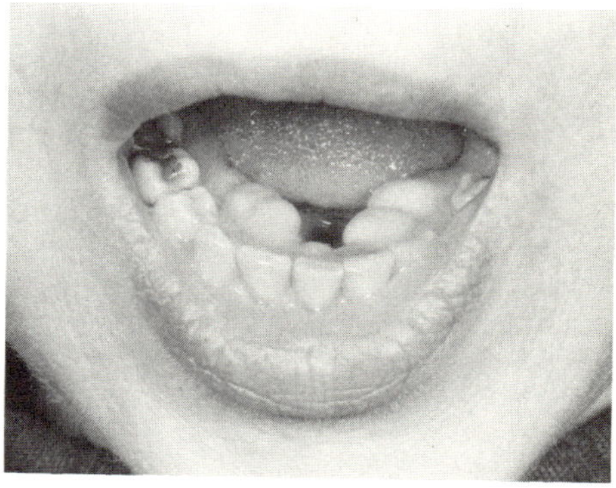

Fig. 1.19. Torus mandibularis, multilobulated variety.

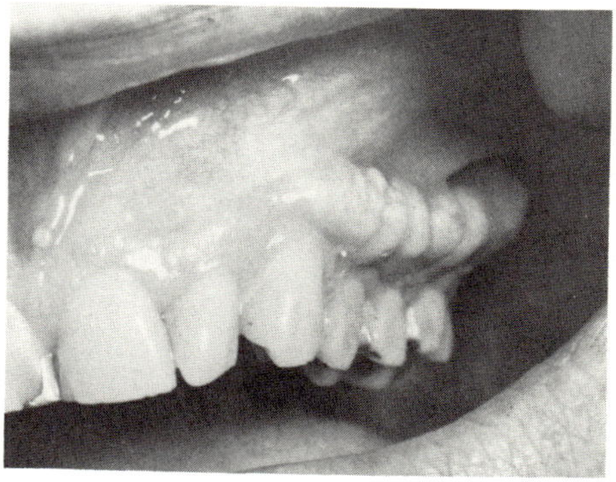

Fig. 1.20. Maxillary exostosis.

mensions of the infant. Eruption of the primary dentition starts at 6 months. The secondary, succedaneous, or permanent dentition is composed of 32 teeth, 16 in each arch. Permanent teeth start erupting at the age of 6 years with the first mandibular molars, and the rate of eruption of the remaining teeth parallels the bone growth. Accurate dates for calcification and eruption of both dentitions are given in Table 1.1.

A comprehensive analysis of dental and paradental anatomy is beyond the scope of this chapter. Figure 1.18 schematically illustrates a tooth and its relationship to the alveolar bone and gingival mucosa. The relationship between maxillary and mandibular dental arches is achieved by occlusion of the teeth. Figures 1.21–23 illustrate examples of Class I, II, and III occlusions, respectively. Alterations in number, shape, color, size, and degree of calcification of teeth occur as isolated phenomena or as part of complex syndromal associations of varied etiology.

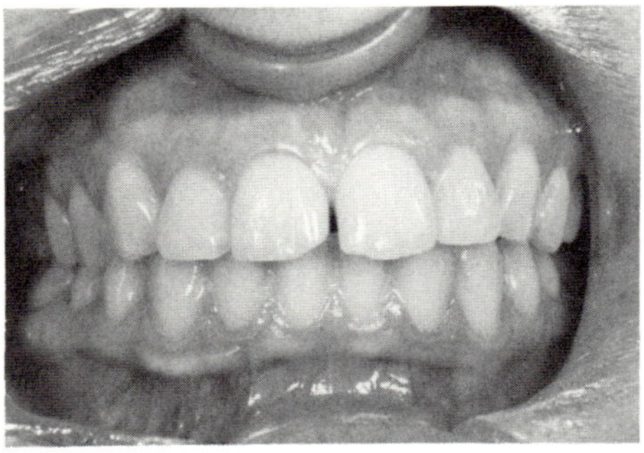

Fig. 1.21. Class I occlusion.

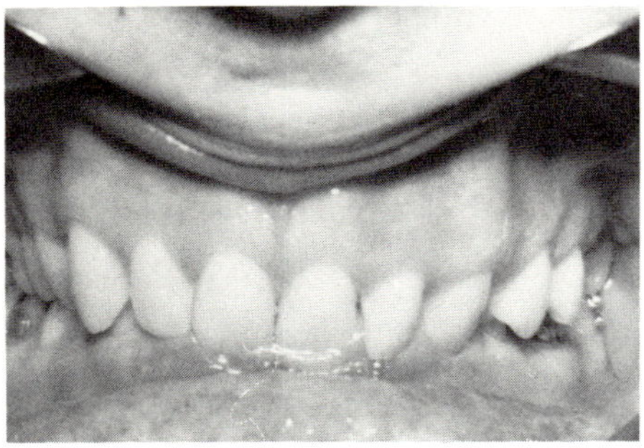

Fig. 1.22. Class II occlusion.

1.3 Radiologic Interpretation of Some Oral and Paraoral Structures

Only a brief summary of some intraoral radiologic landmarks will be presented here. Figure 1.24A is an example of a "bite-wing" radiograph which is generally used to study tooth crowns and contact points between teeth. The enamel (E), the most radiopaque tissue, covers the entire crown. Superimposition of teeth produces a more pronounced

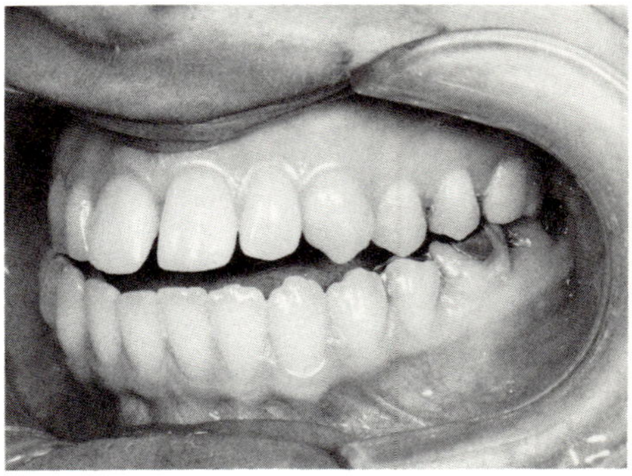

Fig. 1.23. Class III occlusion.

radiopacity. The dentin (D) is less radiopaque and the cementum (calcified tissue similar to bone covering the root) can not be radiologically differentiated from the dentin. The center of the tooth is occupied by a radiolucent area corresponding to the pulp (P). The alveolar bone (AB) is noted between the teeth. The shape of the alveolar crest (AC), the alveolar bone between the teeth, varies normally from a triangle to a slight plateau.

Figure 1.24B is an intraoral periapical radiograph taken at the level of the mandibular molars. This type of film is used to study root and periapical areas in addition to the tooth crown. The alveolar bone is nicely illustrated here. Note that there is a thin space between root and bone; this is the periodontal ligament. The bone that lines the tooth socket, known as lamina dura (LD), is denser than the rest of the alveolar bone, as demonstrated by its increased radiopacity. Destruction of the lamina dura is associated with a great number of pathological processes. Pulp chambers can be readily identified in the radiograph. Areas of increased density in the crowns of the first and second molars represent metallic restorations after treatment of caries.

Figure 1.25 is shown here for comparison with the previous normal radiograph. This film was taken at the level of the primary molars in a five-year-old child. Note that the enamel, when present, has neither a uniform density nor a marked

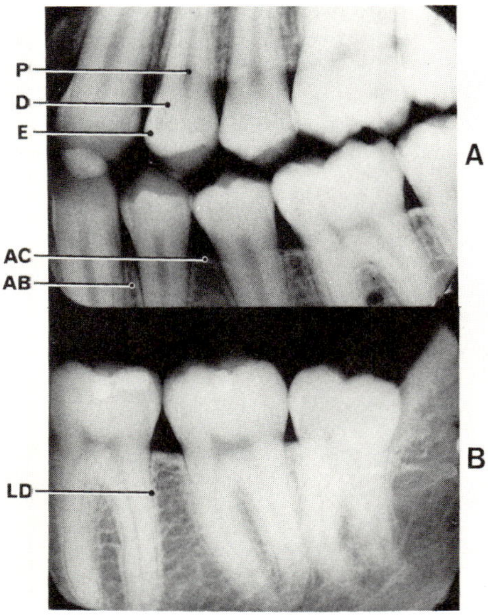

Fig. 1.24A. Example of "bite-wing radiograph. B. Intraoral periapical radiograph.

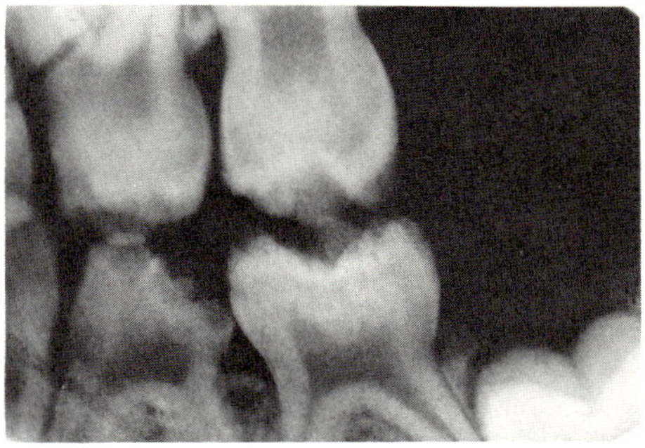

Fig. 1.25. Radiograph showing amelogenesis imperfecta.

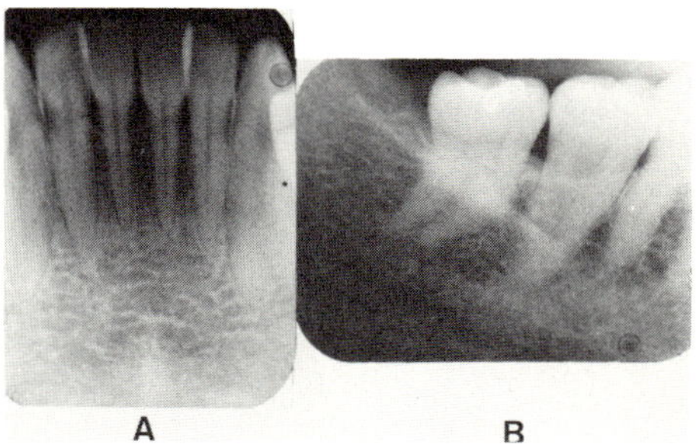

Fig. 1.26A. Radiograph showing alveolar bone type I. B. Radiograph showing alveolar bone type II.

radiopacity. Much of the enamel is absent. This disorder is amelogenesis imperfecta.

Figure 1.26A is a radiograph taken at the level of the mandibular permanent incisors. The bone trabeculae have a uniform horizontal arrangement known as alveolar bone type I. Figure 1.26B, taken at the level of the mandibular permanent molars of another patient, shows an irregular arrangement of bone trabeculae known as alveolar bone type II. Several other patterns or variations from these two basic forms of trabecular arrangement of bone are recognized as within the normal range.

Figure 1.27 represents the right half of a panoramic radiograph. The left half, not illustrated here, is essentially identical. This film illustrates the adult mandibular ramus, condyle, and coronoid process. The area of decreased radiopacity observed in the center of the ramus and running vertically represents the mandibular canal. Note that both maxillary and mandibular third molars have not completed their eruption. These are impacted or retained teeth. The area of radiolucency around the crown of the impacted mandibular molar represents the follicular sac. Several molars have metallic restorations. The contour of the maxillary sinus is noted above the maxillary molars. This type of radiograph is useful for scanning procedures; minute details are generally not properly identifiable because of distortion or superimposition of images.

Figure 1.28 is part of a panoramic radiograph from a 4-year-old child.

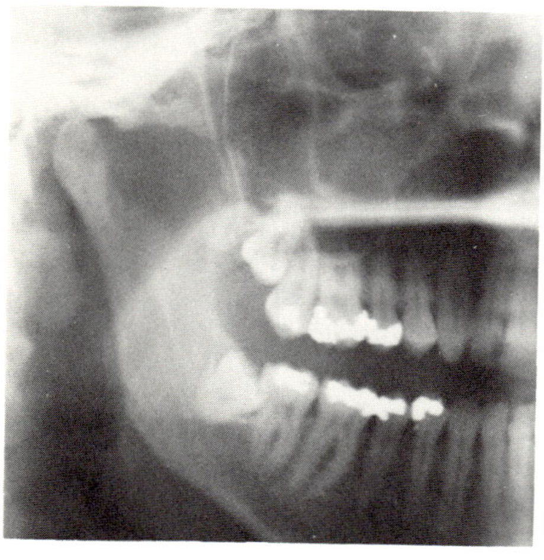

Fig. 1.27. Panoramic radiograph of adult mandibular ramus, condyle, and coronoid process.

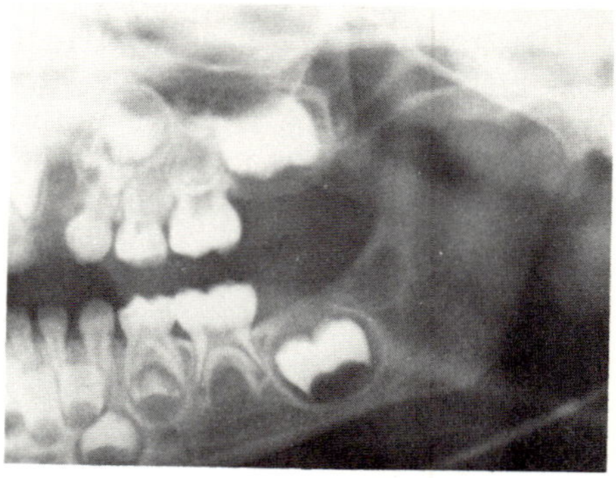

Fig. 1.28. Panoramic radiograph of 4-year-old child with cleft palate.

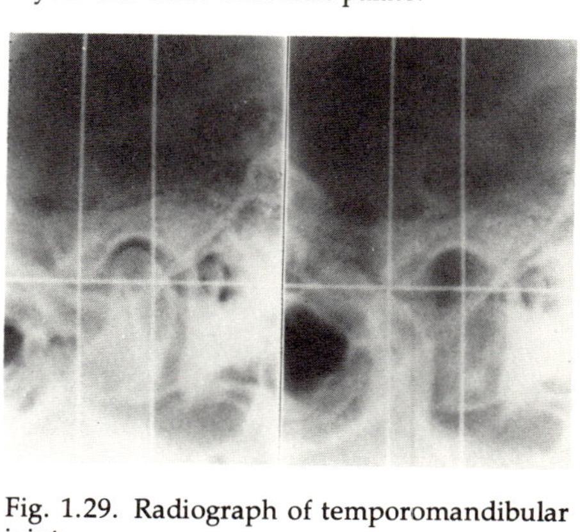

Fig. 1.29. Radiograph of temporomandibular joint.

Note that the maxillary lateral incisor is absent, its place being occupied by a wide space. The child had unilateral cleft palate; the wide space represents the area of clefting. The primary canine tooth is seen to one side of the cleft. The mandible contains several developing teeth buds. Note that the germ of the mandibular permanent first molar has completed the crown formation. The radiolucent space around the entire tooth germ represents the dental or follicular sac. The radiolucent rounded area to the right of this molar represents the tooth bud of the second permanent molar which has not yet begun to calcify.

Figure 1.29 is a composite radiograph illustrating the temporomandibular joint. To the left, with the mouth closed, the condyle is located within the glenoid fossa. The space between these two structures is occupied by the articular meniscus. In front of the condyle, the tuberculum temporalis can be seen. In back of the condyle, the auditory meatus and a distorted image of the mastoid process can be recognized. The radiograph to the right illustrates the temporomandibular joint of the same patient with the mouth open. Note that the condyle is now anterior and caudal to the tuberculum temporalis.

TABLE 1.1 Chronology of Human Dentition

		Tooth	Mean C-R Range (mm) of initial calcification	Calcification of enamel begins in utero
Primary dentition	Maxillary	Central incisor	106	14 weeks
		Laternal incisor	130	16 weeks
		Canine	140	17 weeks
		First molar	127	15.5 weeks
		Second molar	173	19 weeks
	Mandibular	Central incisor	106	14 weeks
		Lateral incisor	130	16 weeks
		Canine	140	17 weeks
		First molar	126	15.5 weeks
		Second molar	160	18 weeks
		Tooth	Formation of enamel matrix and dentin begins	
Permanent dentition	Maxillary	Central incisor	3–4 mo	
		Lateral incisor	10–12 mo	
		Canine	4–5 mo	
		First premolar	1½–1¾ yr	
		Second premolar	2–2¼ yr	
		First molar	At birth	
		Second molar	2½–3 yr	
		Third molar	7–9 yr	
	Mandibular	Central incisor	3–4 mo	
		Lateral incisor	3–4 mo	
		Canine	4–5 mo	
		First premolar	1¾–2 yr	
		Second premolar	2¼–2½ yr	
		First molar	At birth	
		Second molar	2½–3 yr	
		Third molar	8–10 yr	

From Logan WHC, Kronfeld R: *JADA* 20:379, 1933; Modified from data of Kraus B, Jordon RE, *The Human Dentition Before Birth*, Philadelphia, Lea & Febiger, 1965.

Amount of enamel matrix formed at birth	Enamel completed	Emergence into oral cavity	Root completed
Five-sixths	1½ mo	7½ mo	1½ yr
Two-thirds	2½ mo	9 mo	2 yr
One-third	9 mo	18 mo	3¼ yr
Cusps united	6 mo	14 mo	2½ yr
Cusp tips still isolated	11 mo	24 mo	3 yr
Three-fifths	2½ mo	6 mo	1½ yr
Three-fifths	3 mo	7 mo	1½ yr
One-third	9 mo	16 mo	3¼ yr
Cusps united	5½ mo	12 mo	2¼ yr
Cusp tips still isolated	10 mo	20 mo	3 yr
Amount of enamel matrix formed at birth	Enamel completed	Emergence into oral cavity	Root completed
	4–5 yr	7–8 yr	10 yr
	4–5 yr	8–9 yr	11yr
	6–7 yr	11–12 yr	13–15 yr
	5–6 yr	10–11 yr	12–13 yr
	6–7 yr	10–12 yr	12–14 yr
Sometimes a trace	2½–3 yr	6–7 yr	9–10 yr
	7–8 yr	12–13 yr	14–16 yr
	12–16 yr	17–21 yr	18–25 yr
	4–5 yr	6–7 yr	9 yr
	4–5 yr	7–8 yr	10 yr
	6–7 yr	9–10 yr	12–14 yr
	5–6 yr	10–12 yr	12–13 yr
	6–7 yr	11–12 yr	13–14 yr
Sometimes a trace	2½–3 yr	6–7 yr	9–10 yr
	7–8 yr	11–13 yr	14–15 yr
	12–16 yr	17–21 yr	18–25 yr

CHAPTER 2

Some Inherited Conditions Affecting Only Calcified Dental Tissue

2.1 Amelogenesis Imperfecta

Hereditary defects in enamel, unassociated with other generalized defects, are referred to as amelogenesis imperfecta. Classification of these defects has required clinical, histologic, and genetic criteria. Utilizing the clinical and histologic criteria as major divisions, Witkop and Sauk *(1971)* classified amelogenesis imperfecta into hypoplastic, hypocalcified, and hypomaturation types.

In general, hypoplastic types of amelogenesis imperfecta are those in which the enamel has not attained a normal thickness. In enamel which has attained normal thickness, subnormal hardness differentiates hypocalcified varieties from hypomaturation amelogenesis imperfecta. Hypomaturation amelogenesis imperfecta contains large amounts of enamel matrix, allowing the tip of a dental explorer to penetrate under pressure, while hypocalcified enamel is of such a consistency that it can be scraped away during prophylaxis.

Further subclassification of enamel defects utilizes a combination of clinical and histologic appearances and modes of inheritance (see Table 2.1).

References

General

Witkop CJ, Rao, S: Inherited defects in tooth structure. *Birth Def* 7(7):153–184, 1971.

Witkop CJ Jr, Sauk JJ: Defects of enamel, in Stewart RE, Prescott J, (eds) *Oralfacial Genetics.* St. Louis, Mo., CV Mosby, in press.

Hypoplastic Amelogenesis Imperfecta

Darling, AI: Some observations on amelogenesis imperfecta and calcification of the dental enamel. *Proc Roy Soc Med* 49:759–765, 1956.

Frank, RM, Bolender, C: Amelogenesis imparfaite et retentions totales multiples des dents permanentes. *Rev Stomat* 63:23–36, 1962.

Sauk, JJ Jr, et al: The surface of genetically determined hypoplastic enamel in human teeth. *Oral Surg* 34:60–68, 1972.

Winter, GB: Hereditary and idiopathic anomalies of teeth number, structure and form. *Dent Clin N Am* 13:355–373, 1969.

Witkop, CJ Jr: Hereditary defects in enamel and dentin. *Acta Genet Stat Med* 7:236–239, 1957.

Witkop, CJ Jr, Sauk, JJ Jr: *Dental and oral manifestations of hereditary disease. Amer Acad Oral Path* Washington, DC, 1971.

Hypomaturation Amelogenesis Imperfecta

Sauk, JJ Jr, et al: Electron optic micro analysis of two gene products in enamel of females heterozygous for X-linked hypomaturation amelogenesis imperfecta. *Amer J Hum Genet* 24:267–276, 1972.

Winter, GB, Brook, AH: Enamel hypoplasia and anomalies of the enamel, in Poole, AE, Symposium on Genetics. *Dent Clin N Am* 19:3–24, 1975.

Winter, GB, et al: Hereditary amelogenesis imperfecta. A rare autosomal dominant type. *Brit Dent J* 127:157–164, 1969.

Witkop, CJ Jr, et al: Autosomal recessive pigmented hypomaturation amelogenesis imperfecta. *Oral Surg* 36:367–382, 1973.

Hypocalcified Amelogenesis Imperfecta.

Sauk, JJ, Jr, et al: Electron optic analysis of hypomineralized amelogenesis imperfecta in man. *Arch Oral Biol* 12:771–779, 1972.

Schulze, C: Über einen Fall von Hypoplasie, die Hartsubstanzen bei Zähnen im Bereich des rechten Oberkiefers (Odontodysplasia). *Deutsch Zahnärztl Z* 11:14–25, 1956.

2.2 Coronal Dentin Dysplasia

Dentin dysplasia type II was first completely delineated from other dentinal conditions by Shields and coworkers in 1973. The condition is characterized by (1) amber-translucent primary teeth, (2) obliteration of primary tooth pulp chambers, (3) normally colored permanent teeth, and (4) radicular extension of pulp chamber in permanent teeth. Dentin dysplasia type II is inherited as an autosomal dominant condition.

Facies. There are no characteristic facial features.

Oral Structures. Although both dentitions are affected, the pattern is different (Fig. 2.8). Primary teeth have a translucent-amber color and show obliteration of pulp chambers by abnormal dentin. These teeth closely resemble dentinogenesis imperfecta type II. The permanent teeth have normal coloration; however, there is a radicular extension of the pulp chambers containing numerous pulp stones.

TABLE 2.1 Classification of Amelogenesis Imperfecta

		Dentition Affected		
		Primary	Secondary	Color of Enamel
HYPOPLASTIC	1. Pitted, autosomal dominant	+	+	Initially yellow-white, becomes black pockmarked
	2. Local, autosomal dominant	+	+	Yellow-white to chalky white
	3. Smooth autosomal dominant (Figs. 2.1, 2.2)	−	+	Yellow on eruption later become: opaque white to brownish
	4. Rough autosomal dominant	+	+	Yellow-white on eruption
	5. Rough autosomal recessive	+	+	Yellow, resembling dentin
	6. Smooth, X-linked (dominant) (Fig. 2.3)	+	+	Yellow-brown
HYPOMATURATION	1. Hypomaturation-hypoplastic with taurodontism, autosomal dominant	+	+	Shiny-opaque white with irregular areas of yellow-brown mottling
	2. X-linked recessive (Figs. 2.4, 2.5)	+	+	Primary teeth of males show opaque white. Permanent teeth show yellow-white color which stains with age. Females show alternating vertical bands of white opaque enamel
	3. Pigmented-autosomal recessive	+	+	Milky to shiny agar brown
	4. Snow-capped teeth	+	+	Opaque white
HYPOCALCIFIED	1. Autosomal dominant (Figs. 2.6, 2.7)	+	+	Newly erupted teeth are dull, lusterless, opaque white, honey colored or yellow-orange-brown
	2. Autosomal recessive	+	+	Same as dominant form

Defect & Surface Affected	Histology	Miscellaneous
Random pinpoint pits on labial and lingual	Incremental lines of Retzius bend under bottom of pits, bottom of pits may be hypocalcified	None
Buccal middle ⅓ of enamel as horizontal row of pits or linear depression	Disoriented enamel rods, bending of incremental lines toward dentinoenamel junction with voids in prism sheath and within rods.	None
Thin-hard-glossy with smooth surface on buccal and lingual surfaces	Short-thick enamel rods may be covered with a laminated calcified layer	Pulpal calcifications may be present in erupted and unerupted teeth. Multiple unerupted teeth undergoing resorption are common
Thin-rough-hard. Buccal and lingual surface involved	Absence of enamel rod structure. Enamel consists of a horizontally laminated highly calcified structure	Impacted and partly resorbed teeth are rare but have been reported
Rough granular enamel on labial and lingual surfaces.	Enamel has a vitreous lamellar or globular appearance	Numerous teeth are missing in erupted dentition and are manifest radiographically as unerupted teeth undergoing resorption
Shiny-thin occlusal and incisal abrasion	Enamel may be homogenous with indistinct rods or rods may be evident with reduction in distance between incremental lines	Females show vertical banding of hypoplastic and normal enamel consistent with Lyonization effect of genes on the X chromosome in heterozygous females. Anterior open bite is common.
Mottling and pitting of labial surfaces	Enamel is porous with opaque globular spaces	This condition may be an incomplete expression of the tricho-dento-osseous syndrome.
Translucent mottling in primary teeth of males on labial and lingual surfaces. Enamel in secondary dentition of males is normal thickness and may be penetrated with an explorer.	Enamel rod sheaths may be lacking, filled with pigmented debris which is an eosinophilic staining (hematoxylin-eosin) material	Females show vertical banding of hypomature and normal enamel consistent with Lyonization effect of genes on the X-chromosome in heterozygous females.
Labial and lingual surfaces show normal thickness but hypomature enamel	Interrod spaces are present and contain a brown pigment in addition to pink staining material (Masson trichome)	Unerupted teeth may be present and undergo resorption.
Hypomaturation of incisal or occlusal ⅓	Surface of enamel below first 1 mm shows disoriented enamel crystals in enamel rod sheaths	None
Labial and lingual surfaces are covered with cheesy soft enamel	Enamel matrix in ground sections is normal but lacks calcification	Anterior open bite and excessive calculus formation are common.
Same as dominant form	Same as dominant form	Clinically, radiographically, and histologically this recessive form is more severe than autosomal dominant hypocalcified amelogenesis imperfecta.

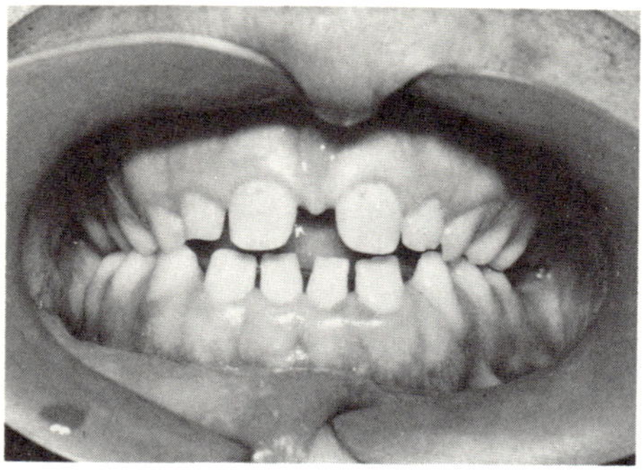

Fig. 2.1. Generalized hypoplastic enamel. Note prominent interdental spaces.

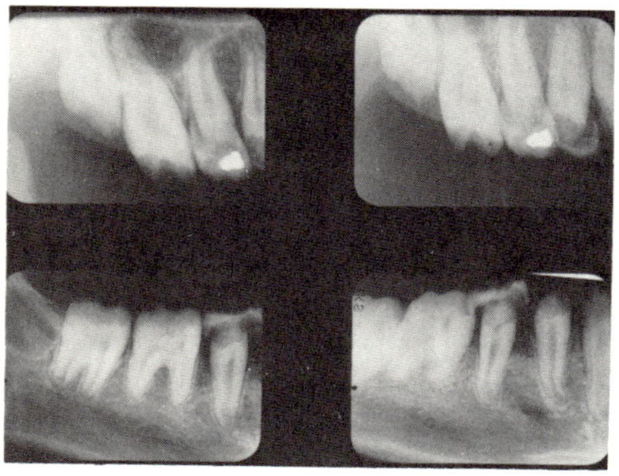

Fig. 2.2. Radiograph showing very thin enamel.

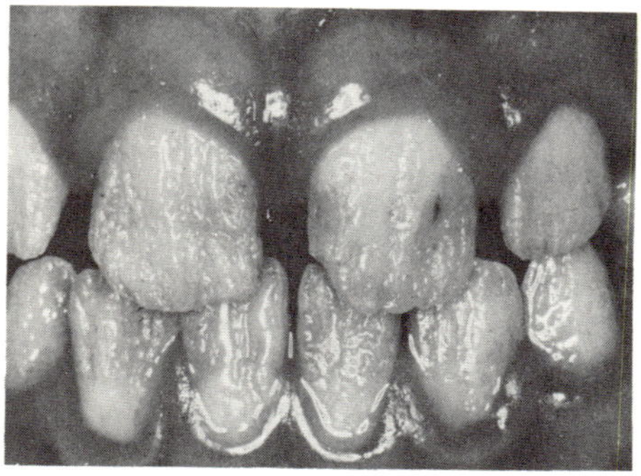

Fig. 2.3. Alternating vertical pitted hypoplastic enamel in this form of amelogenesis imperfecta demonstrates both pitted-type of enamel hypoplasia and Lyonization effect in an X-linked trait.

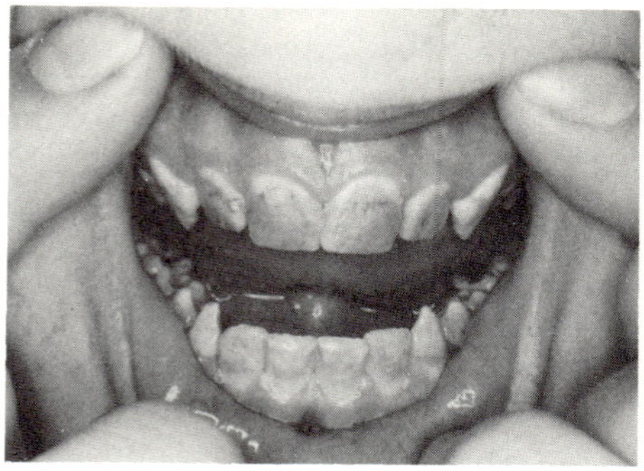

Fig. 2.4. Enamel is of normal thickness but it is soft and has an agar brown color.

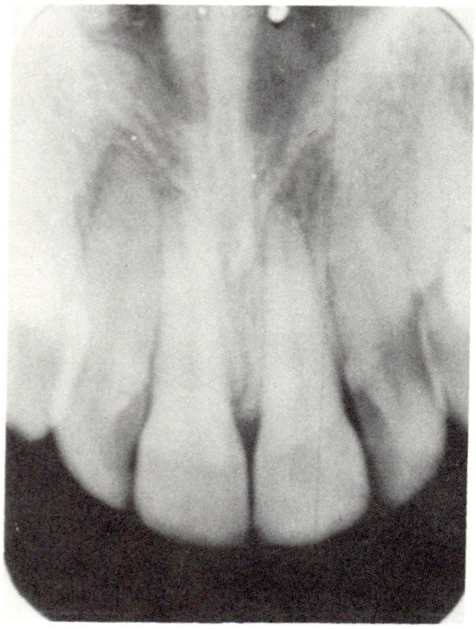

Fig. 2.5. Radiograph does not distinguish enamel from dentin.

Systemic Features. None.

Differential Diagnosis. Dentinogenesis imperfecta type II (hereditary opalescent dentin) and pulpal dysplasia should be considered in the differential diagnosis.

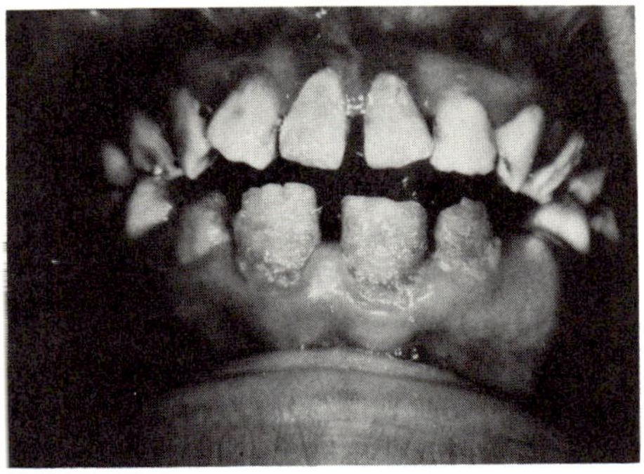

Fig. 2.6. Grossly hypocalcified enamel with consequent enamel loss.

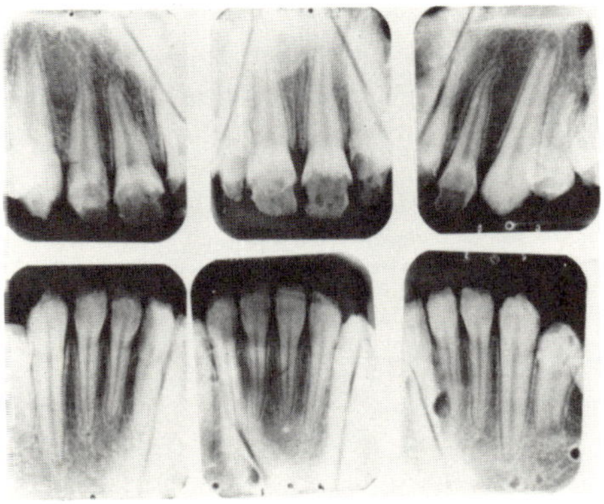

Fig. 2.7. Radiograph showing moth-eaten appearance in the enamel.

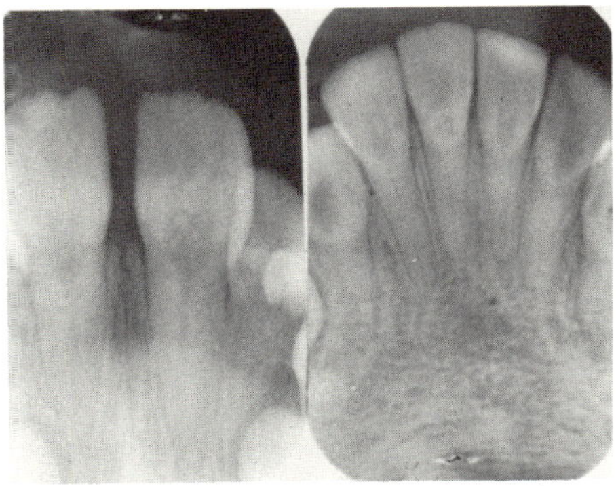

Fig. 2.8. Large rounded pulp chambers containing pulp stones and thin narrow root canals are characteristic radiologic findings in coronal dentin dysplasia.

Laboratory Aids. Roentgenographic examination of primary and secondary teeth establishes the diagnosis.

Synonym. Dentin dysplasia type II.

References

Shields EP, et al: A proposed classification for heritable human dentin defects with a description of a new entity. *Arch Oral Biol* 18:543–553, 1973.

2.3 Hereditary Opalescent Dentin

Barrett in 1883 and Talbot in 1893 were among the first to describe this condition. Dentinogenesis imperfecta is characterized by (1) bluish brown teeth, (2) bulbous crowns, (3) absence of pulp chambers and canals, and (4) enamel hypoplasia (20%). The condition is inherited in an autosomal dominant mode with high penetrance.

Facies. The facies is not characteristic, except that a closed vertical dimension may result from tooth fractures and attrition.

Oral Structures. The teeth may vary in color from opalescent brown to brownish blue. Although both dentitions are affected, the primary dentition is usually more severely affected. The dentin is soft and the enamel is often dislodged, resulting in exposed dentin and rapid attrition. The progressive attrition may be so severe that the teeth are worn down to the alveolar process, thus initiating fibrous and bony hyperplasia. Roentgenographic examinations reveal teeth with bulbous crowns, thin roots, and reduction or absence of pulp chambers and canals (Fig. 2.9). Periapical radiolucencies may be noted; however the frequency is less than that for radicular dentin dysplasia (Fig. 2.10).

Histologically the enamel is usually normal; however 20% of the teeth may have regions of hypomature enamel. The dentinoenamel junction is variable and may show reduced scalloping. Except for mantle dentin, the majority of the dentin is amorphous and contains increased water and organic periodic acid-Schiff staining material. The dentinal tubules are of irregular size and shape and present a disorganized pattern between zones of interglobular dentin.

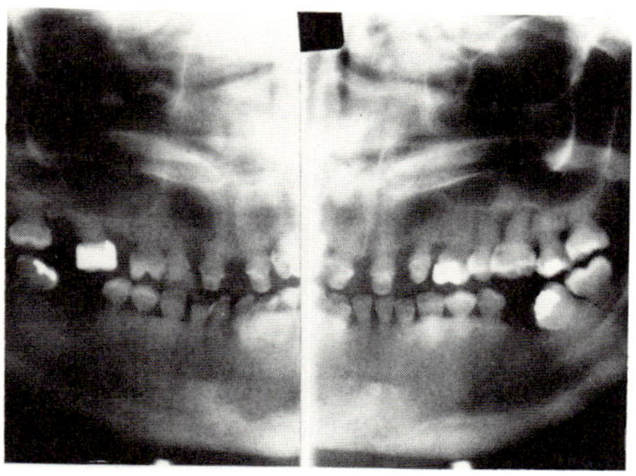

Fig. 2.9. Radiograph from a 32-year-old female with hereditary opalescent dentin. Note short, almost absent roots and absence of pulp chambers.

Systemic Features. None.

Differential Diagnosis. Dentinogenesis imperfecta, associated with osteogenesis imperfecta, may present similar tooth changes.

Laboratory Aids. None.

Synonyms. Detinogenesis imperfecta, dentinogenesis imperfecta type II.

References

Shields EP, et al: A proposed classification for heritable human dentin defects with a description of a new entity. *Arch Oral Biol* 18:543–553, 1973.

Witkop CJ Jr, Rao S: Inherited defects in tooth structures. *Birth Def* 7(7):153–184, 1971.

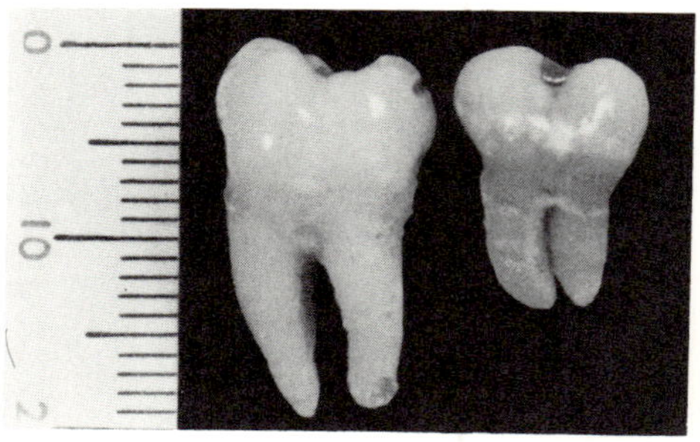

Fig. 2.10. To the left, an extracted normal second mandibular molar, compared to the corresponding tooth on the right from the previous patient.

2.4 Radicular Dentin Dysplasia

Radicular dentin dysplasia was probably first described by Ballschmiede in 1920. The condition is characterized by (1) clinically normal crown forms, (2) abnormal root shapes, and (3) absence or partial absence of pulp chamber and canals. The condition is inherited in an autosomal dominant mode and occurs with a frequency of about 1 in 100,000.

Facies. There are no characteristic facial features for the condition.

Oral Structures. Both primary and secondary dentitions are affected. Tooth color is usually within normal limits; however, brownish and opalescent teeth have been reported. The teeth are often malaligned and are easily exfoliated with minor trauma. Radiographic examination reveals normal crown shapes; however, the roots are blunt, shortened, bulged, or absent (Fig. 2.11). The pulp chambers and canals are absent in the primary dentition. However in the secondary dentition, the pulp chambers are often partially present and appear as coronal demilune shadows in radiographs.

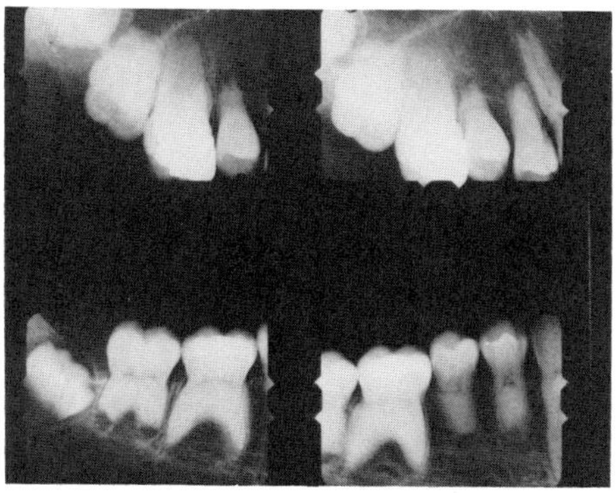

Fig. 2.11. Radiograph showing abnormal roots, absence of pulp chambers, and periapical radiolucencies.

Histologic examination reveals that the enamel and dentin in the crowns of these teeth are normal. The demilune shadows on radiographs represent the existing pulp chamber. Below these areas are zones of tubular and osteodentin. The apices of these teeth are frequently surrounded by radiolucencies that histologically resemble radicular cysts.

Systemic Features. None.

Differential Diagnosis. Coronal dentin dysplasia (dentin dysplasia type II) and calcinosis universalis should be included in the differential diagnosis.

Laboratory Aids. Roentgenographic examination is often useful in making the diagnosis.

Synonyms. Dentin dysplasia type I, rootless teeth, dentinal dysplasia.

References

Witkop CJ Jr: Hereditary defects of dentin. *Dent Clin N Am* 19:25–45, 1975.

Witkop CJ Jr, Rao S: Inherited defects in tooth structure. *Birth Def* 7(7):153–184, 1971.

CHAPTER 3

Systemic Inherited Disorders with Dental Involvement

3.1 Acroosteolysis

Acroosteolysis, which has an autosomal dominant mode of inheritance, is characterized by (1) short stature, (2) disintegration of the terminal phalanges of fingers and toes, (3) abnormal skull shape, and (4) premature loss of teeth.

Facies. The face presents coarse features accentuated by a low frontal hairline and a markedly long nose. The ears are generally flared (Fig. 3.1).

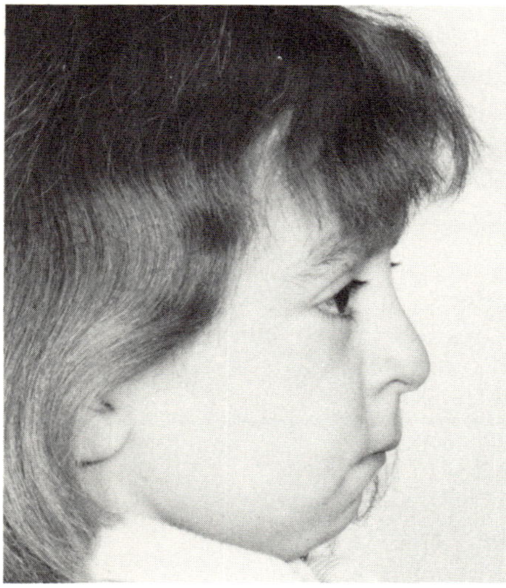

Fig. 3.1. Note small receded mandible and mid-facial hypoplasia.

Oral Structures. A constant component of the syndrome is premature loss of teeth with associated reabsorption or atrophy of the maxillary and mandibular alveolar bone (Fig. 3.2). Other oral findings have included markedly short molar roots, prognathism, and a small receded mandible.

Systemic Features. Adult height is below 155 cm (5 ft 1 in); intelligence is within normal limits. Severe

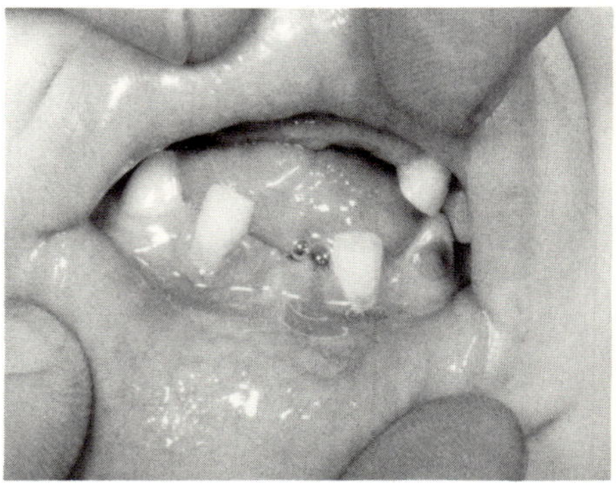

Fig. 3.2. Intraoral view demonstrating early loss of primary teeth.

kyphosis, osteoporosis, and compression of thoracic vertebrae with a "fish-bone" radiological appearance account in part for the reduced height. The most striking skeletal alteration is acroosteolysis of the distal portion of the terminal phalanges of fingers and toes (Fig. 3.3). Clubbing, especially of the fingers, is a typical clinical finding. Hyperextensibility of finger joints and occasional pain over the interphalangeal joint areas are also present. The skull is dolichocephalic with marked occipital protuberance. Wormian bones, wide-open sutures, depression of anterior fontanel, absent frontal sinuses, and large sella turcica are additional roentgenographic findings (Fig. 3.4). Valgus deformity can be seen in knees and elbows. Multiple fractures, especially of the fingers, long bones, and spine, are a frequent complication.

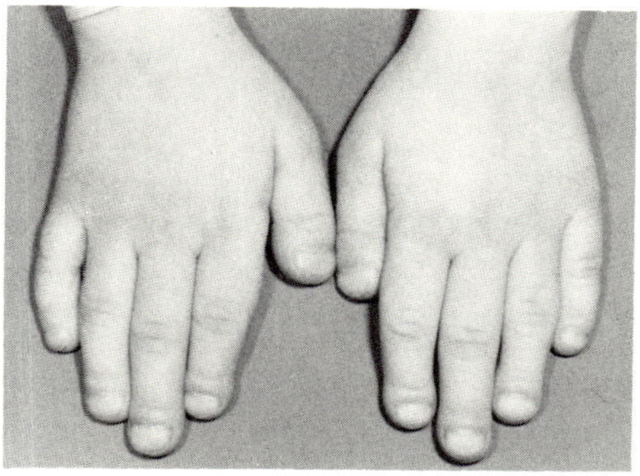

Fig. 3.3. Note abbreviation of terminal phalanges.

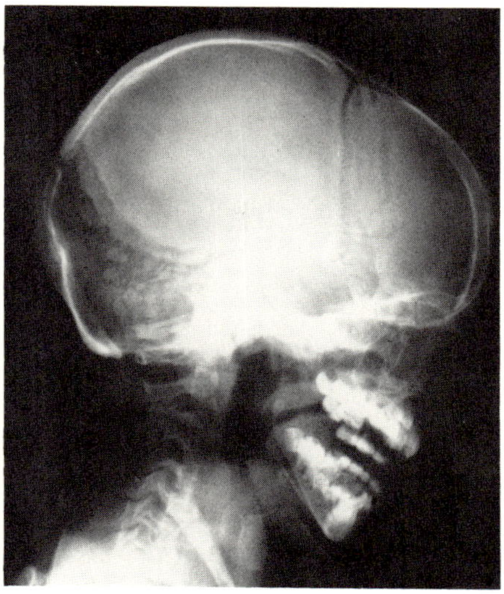

Fig. 3.4. Note bathrocephaly and numerous Wormian bones in suture lines.

Differential Diagnosis. A great variety of conditions are associated with acroosteolysis, such as pyknodysostosis, progeria, leprosy, and vinyl chloride industrial toxicity.

Laboratory Aids. There is a single report of acroosteolysis associated with increased levels of serum alkaline phosphatase and lactic dehydrogenase.

Synonyms. Hajdu-Cheney syndrome, arthrodento-osteo dysplasia.

References

Cheney WD: Acro-osteolysis. *Am J Roentgenol* 94:595–607, 1965.

Herrmann J, et al: Arthro-dento-osteo Dysplasia (Hajdu-Cheney Syndrome) *Z Kinderheilkd* 114:93–110, 1973.

Matisonn A, Zaidy F: Familial acro-osteolysis. *S Afr Med J* 47:2060–2063, 1973.

3.2 Amelocerebrohypohidrosis Syndrome

This condition was first described by Kohlschütter and coworkers in 1974. The syndrome is characterized by (1) severe seizures, (2) progressive mental retardation, (3) muscular spasticity, (4) hypohidrosis, and (5) enamel hypoplasia. Present evidence supports either an X-linked or autosomal recessive mode of inheritance.

Facies. No characteristic facial features.

Oral Structures. There is marked hypoplasia of enamel, resulting in complete absence, except for small zones, of thin enamel at cervix of the tooth crowns. The enamel defect is generalized and involves all teeth in both primary and secondary dentitions.

Systemic Features. Affected individuals appear to be completely normal until the onset of seizures, which may occur as early as the end of the first year of life. Subsequent to the onset of severe seizures, the patients exhibit muscular spasticity and progressive mental retardation. Histologic examination of the brain has revealed reduced numbers of neurons, atrophy of glial cells, and ballooning of axons. Patients demonstrating hypohidrosis reveal decreased numbers of sweat and sebaceous glands on biopsy. The sweat contains mild elevation of sodium and chloride and marked elevation of potassium.

Differential Diagnosis. The differential diagnosis should include the various types of amelogenesis imperfecta and ectodermal dysplasia.

Laboratory Aids. None known.

Synonyms. Epilepsy, mental deterioration, and amelogenesis imperfecta.

References

Kohlschütter A, et al: Familial epilepsy and yellow teeth—a disease of the CNS associated with enamel hypoplasia, *Helv Paediatr Acta* 29:283–294, 1974.

3.3 Cryptodontic Brachymetacarpalia

This syndrome, first described by Gorlin and Sedano (1971), consists of (1) shortened metacarpals and metatarsals, (2) short thumbs, (3) short, straight clavicles, and (4) multiple impacted teeth. The clinical features present variable expressivity. The syndrome is inherited as an autosomal dominant condition. Affected individuals have a marked similarity to patients with pseudohypoparathyroidism, but in cryptodontic brachymetacarpalia the somatic and mental growth is normal, and cataracts and ectopic calcification are absent. Serum calcium and phosphorus levels are normal, as is the response to parathormone (Ellsworth-Howard test). For several years debate has been carried on concerning whether the mode of inheritance of pseudohypoparathyroidism and pseudo-pseudohypoparathyroidism is X-linked dominant or autosomal dominant. The vast majority of investigators have held to the former, but the existence of cases with apparent male-to-male transmission has caused confusion. Recent review of the literature of those cases of pseudopseudo- and pseudohypoparathyroidism in which male-to-male transmission has been reported has suggested that some cases represent examples of cryptodontic brachymetacarpalia.

Facies. There is no characteristic facies.

Oral Structures. Multiple impaction of teeth is a constant feature; several teeth in both dentitions remain unerupted (Fig. 3.5).

Systemic Features. Somatic and mental growth are normal. Patients have one or more shortened metacarpals (Fig. 3.6). Skeletal anomalies also include shortened metatarsals, short thumbs, and straight, shortened clavicles. The rest of the skeleton is normal.

Differential Diagnosis. As mentioned earlier, pseudopseudo- and pseudohypoparathyroidism are the main conditions to be considered in the differential diagnosis. Cleidocranial dysplasia also should be included.

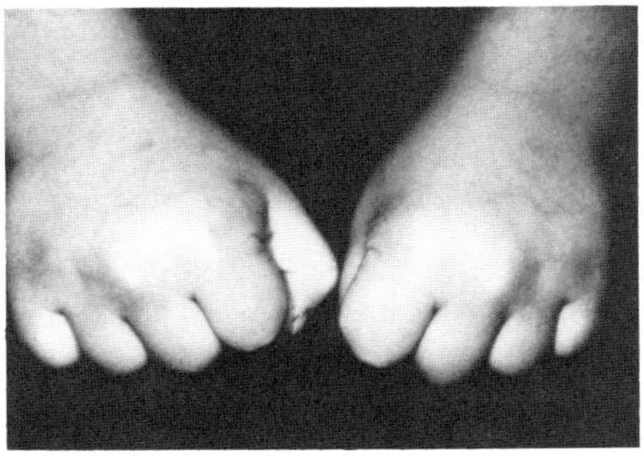

Fig. 3.6. Shortening of metacarpals is manifested by absence of several knuckles. The patient's father had a similar abnormality.

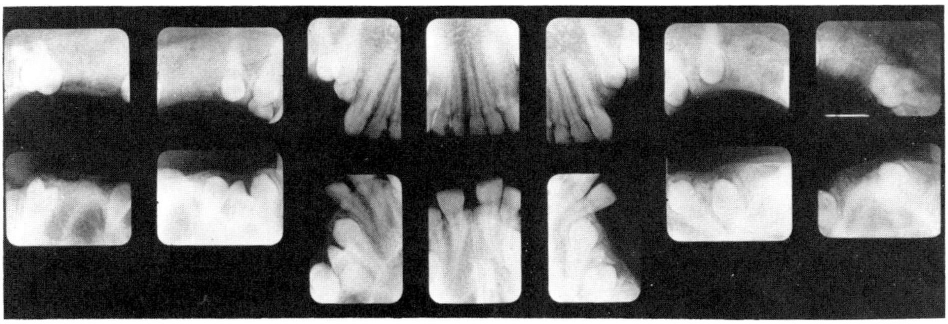

Fig. 3.5. Oral roentgenograms demonstrate that several bicuspid and molar teeth have failed to erupt.

Laboratory Aids. Serum calcium, phosphorus, and the Ellsworth-Howard test are all within normal values.

References

Goeminne L: Albright's hereditary poly-osteochondrodystrophy, (pseudo-pseudohypoparathyroidism with diabetes, hypertension, arteritis and polyarthrosis). *Acta Genet Med* 14:226–281, 1965.

Gorlin RJ, Sedano HO: Cryptodontic brachymetacarpalia. *Mod Med* 39:166–167, 1971.

Gorlin RJ, Sedano HO: Cryptodontic brachymetacarpalia. *Birth Def* 7(7): 200–203, 1971.

Temtamy S, McKusick VA: Synopsis of hand malformations with particular emphasis on genetic factors. *Birth Def* 5(3):125–184, 1969.

3.4 Hypodontia and Nail Dysgenesis

The syndrome of hypodontia and nail dysgenesis was first reported in 1969 by Redpath and Winter. The condition is characterized by (1) fine hair, (2) oligodontia, and (3) hypoplasia or koilonychia of fingernails and toenails. Present evidence suggests an autosomal dominant mode of inheritance; however an autosomal recessive form may also exist, suggesting genetic heterogeneity.

Facies. No characteristic facies.

Oral Structures. Oligodontia is a constant finding with the mandibular incisors, second molars, and maxillary canines being the most frequently missing teeth (Fig. 3.7).

Systemic Features. Mental development and somatic growth are both within normal limits. Affected individuals often present with thin, fine hair of normal distribution. The skin

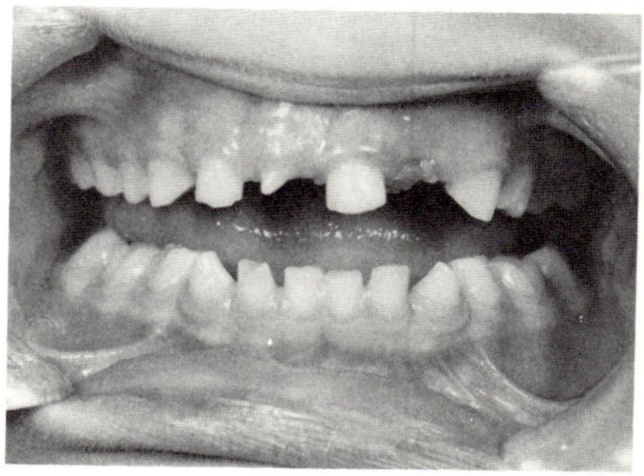

Fig. 3.7. Note pegging of anterior teeth. Several teeth are absent.

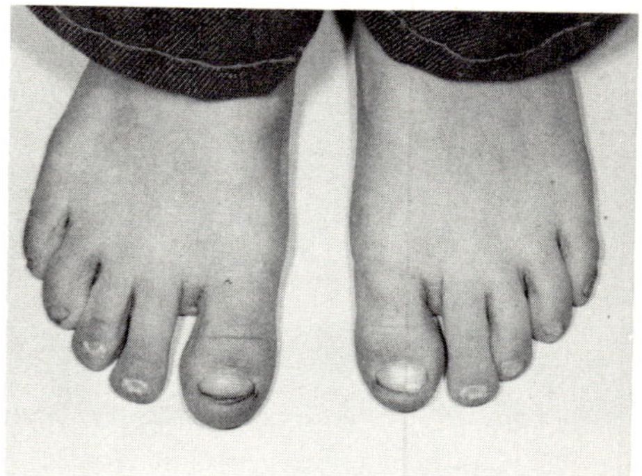

Fig. 3.8. Nails are small and dysplastic.

may appear fine and dry; however, an o-phthaldialdehyde sweat test is usually normal and patients rarely show an intolerance to heat. The nails of the fingers and especially the toes may reveal hypoplasia or koilonychia or both (Fig. 3.8); the latter has been reported infrequently.

Differential Diagnosis. The various forms of ectodermal dysplasia should be included in establishing a diagnosis (see Table 7.1).

Laboratory Aids. The o-phthaldialdehyde sweat test of Redpath and Winter may be used to differentiate this syndrome from some forms of ectodermal dysplasia.

Synonym. Witkop syndrome.

References

Giansanti JS, et al: The "tooth and nail" type of autosomal dominant ectodermal dysplasia. *Oral Surg* 37:576–582, 1974.

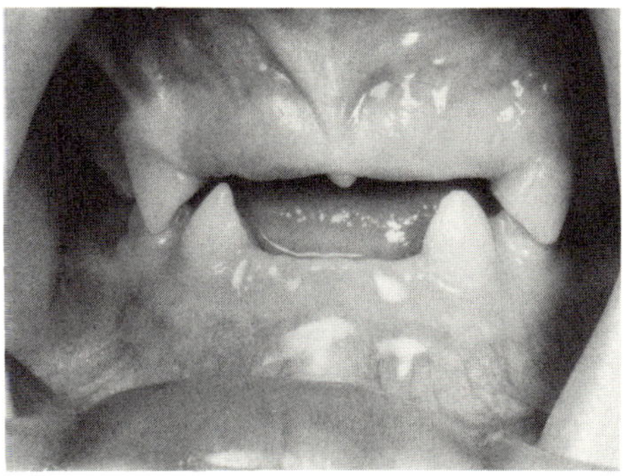

Fig. 3.9. Partial anodontia as a result of spontaneous tooth exfoliation.

Hudson CD, Witkop CJ Jr: Autosomal dominant hypodontia with nail dysgenesis. *Oral Surg* 39:409–423, 1975.

Redpath TH, Winter GS: Autosomal dominant ectodermal dysplasia with significant dental defects. *Br Dent J* 126:123–128, 1969.

3.5 Hypophosphatasia (Phosphoethanolaminuria)

The condition, first described by Rathbun in 1948, is characterized by (1) skeletal abnormalities, (2) decreased level of serum alkaline phosphatase, (3) presence of phosphoethanolamine in urine and plasma, and (4) premature loss of teeth, which may be the initial manifestation of the disease. This condition is inherited in an autosomal recessive manner. The heterozygous carrier can be detected by the presence of low serum alkaline phosphatase levels, as well as the presence of slightly elevated levels of urinary phosphoethanolamine.

Facies. There is no characteristic facies for the disorder.

Oral Structures. Spontaneous premature shedding of primary teeth, especially the mandibular incisors, is a characteristic finding and, in some cases, the only manifestation of the disease (Fig. 3.9). Shedding also can occur after slight trauma and without evidence of gingival or periodontal disease or both. Primary molars and the permanent dentition are rarely affected. Complete lack of cementum is observed in exfoliated teeth, with consequent lack of periodontal fiber attachment (Fig. 3.10). Enlarged pulp chambers have also been noted in the primary dentition (Fig. 3.11).

Systemic Features. Patients reveal diminished somatic growth but normal mental development. Severe manifestations of the condition in the neonatal period account for a 60%–70% mortality rate. Severely affected infants may present dyspnea, cyanosis, growth retardation, vomiting, and renal calcinosis. The cause of death is most often due to renal damage from hypercalcemia or from cardiac and pulmonary failure. The most significant defect in the condition is lack of formation of mature bone; therefore, the clinical manifestations of surviving individuals are rachitic-like changes: bowing of long bones, fractures, and pseudofractures. Irregular areas of ossification at the metaphyseal ends of long bones are often noted. Premature synostosis of the skull may develop in patients surviving the neonatal period, resulting in oxycephaly or increased intracranial pressure or both. Roentgenographically, the skull may have a "beaten-silver" appearance as a result of the mineralization defect.

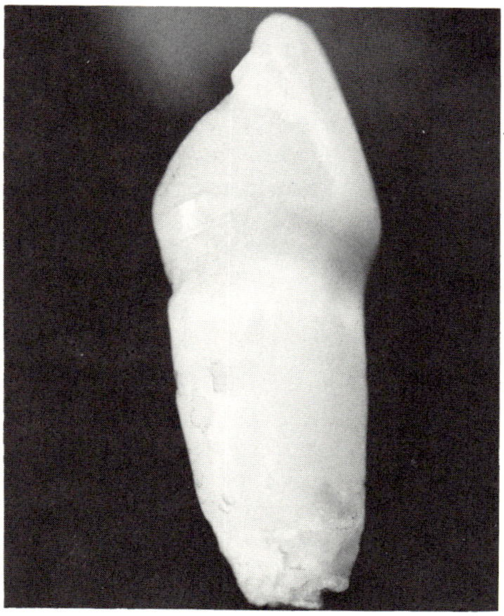

Fig. 3.10. Note absence of cementum.

Differential Diagnosis. Differential diagnosis should include other conditions resulting in premature tooth loss: osteomyelitis, leukemia, agranulocytosis, acrodynia, reticuloendotheliosis, juvenile periodontosis, cyclic neutropenia, Papillon-Lefèvre syndrome, dentin dysplasia, odont-

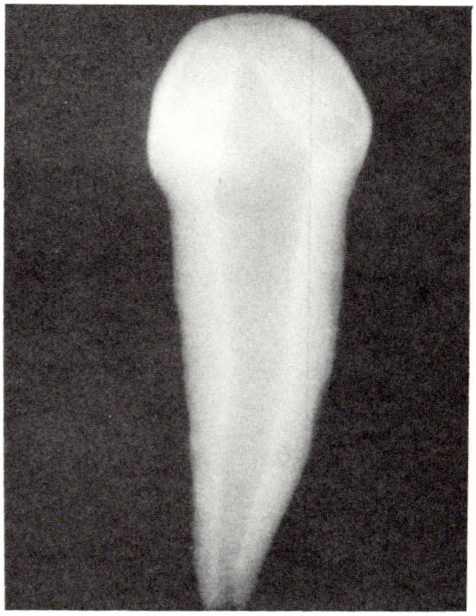

Fig. 3.11. Radiograph of an exfoliated tooth showing enlarged pulp chamber, a variable finding in patients affected with hypophosphatasia.

ogenesis imperfecta, dentinogenesis imperfecta, vitamin D deficiency, and vitamin D-resistant rickets. Dominantly inherited forms of the condition also exist but are without oral manifestations.

Laboratory Aids. Decreased level of serum alkaline phosphatase is found in addition to increased levels of plasma and urinary phosphoethanolamine.

References

Mehes K, et al: Hypophosphatasia; screening and family investigation in an endogamous Hungarian village. *Clin Genet* 3:60–66, 1972.

Pimstone B, et al: Hypophosphatasia; genetic and dental studies. *Ann Intern Med* 65:722–729, 1966.

Rathbun JC: Hypophosphatasia, a new developmental anomaly. *Amer J Dis Child* 75:822–831, 1948.

Warshaw JB, et al: Serum alkaline phosphatase in hypophosphatasia. *J Clin Invest* 50:2137–2142, 1971.

3.6 Hypophosphatemic Vitamin D-Resistant Rickets

This common disorder is inherited in an X-linked dominant mode and consists of (1) hypophosphatemia associated with diminished renal tubular resorption of inorganic phosphate, (2) rickets or osteomalacia in some patients, (3) resistance to the usual doses of vitamin D, and (4) absence of other abnormalities. The hypophosphatemia is due to defective reabsorption and increased excretion of phosphate by the renal tubules. The rickets is secondary to the biochemical abnormality.

Facies. Usually no significant facies.

Oral Structures. The most common oral findings include multiple gingival and periapical abscesses without concurrent evidence of caries or tooth fractures. Roentgenologic examination may reveal large pulp chambers with pulp horns extending to the dentinoenamel junction (Figs. 3.12–13). Attrition or cracks of the enamel thus result in pulpal exposures. Microradiographs of dentin reveal poorly mineralized circumpulpal dentin, while the enamel appears normal or hypercalcified. Regional lymphadenitis may be evident in cases of long duration.

Systemic Features. Four different types of affected individuals can be recognized: (1) asymptomatic hypophosphatemia, (2) hypophosphatemia in adults with inactive postrachitic deformities, (3) hypophosphatemia in adults with deformities and active osteomalacia, and (4) hypophosphatemia with resistant rickets in childhood. The clinical findings differ in the four types. Hypophosphatemic adults may not present any stigmata with the exception of low inorganic phosphate. If evidence of rickets is present in childhood, short stature and bowing of legs persist in adulthood. In addition, a few adults will show evidence of osteomalacia characterized by pseudofractures and slightly elevated levels of serum alkaline phosphatase. Massive doses of vitamin D will reverse these changes. Only a few patients will present muscular weakness, atonia, craniostenosis, and convulsions.

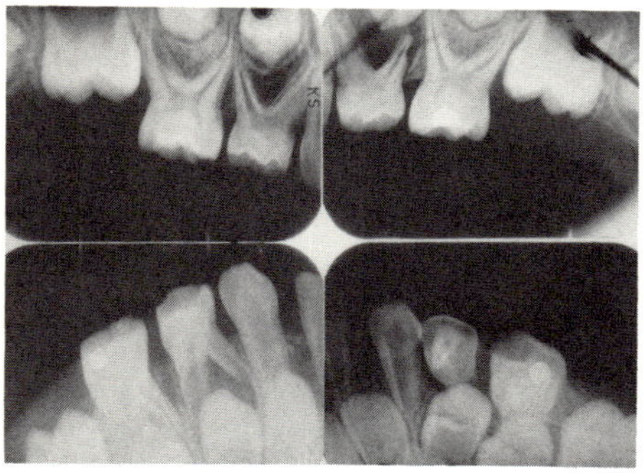

Fig. 3.12. Primary dentition shows large pulp chamber and high pulp horns extending to the dentinenamel junction.

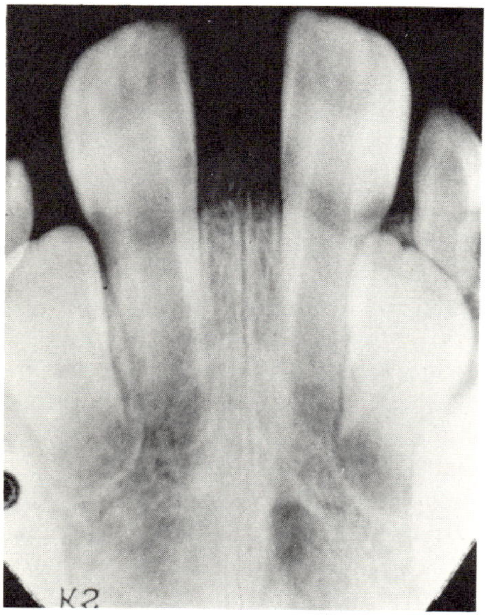

Fig. 3.13. Enlarged pulp chamber in hypophosphatemic vitamin D-resistant rickets.

Differential Diagnosis. Vitamin D-dependent rickets, nutritional rickets, and hypophosphatasia all should be considered in the differential diagnosis.

Laboratory Aids. The serum calcium is normal, alkaline phosphatase is normal or slightly elevated, and inorganic phosphate is low but must be compared to age-matched controls.

Synonym. Vitamin D-resistant rickets.

References

Condon JR, et al: Pathogenesis of rickets and osteomalacia in familial hypophosphatemia. *Arch Dis Child* 46:269–272, 1971.

Sauk JJ Jr, Witkop CJ Jr: Electron optic analysis of human dentin in

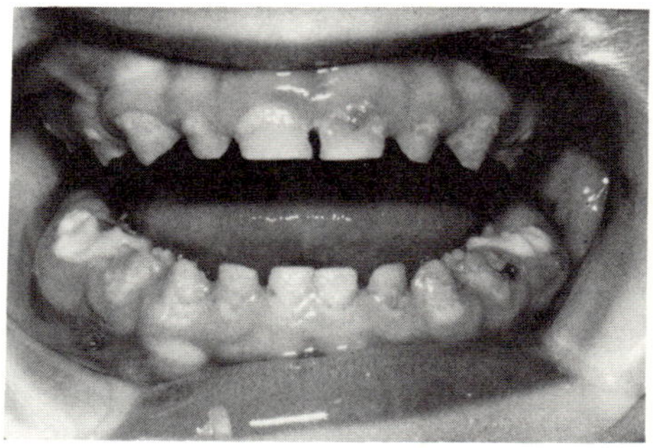

Fig. 3.14. Hypoplastic and hypocalcified enamel is present on both anterior and posterior teeth.

hypophosphatemic vitamin D-resistant rickets (report of a kindred with consanguinity). *Oral Surg* 2:203–214, 1973.

Short E, et al: Familial hypophosphatemic rickets: Defective transport of inorganic phosphate by intestinal mucosa. *Science* 179:700–702, 1973.

3.7 Hypoplastic-Hypocalcified Enamel, Onycholysis, and Functional Hypohidrosis

This syndrome was first described by Witkop and collaborators (1975) and consists of (1) hypoplastic-hypocalcified enamel, (2) onycholysis, (3) seborrheic dermatitis of the scalp, and (4) xerosis and functional hypohidrosis. The condition is inherited in an autosomal dominant manner.

Facies. The scalp reveals seborrheic dermatitis and the facial skin is dry and rough.

Oral Structures. The enamel defect affects both the primary and permanent teeth (Fig. 3.14). The enamel is thin, and many teeth do not meet at the contact points, so spaces are seen between teeth. On some teeth the enamel approaches normal hardness, but on others it is soft and can easily be removed from newly erupted teeth by a sharp instrument. Eruption of permanent teeth may be delayed. Oral radiographs may show unerupted teeth undergoing resorption within the alveolus.

Systemic Features. Somatic and mental development are normal. In infancy a few toenails or fingernails may show detachment of the distal one-quarter or one-half of the nail from its bed (Fig. 3.15). By puberty usually all nails are affected. They appear clinically as "dirty nails." The detachment is due to a hyperkeratosis which does not markedly elevate the nail from its bed. All patients in the two kindreds examined have seborrheic dermatitis of the scalp, usually present from early infancy. The skin is dry and rough. Counts of eccrine gland openings on dermal fingerpad ridges are within the normal range, approximately 22–26 openings per linear centimeter. In adults, however, on testing the function of those glands at room temperature or by sweat-eliciting procedures as compared to normal subjects, the affected individuals show less than 10% of the glands functioning.

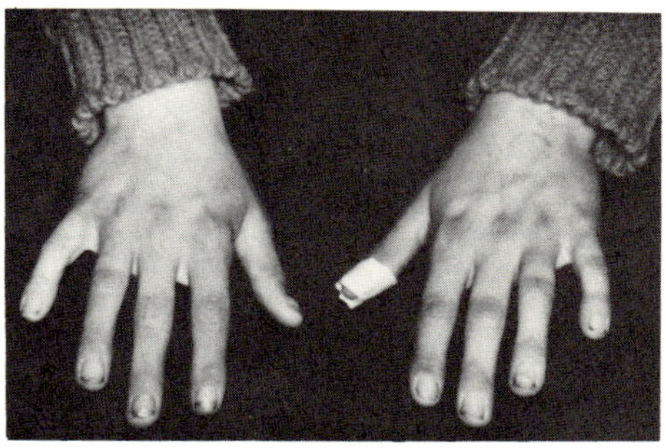

Fig. 3.15. Generalized onycholysis present on digits. Toes were equally affected.

Differential Diagnosis. Ectodermal dysplasias should be included in the differential diagnosis.

Laboratory Aids. Eccrine gland testing can be performed by preparing an alcoholic iodine solution of 150 mg of iodine dissolved in 20 cc of 95% ethanol and 5 cc of castor oil, painted on any glossy finished starch-bonded paper. Most high-quality typing papers are starch-bonded. Sweat prints appear as purple dots. Finger, palm, or other skin sweat prints can be prepared that compare the patient's prints with those of normal controls under a variety of sweat unstimulated or stimulated conditions.

References

Witkop CJ Jr, et al: Hypoplastic enamel, onycholysis and hypohidrosis inherited as an autosomal dominant trait. A new syndrome. *Oral Surg* 39:71–86, 1975.

3.8 Incontinentia Pigmenti

The major components of the syndrome include (1) vesicles, verrucae and pigmented macules of the skin, and (2) anomalies involving eyes, skeletal system, central nervous system and teeth. The mode of inheritance is X-linked dominant, lethal in the male. Thus, nearly all affected individuals are female. Increased numbers of chromosomal breaks in cultured cells have been reported in patients with the syndrome.

Facies. There is no characteristic facies.

Oral Structures. The teeth of both dentitions are affected; delayed tooth eruption, pegged teeth or teeth with conical crowns, and oligodontia are noted almost constantly (Figs. 3.16–17).

Systemic Features. Physical growth is within normal limits. Mental retardation of variable degree has been observed in about 30% of affected patients. Hydrocephalus, spastic and lax paralysis, microcephaly, convulsive episodes, and paresis of eye muscles are seen in about 35% to 40% of affected individuals. The first manifestations of the syndrome appear on the skin of the extremities during the first week of life, as linear or grouped vesicles containing brownish-colored serum. The vesi-

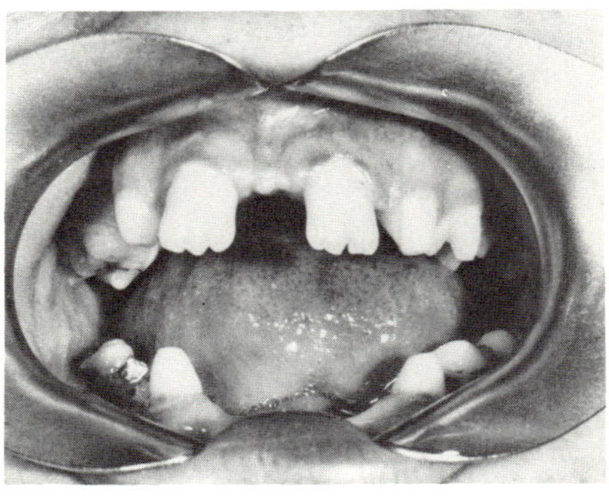

Fig. 3.16. Oligodontia and teeth with conical crown shape.

cles may disappear by the end of the first month. Recurrence is not infrequent and they may be replaced by violaceous papules or inflammatory lesions or both. Pigmented macules, brownish gray in color, with a reticular or whorly pattern, generally present at birth, occur over the trunk and extremities (Fig. 3.18). These pigmented areas are not related to the sites or numbers of vesicles or warty formations. By the second year of life, the pigmentation tends to disappear, but some residuum generally is present throughout life.

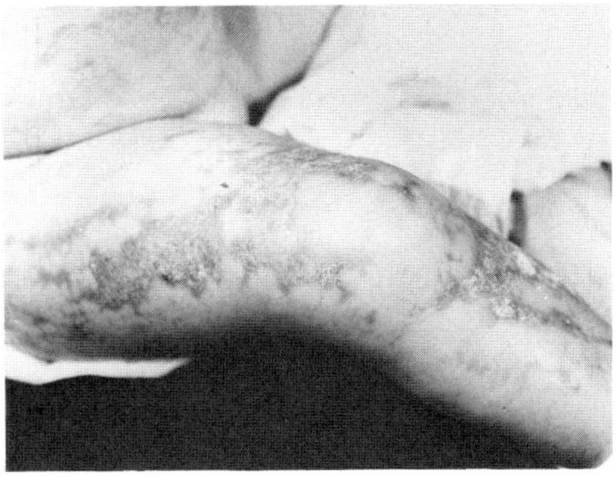

Fig. 3.18. Thigh, ten-month-old female. Note crusting, scarification, bullae, and linear pigmentation.

By the second month of life, hyperkeratotic warty lesions usually appear on the dorsal surface of the digits, knuckles, and joints, and disappear after three or four months. Healing of inflamed areas eventuates in a scleroderma-like appearance. Alopecia areata has been described in 20% to 25% of affected persons. Occasional findings are dystrophic fingernails and breast asymmetry. The most frequent ophthalmologic changes (seen in about 25% to 35% of patients) are cataracts, strabismus, and optic atrophy. The skeleton is affected in about 20% of patients, with syndactyly, supernumerary ribs, hemiatrophy, and shortening of the legs and arms.

Differential Diagnosis. During early childhood several conditions

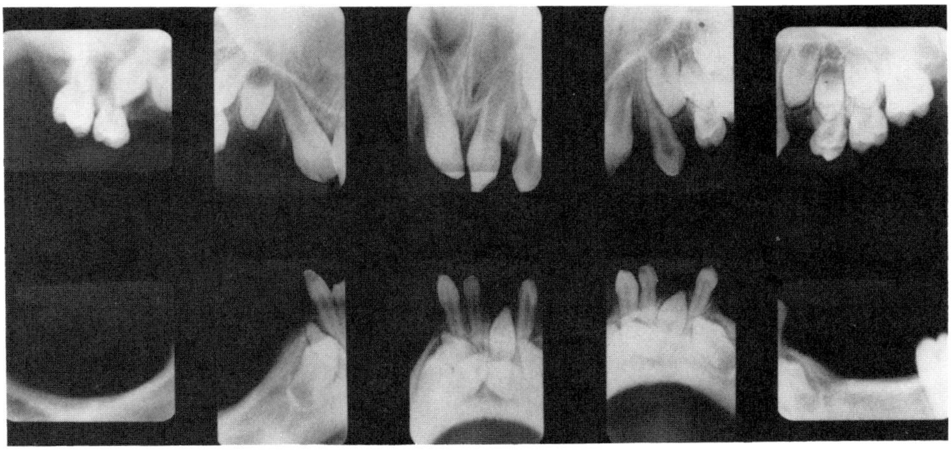

Fig. 3.17. Roentgenograms from another patient with incontinentia pigmenti showing oligondontia, impacted teeth, and teeth with peg-shaped crown.

should be considered, such as congenital syphilis, epidermolysis bullosa, dermatitis, and Naegeli syndrome. With eruption of the malformed teeth, other conditions can be added to the differential diagnosis, such as chondroectodermal dysplasia and the various ectodermal dysplasias.

Laboratory Aids. Chromosomal breaks in cultured cells and increased blood eosinophilia, the latter especially elevated during the vesicular phase of the syndrome, may aid in the diagnosis.

Synonym. Bloch-Sulzberger syndrome.

References

Cantu JM, et al: Chromosomal instability in incontinentia pigmenti. *Ann Génét* 16:117–119, 1973.

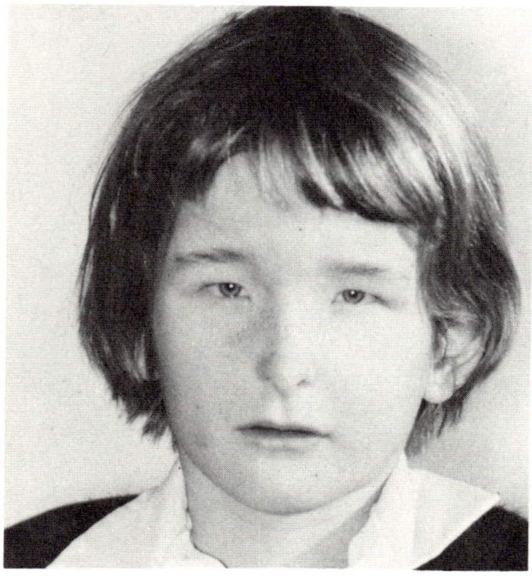

Fig. 3.19. Note microphthalmia and thin elongated nose with flaring of the alae.

Iancu T, et al: Incontinentia pigmenti. *Clin Genet* 7:103–110, 1975.

Russell DL, and Finn SB: Incontinentia pigmenti (Bloch-Sulzberger syndrome): A case report with emphasis on dental manifestations. *J Dent Child* 34:494–500, 1967.

3.9 Oculodentoosseous Dysplasia

The condition was first recognized by Lohmann (1920); however, not until 1957 did Meyer-Schwickerath and collaborators suggest the term oculodentodigital dysplasia (ODD) to describe a syndrome consisting of (1) a thin nose with hypoplastic alae and narrow nostrils, (2) microcornea with iris anomalies, (3) syndactyly and camptodactyly of the fourth and fifth fingers, and (4) enamel hypoplasia similar to amelogenesis imperfecta. The condition is rare, only about 40 cases having been reported. The syndrome exhibits autosomal dominant inheritance with variable expressivity.

Facies. Patients present a characteristic facies with small sunken eyes and true ocular hypertelorism. Epicanthal folds are frequent. Microcornea is the most constant eye anomaly, the corneal diameter generally being less than 10 mm. Other eye abnormalities are microphthalmus (Fig. 3.19), secondary glaucoma, congenital cataract, persistence of pupillary membrane, disk coloboma, synechia, strabismus, and optic atrophy. The eyelid aperture is reduced in width to about 24 to 25 mm. In most cases vision is essentially normal. Several patients have proved to be microcephalic. The ears generally present malformed pinnae. Conduction deafness has been noted in some patients. The nasal alae are hypoplastic, and the nostrils are slit-like.

Oral Structures. The teeth are usually yellow on eruption. Both dentitions may be affected by a generalized enamel hypoplasia, similar to that seen in amelogenesis imperfecta (Figs. 3.20–21). Thickening of the mandibular alveolar ridge has been reported.

Systemic Features. Somatic growth and mental development are within normal limits. The most frequent skeletal anomaly is syndactyly of the fourth and fifth fingers (the third finger may rarely be involved) with camptodactyly and ulnar clinodactyly. Roentgenograms show the middle phalanx of these fingers to be cube-shaped. There is aplasia or hypoplasia of the middle phalanx of one or more toes, which are otherwise clinically normal. Syndactyly of the third and fourth toes is an occasional finding. The femurs present a mild broadening of the metaphyseal area. The hand and feet bones are generally osteoporotic. Dry, thin, and sparse hair that fails to grow to normal length has been noted in several patients.

Differential Diagnosis. Trisomy 13, as well as the various forms of amelogenesis imperfecta, should be included in the differential diagnosis.

Laboratory Aids. None known.

Synonyms. ODD syndrome, oculodentodigital syndrome.

References

Dudgeon J, Chisolm JA: Oculo-dento-digital dysplasia. *Trans Ophthalmol Soc UK* 94:203–210, 1974.

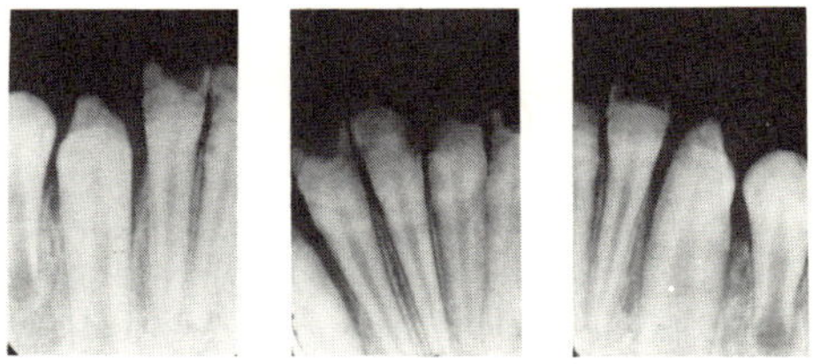

Fig. 3.20. Intraoral radiograph from another patient with the syndrome demonstrating marked enamel hypoplasia.

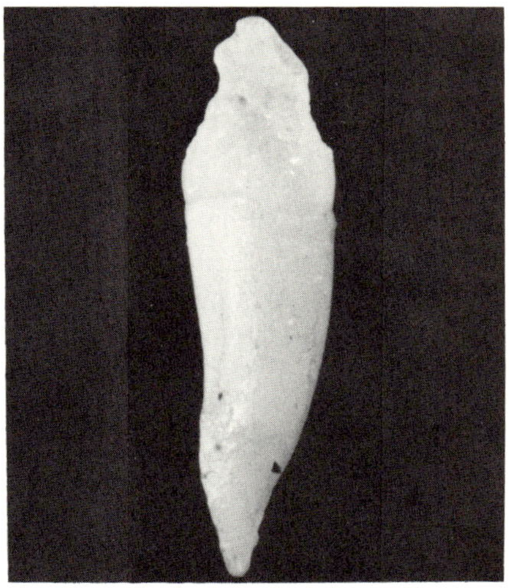

Fig. 3.21. Extracted tooth from a patient with oculodentoosseous dysplasia with enamel hypoplasia.

Gillespie FD: A hereditary syndrome: 'Dysplasia oculodentodigitalis'. *Arch Ophthalmol* 71:187–192, 1964.

Gorlin RJ, et al: Oculo-dento-digital dysplasia. *J Pediatr* 63:69–75, 1963.

Lohmann W, Beitrag zur Kenntnis des reinen Mikrophthalmus. *Arch Augenheilkd* 86:136–141, 1920.

Meyer-Schwickerath G et al: Mikrophthalmussyndrome. *Klin Monatsbl Augenheilkd* 131:18–30, 1957.

3.10 Otodental Syndrome

Otodental syndrome is an autosomal dominant condition, characterized by gigantic globe-shaped teeth and a high-frequency sensorineural hearing loss.

Facies. No characteristic facial features.

Oral Structures. The crowns of canine, bicuspid, and molar teeth have a globe-like shape (Fig. 3.22). The teeth are large, bulbous, and often lack definite cusp formation (Fig. 3.23). Yellow-white spots have been noted on focal areas of the enamel. The pulp chambers are large and may be duplicated (Fig. 3.24).

Systemic Features. A high-frequency hearing loss, with hearing thresholds of 6,000 to 8,000 cycles per second of greater than 50 decibels, has been described; however, variable expressivity of this trait has been noted.

Differential Diagnosis. Dentinal dysplasia, dentinogenesis imperfecta, and trichoosseousdental syndrome should be included in the differential diagnosis.

Laboratory Aids. None known.

Synonyms. Otodental syndrome with high-frequency hearing loss, otodental dysplasia.

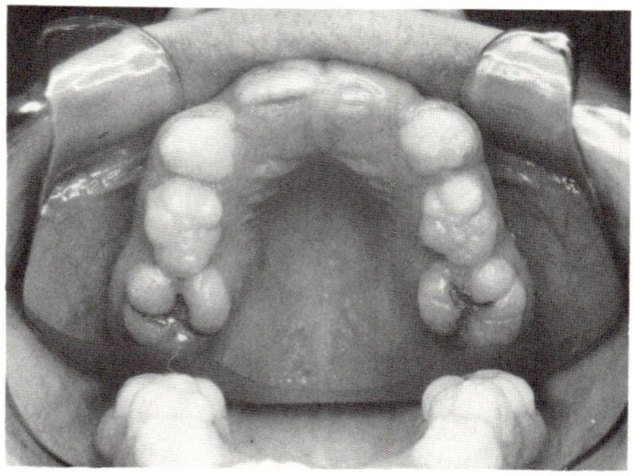

Fig. 3.22. Note grossly enlarged globe-shaped molars and premolars.

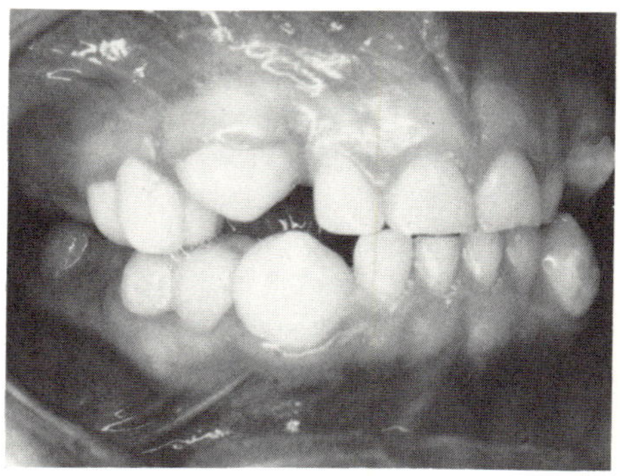

Fig. 3.23. The cuspid teeth are large and bullous in shape, but the central and lateral incisors are not affected.

References

Levin LS, et al: Otodental dysplasia: A new ectodermal dysplasia. *Clin Genet* 8:136–144, 1975.

Witkop CJ, et al: Globodontia in the otodental syndrome. *Oral Surg* 41:472–483, 1976.

3.11 Pseudohypoparathyroidism and Pseudopseudohypoparathyroidism

Albright and coworkers (1942) described pseudohypoparathyroidism (PHP), a hypocalcemic syndrome having clinical and biochemical similarity to hypoparathyroidism but failing to respond to administered parathormone by normal phosphorus diuresis. Later, a normocalcemic variant of PHP called pseudopseudohypoparathyroidism (PPHP) was described. The occurrence of both PHP and PPHP in the same kindred and demonstration of the transformation of PHP to PPHP suggest that PHP and PPHP are different forms of the same condition. The syndrome appears to be inherited as an X-linked dominant condition. Lack of an end-organ receptor for parathyroid hormone (PTH) resulting in failure of cyclic AMP elevation appears to be the biochemical basis for the syndrome.

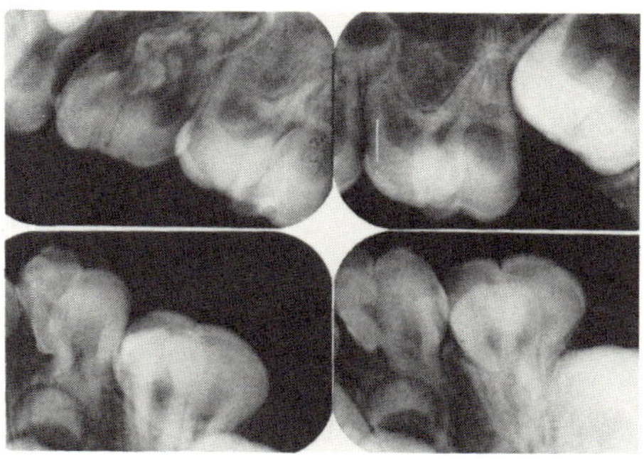

Fig. 3.24. Radiograph showing bizarre multiple fusions and pulp stones.

Facies. The head is round and the facies is mask-like. Cataracts may or may not be present.

Oral Structures. The crowns of the teeth have a normal shape; however, the enamel may be covered with large pits (Fig. 3.25). Roentgenograms reveal retarded root development with large root canals. The dentin at the apical foramina is usually distorted and thick. Dagger-shaped pulp stones can be noted near the

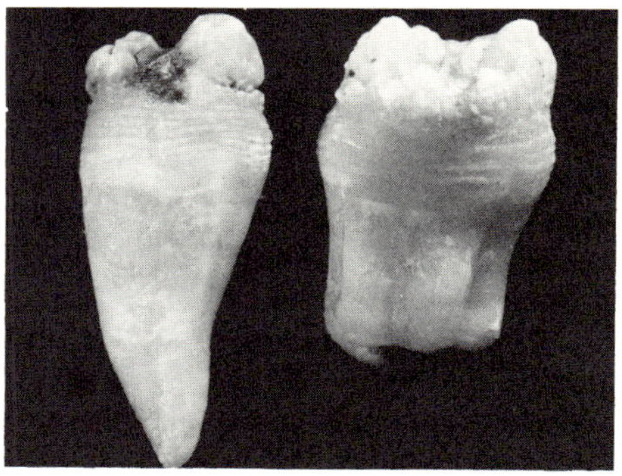

Fig. 3.25. Extracted teeth showing enamel hypoplasia.

pulp horns in primary and secondary teeth (Fig. 3.26).

Systemic Features. Patients with PHP are usually short, 137–152 cm at maturity. About 60% exhibit moderate obesity which has persisted from early childhood. Patients with PPHP have a tendency to be taller and less obese. Mental retardation has been noted in about 65% of patients with PHP but in less than one-half of those with the normocalcemic disorder. Roentgenologic examination of the skull may show calcifications in the basal ganglia. Thickening of the calvaria (in one-third of patients) and premature suture closure are common.

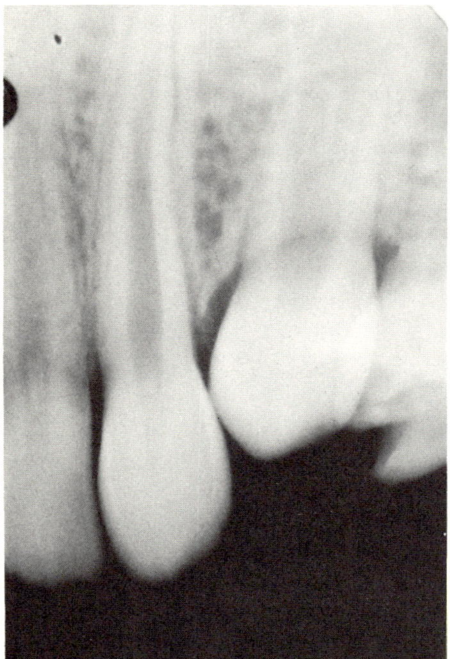

Fig. 3.26. Intraoral radiograph from patient with PHP showing dagger-shaped pulpar calcifications.

Shortening of one or more fingers or toes due to abbreviation of the corresponding metacarpals or metatarsals has been noted in about 70% of patients. Shortened metacarpals are manifested by absence of knuckles, ie, a dimple in the place of the metacarpal head when the patient makes a fist (Fig. 3.27). The fourth and fifth metacarpals are nearly always affected; less often the first, third, and second metacarpals are affected, in that order. The fourth and, less often, the third metatarsal are shortened. The phalanges are also shortened with cone-shaped epiphyses. The radius may be mildly to severely curved with displacement of the distal epiphyses and carpal bones. Calcifications are often found in subcutaneous tissues of the scalp and along extremities, especially in periarticular areas of the hands and feet.

Differential Diagnosis. Idiopathic hypoparathyroidism, basal ganglion calcification syndrome, nevoid basal cell carcinoma syndrome, Gardner syndrome, and Turner syndrome may all be included in the differential diagnosis.

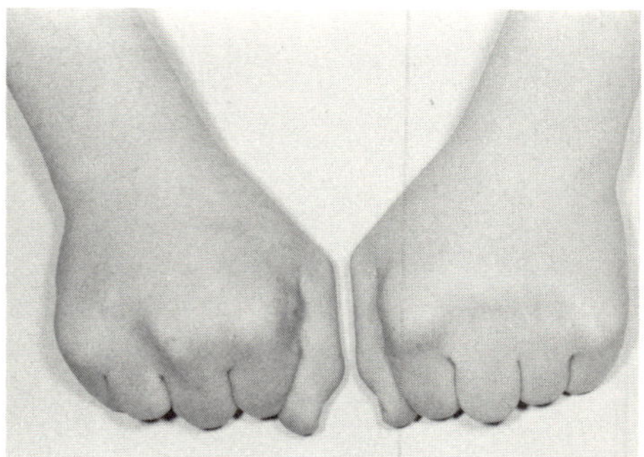

Fig. 3.27. Note characteristic absence of knuckles in a patient with PHP.

Laboratory Aids. Hypocalcemia, hyperphosphatemia, diminished renal excretion of phosphate, and lack of renal response to exogenous administration of parathormone characterize this disorder.

Synonym. Albright hereditary osteodystrophy.

References

Albright F, et al: Pseudohypoparathyroidism—an example of "Seabright-Bantam syndrome." Report of three cases. *Endocrinology* 30:922–932, 1942.

Aurback GD, et al: Polypeptide hormones and calcium metabolism. *Ann Intern Med* 70:1243–1265, 1969.

Chase LR, et al: Pseudohypoparathyroidism: Defective excretion of 3′–5′-AMP in response to parathyroid hormone. *J Clin Invest* 48:1832–1844, 1969.

Witkop CJ Jr: Gardner's syndrome and other osteognathodermal disorders with defects in parathyroid functions. *J Oral Surg* 26:639–642, 1968.

3.12 Rothmund-Thomson Syndrome

Rothmund in 1868 and Thomson in 1923 described the same syndrome consisting of (1) poikiloderma appearing from the third to the sixth month of life, (2) bilateral cataracts which appear from the fourth to the seventh year, and (3) hypogonadism. The syndrome is inherited as a recessive condition, but over 70% of patients have been females. This syndrome might represent another example of genetic heterogeneity. Most patients have been from Switzerland and Austria.

Facies. Affected patients generally have a large head with frontal bossing and a broad depressed nasal bridge. At approximately the third to the sixth month of life, the skin of the cheeks and ears becomes red and swollen. This inflammatory phase is

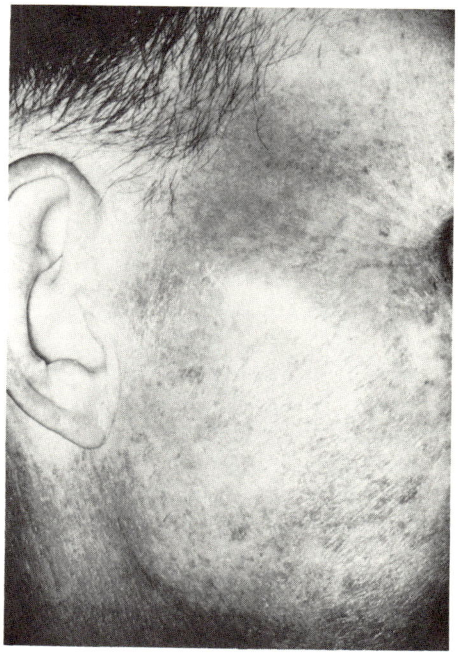

Fig. 3.28. Areas of pigmentation and depigmentation over the facial skin in a patient with the Rothmund-Thomson syndrome.

of short duration but leaves behind areas of various combinations of increased pigmentation, depigmentation, erythema, and atrophy (Fig. 3.28). Blister formation on the facial skin due to sunlight sensitivity is seen in about 35% of affected individuals. The eyebrows and lashes frequently are absent or severely diminished. The facial appearance is completed with the presence of bilateral cataracts, generally appearing between the fourth and the seventh year of life.

Oral Structures. Oral manifestations are very infrequent in this condition. A number of cases of the Rothmund-Thomson syndrome have been reported with dental findings such as microdontia, enamel hypoplasia, delayed abnormal eruption, hypodontia, and supernumerary teeth. Bifid uvula also has been seen in a few cases.

Systemic Features. Mental development is slightly below normal. Microcephaly has also been observed. Over half of the patients are markedly diminished in height and have short terminal phalanges. The dwarfism is proportional. The limbs are often slender or delicate, and acrocyanosis may be severe. Absence of thumbs, rudimentary ulna and radius, bipartite patella, and bone sclerosis have been noted in some patients. Cystic areas similar to fibrous dysplasia have been described.

Dermatologic changes similar to those described for the facial skin are also present in the extensor surfaces of the hands, forearms, legs, thighs, and buttocks, but the exposed surfaces are more severely affected (Fig. 3.29). Scalp, pubic, and axillary hair is somewhat sparse and, in some patients, almost absent. Warty hyperkeratoses, generally over the joints, which eventually develop into squamous cell carcinoma, and keratosis palmoplantaris have been described. Nail dystrophy has been noted in 25% of the cases. Hypogonadism is also present in around 25% of patients. Scanty menstruation is common; nevertheless, several affected females have borne children.

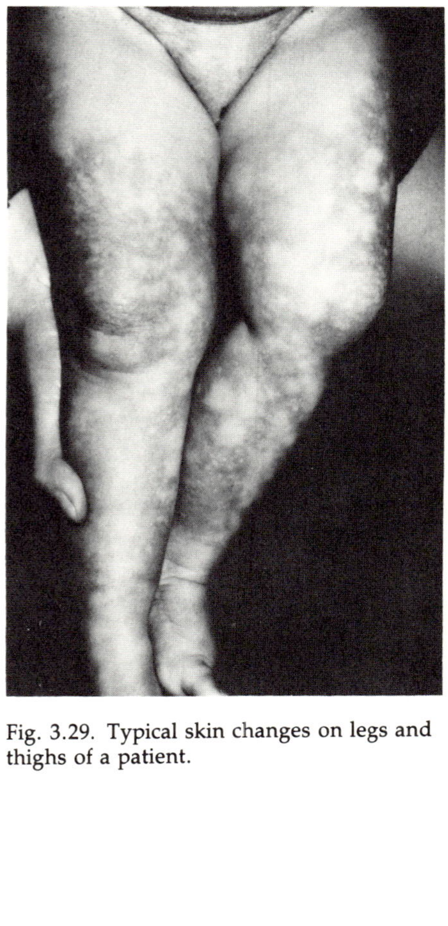

Fig. 3.29. Typical skin changes on legs and thighs of a patient.

Differential Diagnosis. Werner syndrome, Cockayne syndrome, Bloom syndrome, and other photodermatoses should be included in the differential diagnosis. Incontinentia pigmenti also should be considered.

Laboratory Aids. None known.

Synonym. Poikiloderma syndrome.

References

Kraus BS, et al: The dentition in Rothmund's syndrome. *J Am Dent Assoc* 81:894–915, 1970.

Maurer RM, Langford OL: Rothmund's syndrome: A cause of resorption of phalangeal tufts and dystrophic calcification. *Radiology* 89:706–708, 1967.

Silver HK: Rothmund-Thomson syndrome: An oculo-cutaneous disorder. *Am J Dis Child* 111:182–190, 1966.

CHAPTER 4

Systemic Inherited Disorders with Oral or Perioral Soft Tissue Involvement

4.1 Acrodermatitis Enteropathica

Acrodermatitis enteropathica, first recognized as a syndrome by Danbolt and Closs in 1942, is rare, occurs in childhood, and is characterized by (1) skin lesions, (2) hair loss, (3) nail changes, and (4) gastrointestinal disturbances. Acrodermatitis enteropathica generally becomes manifest between three weeks and ten years of age and is only occasionally seen in adults. It seems to improve by puberty. The onset is subtle, followed by episodes of acute exacerbations, alternating with partial remissions. The majority of affected patients used to die of the disease. A history of familial involvement is present in over 65% of cases. Acrodermatitis is inherited as an autosomal recessive condition and is related to an alteration in zinc metabolism.

Facies. Children affected with the syndrome present a marked similarity in facial appearance because of the periorificial location of the skin lesions and the advanced alopecia. Crust formation with psoriasiform appearance is seen on the skin of the face, especially around the eyes, nose, and oral cavity (Fig. 4.1).

Oral Structures. The lips and perioral skin are affected. Pustular formation at the angle of the mouth is almost always complicated with deep fissuring. Intraorally, the changes are confined to the soft tissues and occur in the buccal mucosa, palate, gingiva, and tonsils as reddish white spots, areas of marked edema, erosions, ulcerations, and desquamation. These changes cannot be classified as specific but rather are included under the general term "stomatitis." The majority of affected patients present a superimposed oral infection with candidosis. Many of the clinical oral manifestations could be accounted for by this added infection. Small

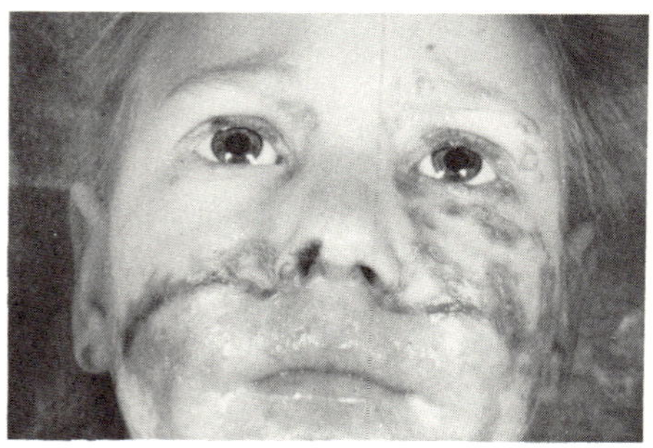

Fig. 4.1. Marked periorificial lesions characterized by erythema and crust formation.

papillomas of the tongue and of the rest of the oral mucosa have also been described. Severe halitosis and pain are always present. Delayed eruption of teeth is seen in some patients.

Systemic Features. Physical development is retarded in around 80% of the patients. Schizoid seizures are present in 40% of affected children, generally during the exacerbations of the condition. Acrodermatitis enteropathica generally starts as a periorificial erythematous skin eruption. After the initial phase, lesions also appear on the cutaneous surface of the buttocks, elbows, hands, and feet, especially between fingers and toes. One of the most common locations is around the bed of the fingernails. The eruption is vesiculobullous, and the vesicles soon rupture, leaving an ulcerated surface. Crust formation follows the ulcerative stage and healing occurs without scarring.

Diarrhea is present in 90% of reported patients, with marked excretion of fat. The stools are large, foul, and green, thus pointing to maladsorption. At times the intestinal symptom is only an occasional loose stool. Alopecia is seen in 98% of cases, in most patients being total. Paronychia with nail dystrophy is observed in 96% of reported cases; complete loss of nails occurs after prolonged involvement. Conjunctivitis, blepharitis, and photophobia are found occasionally.

Differential Diagnosis. Systemic candidosis, Kaposi varicelliform eruption, celiac syndrome, and epidermolysis bullosa should be considered in the differential diagnosis.

Laboratory Aids. Serum zinc levels should be estimated.

Synonym. Danbolt-Closs syndrome.

References

Barnes PM, Monayan EJ: Zinc deficiency in acrodermatitis enteropathica, *Proc R Soc Med* 66:327–329, 1973.

Danbolt N and Closs K: Akrodermatitis Enteropathica. *Acta Derm Venereol (Stockh)* 23:127–169, 1943.

Portnoy B, Molokhia M: Acrodermatitis enteropathica treated by zinc. *Brit J Dermatol* 91:701–703, 1974.

Portnoy B, and Molokhia M: Withdrawal of zinc therapy in acrodermatitis enteropathica. *Brit J Dermatol* 94:112–113, 1976.

4.2 Bloom Syndrome

In 1954, Bloom first described the syndrome consisting of (1) telangiectatic erythema appearing in infancy and affecting principally the face, (2) sensitivity to sunlight, and (3) stunted growth. About 40 patients have been described to date. A most complete survey is that of German (1974), who first pointed out the tendency for these children to exhibit chromosomal breaks and to develop malignancies. The syndrome is inherited in an autosomal recessive manner. It has an increased incidence among Jews of Eastern European extraction. Parental consanguinity, while higher among non-Jews, is no greater among Jews, indicating the rarity of the gene among the former. Cytogenetic studies have demonstrated a consistent tendency to chromosomal breakage and rearrangement in cells cultured in vitro and, consequently, a high incidence of aneuploidy. Immunologic deficiency has been proved in some patients, and familial history of rheumatoid arthritis has been present in a few cases.

Facies. The skull is generally microcephalic, and there is a thin, narrow face. Prominent nose, micrognathia, and flared ears have been described as constant findings. The telangiectatic erythema principally affects the butterfly area of the face, nose, lips, and ears. The eyelashes are commonly lost. Although the acute skin involvement and sunlight sensitivity improve with age, the resultant scarring, depigmentation, and atrophy are permanently disfiguring.

Oral Structures. Chronic cheilitis due to sunlight sensitivity is a constant finding. As mentioned above, micrognathia can also be found. Squamous cell carcinoma of the tongue has been reported.

Systemic Features. Short stature is a predominant feature of the syndrome (Fig. 4.2). Newborns rarely weigh over 2300 gm (5 pounds), and birth length is around 44 cm (17 in; normal mean is 50 cm or 20 in). Dwarfism persists into adulthood, since height rarely exceeds 145 cm (57 in) for the male and 130 cm (51 in) for the female. Many affected individuals present a minor degree of mental retardation. The telangiectatic erythema, due to sunlight sensitivity, appears in any area of exposed skin in early childhood. In addition to the face, the dorsum of the hands and the nape of the neck are most affected. The skin lesions rarely extend

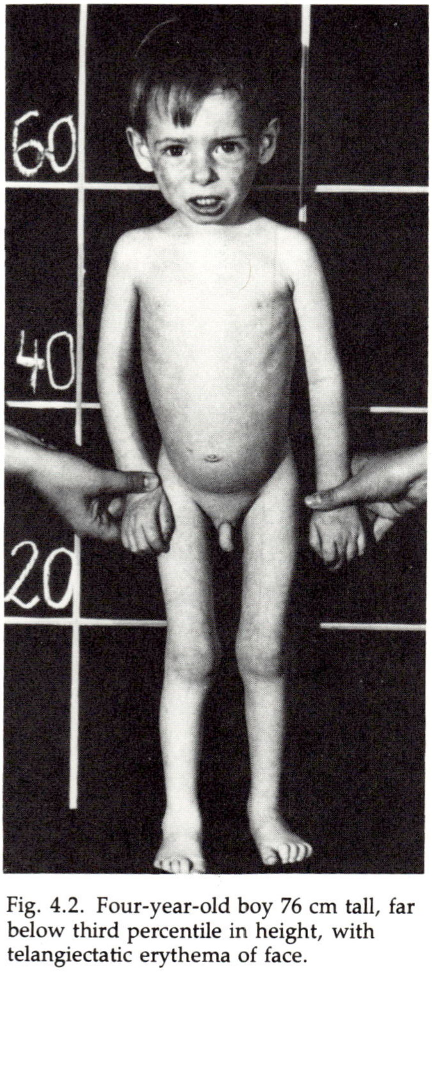

Fig. 4.2. Four-year-old boy 76 cm tall, far below third percentile in height, with telangiectatic erythema of face.

to the trunk. Eye conjunctiva can be similarly affected. Café-au-lait spots are noted in more than half of the cases.

A host of minor anomalies has been described, including high-pitched voice, testicular atrophy or hypoplasia, and urethral stricture. Bloom syndrome is associated with a high incidence of leukemia and lymphoma. Half of the patients with the syndrome who have survived to 21 years of age have subsequently died of malignant neoplasia.

Differential Diagnosis. A varied group of conditions should be included in the differential diagnosis, such as Cockayne syndrome, Louis-Bar syndrome, Fanconi anemia, Rothmund-Thomson syndrome, dyskeratosis congenita, Werner syndrome, and xeroderma pigmentosum syndromes.

Laboratory Aids. Chromosomal breakage and rearrangement can be easily demonstrated in cultured cells from patients with the syndrome. Diminished levels of immunoglobulins IgG, IgA, and IgM are also a constant finding.

Synonyms. Bloom-German syndrome, congenital telangiectatic erythema with growth retardation.

References

Bloom D: Congenital telangiectatic erythema in a Levi-Lorain dwarf. *Arch Dermatol* 69:526, 1954.

German J: Bloom's syndrome. III. Analysis of the chromosome aberration characteristic of this disorder. *Chromosoma* (Berlin) 48:361–366, 1974.

Schroeder TM, German J: Bloom's syndrome and Fanconi's anemia. Demonstration of two distinctive patterns of chromosome disruption and rearrangement. *Humangenetik* 25:299–306, 1974.

4.3 Chédiak-Higashi Syndrome

The Chédiak-Higashi syndrome is manifested by (1) defective pigmentation, (2) large eosinophilic, peroxidase-positive inclusion bodies in myeloblasts and promyelocytes of the bone marrow, (3) neutropenia, and (4) susceptibility to infection and malignant lymphoma. The syndrome is inherited in an autosomal recessive manner. This condition is a disorder of giant lysosomal inclusion bodies that are found in circulating granulocytes and in many other cells of the body. The enormous size of the inclusion bodies reflects an improper handling or distribution of the normal lysosomal enzymes. An accelerated turnover of sphingolipids in leukocytes has been suggested.

Facies. The irides are usually pale and lavender, and the fundi are pale. Horizontal nystagmus and photophobia are common. Papilledema may be present.

Oral Structures. Chronic periodontitis as a result of the neutropenia, and susceptibility to infection are common. Aphthae or gingivitis are present in most affected individuals (Fig. 4.3). Cervical lymphadenopathy is present in most cases.

Systemic Features. Somatic and mental development are within normal limits; however, progressive cranial and peripheral neuropathy, muscle weakness, foot drop, decreased muscle stretch reflexes, headaches, transitory paresis, tremors, emotional lability, EEG abnormalities, and lymphohistiocytic infiltration of central and peripheral nervous systems have been noted. Characteristic cytoplasmic inclusions resembling lysosomes are seen within nerve cells, astrocytes, Schwann cells, etc. Within the neurons of the substantia nigra, the melanin pigment granules are especially large and irregular.

Transillumination of the ocular globe reveals a definite pink coloration. Histologic examination of the eye reveals diminished melanin pigmentation in the iris, choroid, ciliary epithelium, and pigment epithelium of the retina. Affected individuals may also exhibit cutaneous "albinism" characterized by an absence of pigmentation of the areolas and genitals. Scattered pigmented nevi or ephelides are also present on exposed areas of otherwise slate-gray colored skin. Hyperhidrosis, heat rash, marked photosensitivity, and severe and extensive pyoderma may be present (Fig. 4.4). Affected patients have a frosted gray sheen to the scalp hair. Large melanin granules are visible by light microscopy and large melanosomes by electron microscopy.

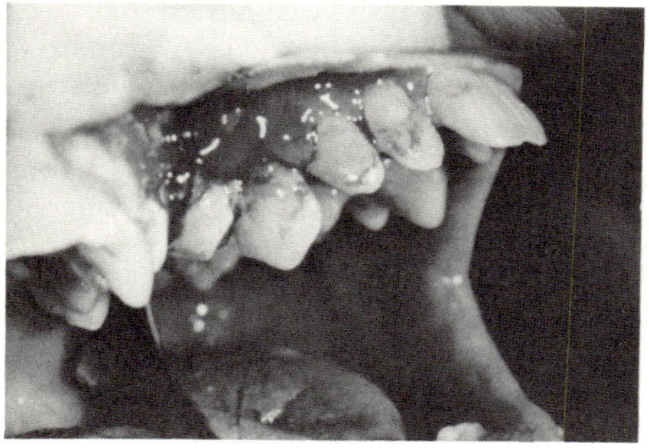

Fig. 4.3. Marked and extensive gingivitis present in a 10-year-old female with Chédiak-Higashi syndrome.

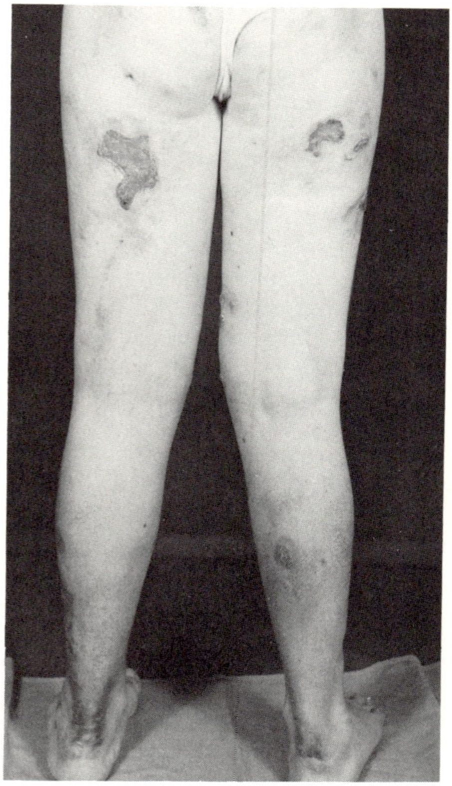

Fig. 4.4. Note extensive and severe pyoderma in patient with Chédiak-Higashi syndrome.

Differential Diagnosis. The differential diagnosis should include tyrosinase-positive albinism, Hermansky-Pudlak syndrome, yellow mutant albinism, cyclic neutropenia, and agranulocytosis of various etiologies.

Laboratory Aids. Demonstration of large eosinophilic peroxidase-positive inclusion bodies in myeloblasts and promyelocytes along with an existing neutropenia is of great value in establishing a diagnosis. Some granulocytes have giant granules (some up to ten times normal size). Anemia has been noted in 80% of cases, thrombocytopenia in 50%, and leukopenia in 40%. The characteristic lymphocytic inclusions have also been found in normal relatives of patients with the Chédiak-Higashi syndrome.

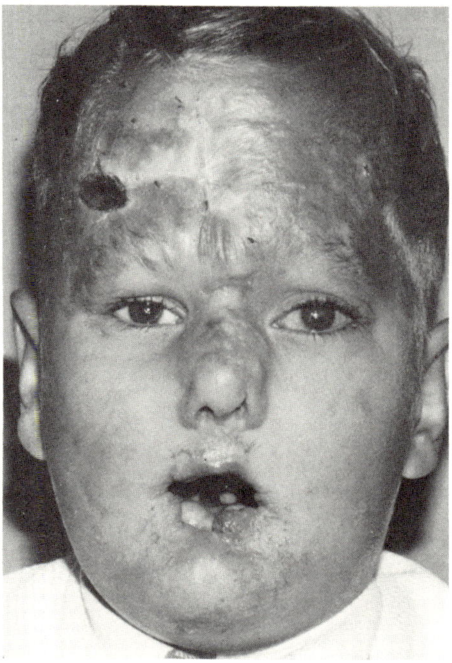

Fig. 4.5. Keloid scar as a result of severe burning without pain. Also note marked destruction of lower lip due to self-chewing.

References

White JG: The Chédiak-Higashi syndrome: a possible lysosomal disease. *Blood* 28:143–156, 1966.

White JG: Chédiak-Higashi syndrome. *Am J Pathol* 72:503–519, 1973.

Windhorst DB, et al: Chédiak-Higashi syndrome: hereditary gigantism of cytoplasmic organelles. *Science* 151:81–83, 1966.

4.4 Congenital Indifference to Pain

The syndrome was described by Dearborn (1931) as characterized by congenital complete indifference to pain, resulting in injury to both soft and hard tissues with subsequent severe scarring. The condition is inherited in an autosomal recessive manner.

Facies. The face does not present any typical features, unless marked mutilation of the lips is present, generally due to self-chewing. Also scarring might be present (Figs. 4.5–6). In such cases the facies will show the same stigmata seen in other syndromes associated with indifference to pain.

Oral Structures. Lack of sensation of pain results in severe oral mutilation, especially of the tongue and lips. Scar formation is a constant sequela. Oral mutilation coincides with tooth eruption and may suggest the diagnosis. Extensive caries occurs without toothache. Some patients painlessly extract their own teeth.

Systemic Features. Physical development is within normal limits. Intelligence ranges from mild mental retardation to normal. There is total absence of reaction to painful stimuli. Deep tendon reflexes are normal. The corneal reflex is absent or diminished, but the thermal, taste, and

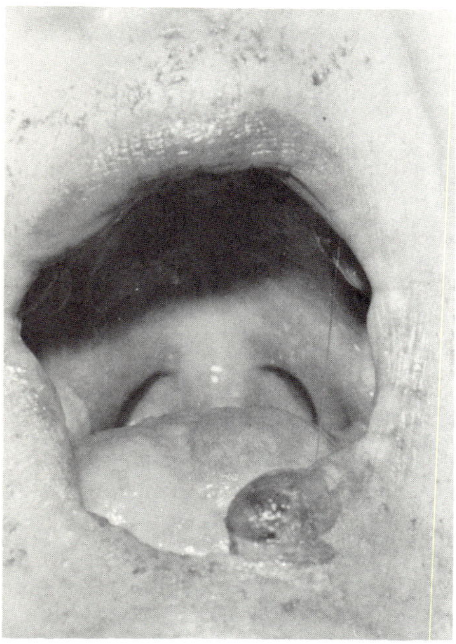

Fig. 4.6. Close-up view of lower lip in same patient shown in Fig. 4.5.

touch reflexes are generally normal or mildly diminished. Osteomyelitis, aseptic necrosis, fracture, Charcot's joint, and distal necrosis with spontaneous resorption of toes and fingers are constant findings. These skeletal alterations are most likely a consequence of the lack of pain sensation; patients cannot recognize trauma due to absence of pain response.

Differential Diagnosis. All other forms of congenital indifference to pain, including the Lesch-Nyhan syndrome and familial dysautonomia, should be considered.

Laboratory Aids. None known.

Synonym. Congenital insensitivity to pain.

References

Appenzeller O, Kornfeld M: Indifference to pain: A chronic peripheral neuropathy with mosaic Schwann cells. *Arch Neurol* 27:322–339, 1972.

Da Costa Maia JC, et al: Isolation of a new urine metabolite excreted in generalized congenital analgesia. *Clin Chim Acta* 12:122–124, 1965.

Dearborn G: A case of congenital general pure analgesia. *J Nerv Ment Dis* 75:612–615, 1931.

Thrush DC: Congenital insensitivity to pain. *Brain* 96:369–386, 1973.

4.5 Cutis Laxa

Cutis laxa is characterized by (1) skin which hangs in loose folds, (2) emphysema, (3) hernia, and often (4) diverticulae of various organs. Although the term "cutis laxa" was initially used to refer to Ehlers-Danlos syndrome or cutis hyperelastica, within the past two decades the name has been restricted to conditions in which the skin hangs in folds. Although it may occur later in life (acquired form) as a postinflammatory cutaneous phenomenon, there appear to be three hereditary forms, the more common form being a severe autosomal recessive type. Parental consanguinity has been noted in several instances, and there have been affected sibs. In the relatively benign autosomal dominant form, patients seldom have more than sagging skin, a deep voice, and inguinal hernia. It is conceivable that several isolated, mildly involved cases represent the dominant form of the disorder. A rare X-linked form of this condition appears to be associated with a deficiency of lysyl oxidase. Most manifestations of the syndrome can be explained on the basis of generalized elastolysis.

Facies. Drooping and ectropion of the eyelids together with sagging facial skin (jowls) and accentuation of the nasolabial and other facial folds produce a "blood-hound" or aged appearance (Fig. 4.7).

Oral Structures. The lack of elasticity produces a marked downward falling of both lips, especially the upper, with pronounced accentuation of labial and labial-medial sulci. Micrognathia and abnormal tooth eruption have been reported.

Systemic Features. Somatic growth has been reported to be retarded in a few instances. Mental development is impaired in a few cases and probably represents a variant of the syndrome. A few children exhibit muscle hypotonia and late closure of the anterior fontanel. Hip dislocation and joint hyperextensibility as well as inguinal, diaphragmatic, and umbilical hernias are not uncommon in the disorder. Diverticulae of the gastrointestinal tract, prolapse of gastric and

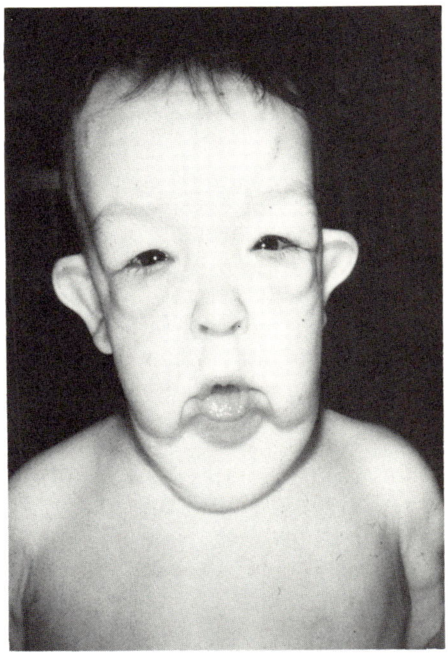

Fig. 4.7. Infant with the autosomal recessive type of cutis laxa. Note sagging facial skin and pronounced downward fall of lips.

rectal mucosae and bladder diverticulae have been described.

The skin of the entire body appears floppy, often hanging in folds. It is not hyperelastic, and there is no fragility or difficulty in healing. The voice is usually deep and resonant in quality, resulting from laxity of the vocal cords. Emphysema has been one of the more common features of the autosomal recessive form, being a result of the generalized elastolysis. This causes right ventricular enlargement, bundle branch block, cor pulmonale, and often death at an early age. Pulmonary stenosis and extremely tortuous blood vessels have been noted.

Differential Diagnosis. The acquired form of cutis laxa should be considered in the differential diagnosis.

Laboratory Aids. With orcein or other elastic fiber stains, biopsy of the skin demonstrates an absence or marked diminution of elastic fibers which normally rise vertically into the papillary bodies and surround the pilosebaceous follicles. Elsewhere in the corium, the elastic fibers are deficient, fragmented, and shortened and undergo granular degeneration. Serum copper values have been reported to be low, and urinary excretion of copper high. The X-linked form of cutis laxa manifests a deficiency of lysyl oxidase in dermal fibroblasts.

Synonym. Generalized elastolysis.

References

Balboni FA: Cutis laxa and multiple vascular anomalies including multiple coarctation of the aorta. *St Francis Hosp Bull* 19:26–35, 1963.

Beighton PH: The dominant and recessive forms of cutis laxa. *J Med Genet* 9:216–221, 1972.

Byers PH, et al: An X-linked form of cutis laxa due to deficiency of lysyl oxidase; the collagen and elastin crosslinking enzyme. *Birth Def,* in press.

Goltz RW, Hult AM: Generalized elastolysis (cutis laxa) and Ehlers-Danlos syndrome (cutis hyperelastica). *South Med J* 58:848–854, 1965.

4.6 Cyclic Neutropenia

Cyclic neutropenia is a form of agranulocytosis characterized by a periodic decrease of neutrophilic leukocytes in the peripheral blood. The clinical features appear and regress spontaneously, only to reappear in a cyclic pattern which is directly associated with the blood picture. The disease lasts throughout life. In some cases spontaneous improvement may occur in adulthood. Cycles have an interval of approximately 21 to 27 days and occasionally several months. An autosomal dominant mode of inheritance is likely, although further evidence is needed to support this theory.

Facies. There is no characteristic facies.

Oral Structures. Oral manifestations include severe ulcerative gingivitis or stomatitis or both (Fig. 4.8). Occasionally ulceration may be observed on the tongue, palate, and labial mucosa (Fig. 4.9). Ulcers are generally round and vary in size from a few millimeters to two or more centimeters, generally with elevated borders and a bleeding base. Pain is a constant feature of these lesions. Loss of alveolar bone results from repeated insults, leading to mobility and early exfoliation of teeth. Oral lesions are generally complicated by infection. Neutropenia usually lasts from two to five days. As the blood count returns to normal, the oral lesions regress. Ulcerations usually heal without scarring, but with successive attacks scarring may occur.

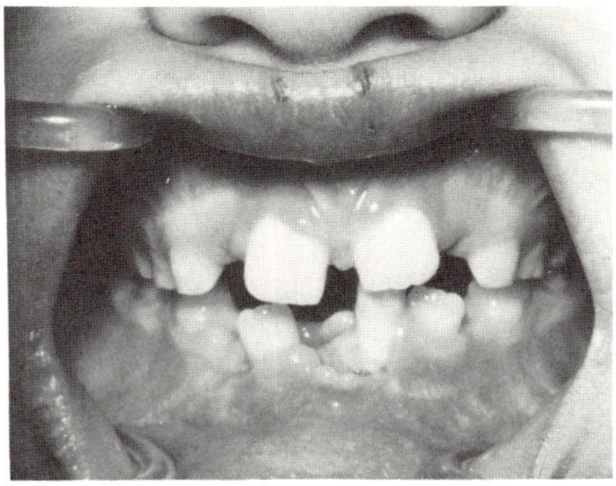

Fig. 4.8. Note malposition of teeth due to early gingival and periodontal destruction.

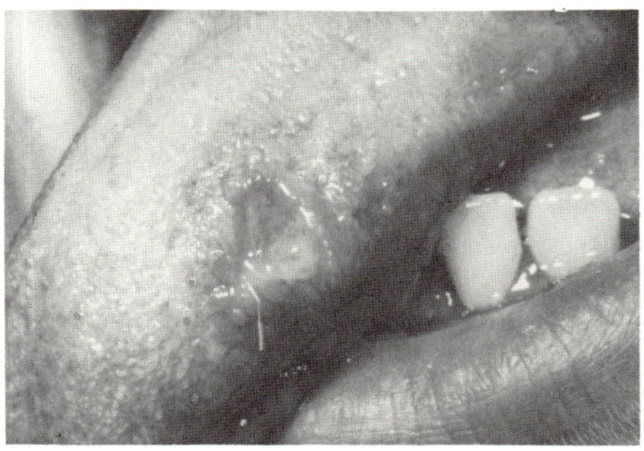

Fig. 4.9. Patient with cyclic neutropenia. Note deep ulceration with elevated erythematous margin on the lateral border of the tongue.

Systemic Features. Physical and mental development are within normal limits. Clinical manifestations generally begin in early childhood with mild fever, malaise, sore throat, oral involvement, and, in some cases, arthritis, headache, and cutaneous manifestations.

Differential Diagnosis. Agranulocytosis, other blood dyscrasias, recurrent aphthous lesions, and periadenitis mucosa necrotica recurrens should be considered in the differential diagnosis. Other conditions producing premature loss of teeth also should be considered.

Laboratory Aids. Hematological examination shows a marked decrease in neutrophils. Within three to five days the peak of the disease is reached and for a period of one to two days neutrophils may be completely absent. Soon after they reappear, and within three to five days, the blood count and differential count are normal.

Synonym. Periodic neutropenia.

References

Kander E, Mauer AM: Neutropenias of childhood. *J Pediatr* 69:147–157, 1966.

Morley AA, et al: Familial cyclical neutropenia. *Brit J Haemat* 13:719–738, 1967.

Sedano HO, Young WG: Nonneoplastic lesions of the oral mucosae, in *Current Diagnosis*. Philadelphia, WB Saunders Co, 5th Ed, 1976.

4.7 Double Lip, Blepharochalasis, and Nontoxic Thyroid Enlargement

The syndrome of (1) blepharochalasis, (2) double lip, and possibly (3) thyroid struma is of unknown etiology, although vasomotor instability, hormonal dysfunction, and autosomal dominant inheritance have been suggested by several authors.

Facies. The typical facies is best appreciated during smiling or talking and is characterized by sagging eyelids and thick double upper lip (Fig. 4.10). The skin of the upper lids is markedly thin and atrophic. The upper lids sag and hang over the palpebral fissure. Angioneurotic edema-like episodes are frequent. The enlargement of the eyelids and lips may occur simultaneously. The lower lids are rarely, if ever, affected.

Oral Structures. The upper lip is characterized by a horizontal duplication, seen only when the patient smiles or talks. The double lip can be present from infancy and is located in the mucosa of the upper lip. The lower lip is almost always normal.

Systemic Features. Thyroid enlargement is variable and not associated with toxic symptoms. The majority of cases presenting thyroid enlargement were reported in Germany during the 1920s and 1930s, in areas of endemic goiter. We have seen cases of Ascher syndrome without thyroid enlargement.

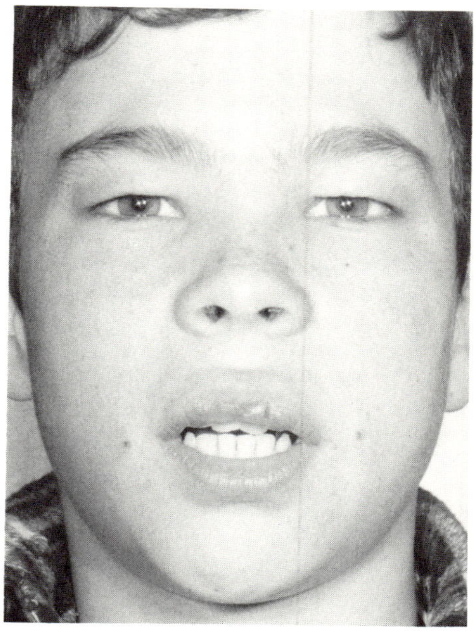

Fig. 4.10. Note blepharochalasis and double lip in a patient with Ascher syndrome.

Differential Diagnosis. Double lip, the Melkersson-Rosenthal syndrome, lip lymphedema, goiter, and vascular neoplasms of the lips should be considered in the differential diagnosis.

Laboratory Aids. Microscopy of the double lip has shown loose connective tissue, hyperplastic minor salivary glands, increased capillarity and perivascular apposition of plasma cells and lymphocytes. Examination of the excessive eyelid tissue has demonstrated prolapsed orbital fat, hyperplastic lacrimal glands and an increased number of capillaries. Elastic fibers also have been studied, but with conflicting results in regard to their absence.

Synonym. Ascher syndrome.

References

Barnett ML, et al: Double lip and double lip with blepharochalasis (Ascher's syndrome) *Oral Surg* 34:727–733, 1972.

Papanayatou PH, Hatziotis JC: Ascher's syndrome. *Oral Surg* 35:467–471, 1973.

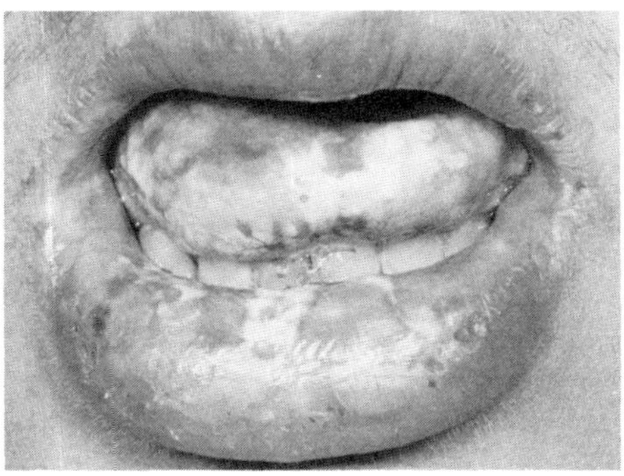

Fig. 4.11. Intraoral view showing marked whitening of lingual and labial mucosae.

4.8 Dyskeratosis Congenita with Pigmentation, Dystrophic Nails, Aplastic Anemia, and Leukoplakia Oris

The syndrome originally described by Zinsser in 1906 consists of (1) reticular atrophy of the skin with pigmentation, (2) nail dystrophy, and (3) oral leukoplakia. The syndrome represents a genetic heterogeneity, and both autosomal and X-linked recessive forms have been well documented in several instances. The majority of affected patients are males, but several examples of the full-blown syndrome have been reported in females. Affected siblings also have been documented.

Facies. The striking facial appearance, which develops with time, is produced by conjunctivitis, blepharitis, loss of scalp hair and lashes, and, as described below, labial and skin changes.

Oral Structures. Around age 5 to 7, numerous flaccid vesicles and bullae start to appear on the oral mucosa. These bullae are short-lived, and after rupture leave areas of ulcerations with peripheral epithelial sloughs. The vesicular eruption is painless and recurrent, with subsequent atrophy of the oral mucosa. This atrophy is most evident on the tongue, due to depapillation of the ventral surface, and results in a smooth, bald tongue similar to that seen in pernicious anemia. The entire oral mucosa becomes thick, fissured, and white (Fig. 4.11). Premalignant changes and frank malignant neoplasms can occur in association with dyskeratosis congenita in the oral mucosae as well as in other mucosal surfaces.

Systemic Features. Mild generalized growth retardation has been reported in the majority of cases. One-third of the affected patients are mildly mentally retarded. The dermatologic changes, mostly affecting the face, neck, and chest, generally develop around puberty and are characterized by moderately large, ill-defined areas, mostly symmetric in distribution and composed of erythema, superficial scaling, telangiectasias, and a prominent reticulated hyperpigmentation (Fig. 4.12). Other manifestations include hyperhidrosis of palms and soles, dystrophic fingernails and toenails (Fig. 4.13), chronic blepharitis, and marked lacrimation due to keratotic plugging with permanent obstruction of the lacrimal points.

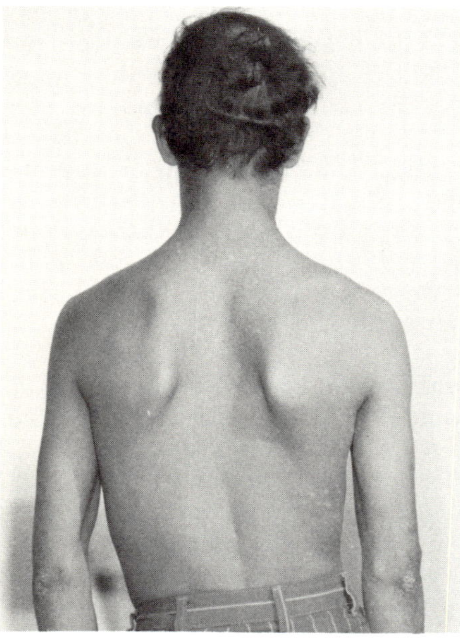

Fig. 4.12. Note whitish, irregular atrophic areas and increased pigmentation.

Differential Diagnosis. The differential diagnosis should include a variety of conditions associated with abnormalities in pigmentation, keratinization, and vesiculobullous eruption, including xeroderma pigmentosum, pachyonychia congenita, white sponge nevus of Cannon, epidermolysis bullosa, and incontinentia pigmenti.

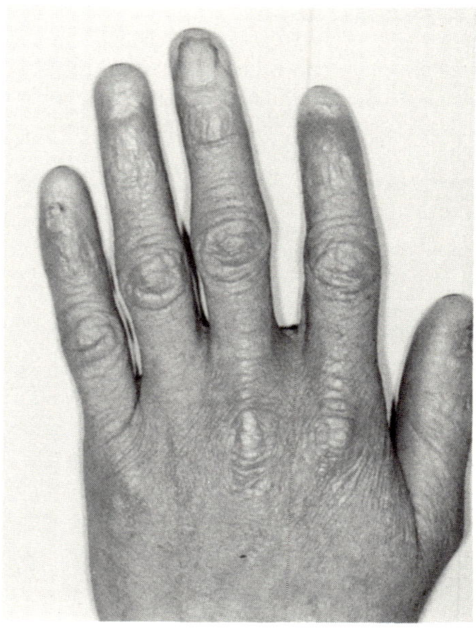

Fig. 4.13. Note dystrophic and absent nails.

Laboratory Aids. Blood analysis for the demonstration of anemia (pancytopenia) might aid in the diagnosis.

Synonyms. Zinsser-Engman-Cole syndrome, dyskeratosis congenita.

References

Cannel H: Dyskeratosis congenita. *Br J Oral Surg* 9:8–20, 1971.

Grekin JN, Schwartz OD: Dyskeratosis congenita with pigmentation, dystrophia unguium and leukokeratosis oris. *Arch Dermatol* 85:124–215, 1962.

Ortega JA, et al: Congenital dyskeratosis. *Am J Dis Child* 124:701–705, 1972.

Sirinavin C, Trowbridge AA: Dyskeratosis congenita: Clinical features and genetic aspects. Report of a family and review of the literature. *J Med Genet* 12:339–354, 1975.

4.9 Fabry Syndrome

The syndrome of (1) angiokeratomata of the skin, (2) pain in the extremities, (3) disturbance in sweat excretion, (4) elevated blood pressure, (5) heart enlargement, and (6) albuminuria was first described by Anderson in England and Fabry in Germany, both in 1898. Sweeley and Klinosky (1963) suggested the name of glycolipid lipoidosis. The condition is inherited in an X-linked recessive manner, with full expression in males and partial expression in heterozygous females. A few homozygous females have also been described. Some heterozygous females manifest the full-blown syndrome. The syndrome is produced by an abnormally high concentration of the glycosphingolipid trihexosyl ceramide in (1) smooth muscle, (2) endothelium, (3) supporting cells of blood vessels in the kidney, skin, gastrointestinal tract, heart, central nervous system, and (4) reticuloendothelial tissue. This lipid apposition is caused by a deficiency of the specific α-galactosidase ceramide trihexosidase catabolizer enzyme for glycosphingolipid.

Facies. The disorder has no characteristic facies. Occasional reports have described affected males with moderate prognathism, prominent lips, and frontal bossing. The facial skin is at times affected with minute angiokeratomas, similar to those seen on the rest of the skin surface,

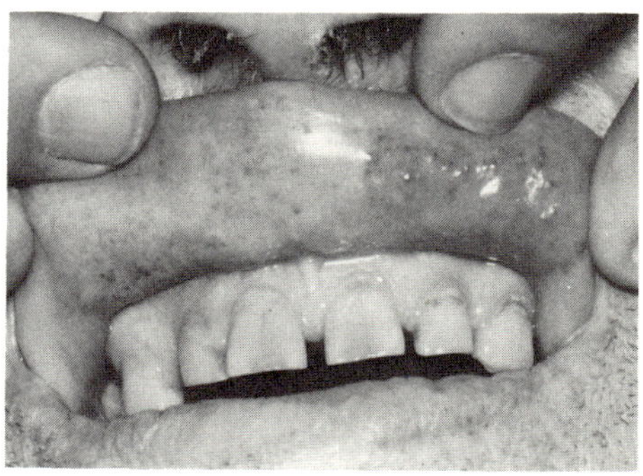

Fig. 4.14. Small pinpoint vascular lesions are seen on the upper lip mucosa. Oral lesions in Fabry syndrome are usually limited to the lips.

as described below. The submental area is generally not affected.

Oral Structures. Most patients present angiokeratomas of the lips smaller than, but otherwise similar to, those of the skin (Fig. 4.14). They are usually located on the lower lip, in the junction of skin and semimucosa on both sides of the midline. The tongue is not affected, and only rarely are other oral tissues involved.

Systemic Features. Angiokeratomas of the skin that do not blanch upon pressure may be present from early childhood, becoming clinically evident at 7 to 10 years of age. The skin lesions manifest as numerous, minute, slightly grouped, round to oval, macular to papular, bluish red to black, blood-filled cavities up to 4 mm in diameter and spread over the iliosacral area, posterior thorax, buttocks, scrotum, thighs, and umbilical area. The ulnar surfaces of the forearms are involved to a lesser degree. Keratosis is often seen covering these lesions. Occasional large lesions are generally raised. In some male patients, the angiokeratomas are absent. Heterozygotic females generally do not have significant numbers of skin lesions. Vascular mottling of palms and soles has also been reported. Elevated temperature and diminution in sweating are frequent.

Pain, usually affecting hands and feet, is the main complaint of affected individuals. The pain is causalgic and may be due to abnormal conduction resulting from defective myelination. It increases in frequency and intensity with age. Swelling of the ankles and around the eyes is first seen during puberty. Most patients present enlargement of the left heart and elevated blood pressure. Gastrointestinal alterations—diarrhea, abdominal pain, nausea, and vomiting—are frequent. Varicose veins and hemorrhoids have been noted in about 25% of affected individuals.

Superficial corneal opacity, resembling that seen in chloroquin intoxication, has been noted in both sexes, but less commonly in female carriers. The fundi may present marked tortuosity of the retinal vessels with dilatation of veins. Varicosities of the palpebral and bulbar conjunctiva are also common.

Differential Diagnosis. Rendu-Osler-Weber syndrome should be considered in the differential diagnosis. Other conditions exhibiting angiokeratosis are generally limited to specific areas of the body and are not widely distributed as in the Fabry syndrome.

Laboratory Aids. Proteinuria has been noted in the majority of patients. Anemia is commonly associated with uremia. Erythrocytes obtained during hemolytic episodes have shown abnormalities in phospholipid composition. Biochemical studies confirm increased levels of trihexosyl ceramide in urine, plasma, or cultured fibroblasts. Biopsy of skin or of bone marrow or microscopic study of urine sediment demonstrates the presence of birefringent lipid inclusions.

Synonyms. Angiokeratoma corporis diffusum universale, angiokeratosis, glycolipid lipoidosis.

References

Desnick RJ, et al: Fabry's disease: enzymatic diagnosis of hemizygotes and heterozygotes: alpha-galactosidase activities in plasma, serum, urine and leukocytes. *J Lab Clin Med* 81:157–171, 1973.

Sweeley CC, et al: Fabry's disease, in JB Stanbury, JB Wyngaarden, and DS Fredrickson (eds), *The Metabolic Basis of Inherited Disease*. New York, McGraw Hill, 1972.

Wallace HJ: Anderson-Fabry disease. *Br J Dermatol* 88:1–24, 1973.

4.10 Familial Dysautonomia

This condition, first recognized by Riley and coworkers in 1949, is characterized by (1) congenital indifference to pain, (2) absence of tears, (3) absence of lingual fungiform papillae, and (4) swallowing difficulties. Genetic studies have shown an autosomal recessive inheritance pattern. Almost all parents are of Ashkenazi Jewish ancestry. An estimation of the frequency of dysautonomia among American Jews, according to McKusick and collaborators (1967), is approximately 1 in 10,000. A similar finding was noted in Israeli Jews of Ashkenazi extraction. No specific enzyme defect has been demonstrated. The carriers do not exhibit any clinical signs of the disorder, but Moses and collaborators (1967) noted a lower urinary level of vanillylmandelic acid (VMA) than in normal adults.

Facies. Characteristically there is an elongated mouth with symmetrical facial drooping (Fig. 4.15). Absence of tears and corneal anesthesia with resultant corneal ulceration and skin blotching complete the facial appearance.

Oral Structures. The tongue shows an almost complete absence of fungiform and circumvallate papillae (Fig. 4.16). Associated with this is a

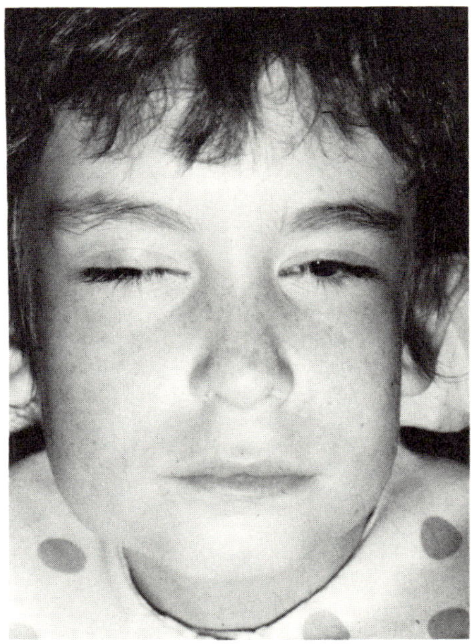

Fig. 4.15. Mouth presents a characteristic horizontal slit-like appearance. Artificial adhesions between the eyelids were created in order to relieve corneal ulceration due to absence of tears.

decreased sensitivity to sweet and bitter tastes. Carriers may exhibit a diminished number of fungiform papillae.

Systemic Features. Stature is small and physical growth and psychomotor development are delayed. The condition becomes evident soon after birth; the child has difficulty in swallowing and regurgitates. Insensitivity to pain (which may result in Charcot joints as the child grows older), motor incoordination, excessive sweating, high fever of unknown etiology, diminished gag reflex, frequent vomiting, breath holding spells that may result in loss of consciousness, and a mild degree of retardation are the most frequent findings during the first three years. There also may be ataxia, scanning and nasal speech, and dysarthria.

Postural hypotension and paroxysmal hypertension may develop later in life. Severe progressive kyphoscoliosis commonly appears around the 8th or 9th year of life. Twenty-five percent of affected individuals succumb by the end of the first decade from pulmonary infection. There is a marked tendency to recurrent bronchopneumonia, probably due to the frequent aspiration of food. Males seem to have a significantly poorer chance of survival up to 6 years of age. Other characteristics include a slight-to-absent reaction to histamine tests and a marked reaction to norepinephrine and related drugs.

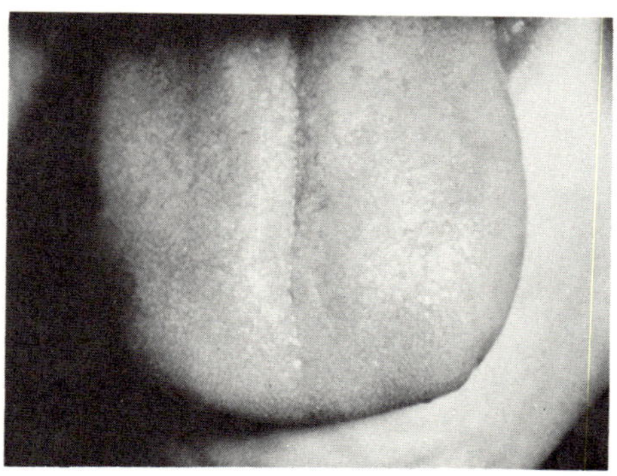

Fig. 4.16. Bald appearance of tongue due to absence of fungiform papillae. Circumvallate papillae also may be absent or scanty.

Differential Diagnosis. All other forms of congenital indifference to pain should be included.

Laboratory Aids. No single test can be recommended, but intradermal injection of histamine will produce a wheal, but without the peripheral axon flare seen in normal individuals. Scratching the skin of these patients will not produce the normal red flare response. Some reports indicate increased urinary ratio of homovanillic acid (HVA) to VMA in patients with the condition, but this finding has not been replicated by some authors.

Synonym. Riley-Day syndrome, dysautonomia.

References

Brunt PW, McKusick VA: Familial dysautonomia: A report of genetic and clinical studies with a review of the literature. *Medicine* 49:343–374, 1970.

McKusick VA, et al: The Riley-Day syndrome: Observations on genetics and survivorship. *Israel J Med Sci* 3:372–379, 1967.

Moses SW, et al: A clinical, genetic and biochemical study of familial dysautonomia in Israel. *Israel J Med Sci* 3:358–369, 1967.

Pearson J, et al: The tongue and taste in familial dysautonomia. *Pediatrics* 45:739–745, 1970.

Riley CM, et al: Central antonomic dysfunction with defective lacrimation. *Pediatrics* 3:468–481, 1949.

4.11 Gingival Fibromatosis with Ear, Nose, Bone, and Nail Defects and Hepatosplenomegaly

Zimmermann in 1928 was the first to describe the syndrome complex. The condition is characterized by (1) gingival fibromatosis, (2) dysplasia of nails, (3) soft bulky cartilage in nose and ears, (4) hepatosplenomegaly, and (5) hypoplastic terminal phalanges. The condition is inherited in an autosomal dominant manner.

Facies. The nose is soft and bulky and the ears are thick and have a floppy appearance. The lips protrude due to the gingival overgrowth (Fig. 4.17).

Oral Structures. The gingival fibromatosis occurs early in childhood and completely covers the teeth and causes the lips to protrude (Fig. 4.18).

Systemic Features. Somatic and mental development are within normal limits. Affected individuals present hypoplasia of terminal phalanges, resulting in clubbed tree-frog-like fingers and toes. In addition there is hyperextensibility of metacarpophalangeal joints. The nails may be dysplastic or absent. Hepatosplenomegaly has been a constant feature.

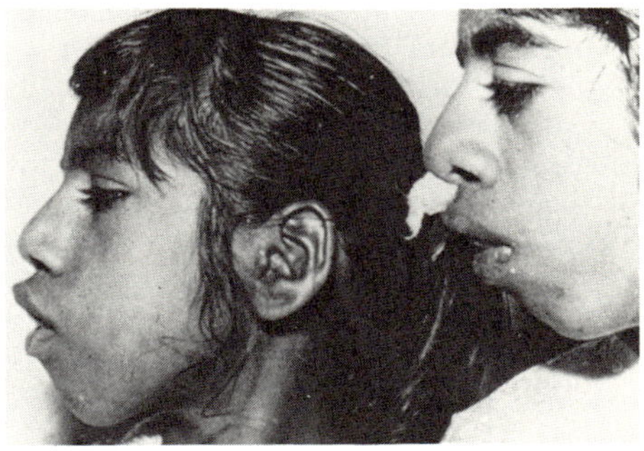

Fig. 4.17. The pinnae and nose are poorly formed as a result of highly pliable cartilage. Gingival enlargement results in protruding lips.

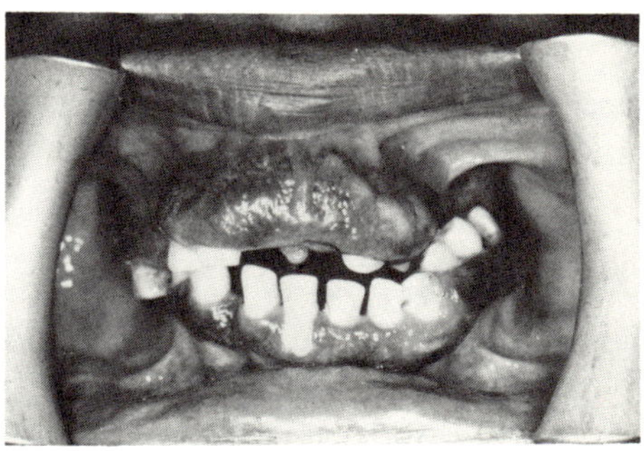

Fig. 4.18. Markedly enlarged maxillary gingiva. The mandibular gingiva appears normal because of recent gingivectomy. Note malposition of mandibular teeth due to gingival hyperplasia.

Differential Diagnosis. Murray syndrome, Cross syndrome, and gingival fibromatosis with or without hypertrichosis should be considered in the differential diagnosis.

Laboratory Aids. None.

Synonym. Zimmermann-Laband syndrome.

References

Alvander G: Elephantiasis gingivae. Report of an affected family with associated hepatomegaly, soft tissue and skeletal abnormalities. *J All-India Dent Assoc* 37:349–352, 1965.

Laband PF, et al: Hereditary gingival fibromatosis. Report of an affected family with associated splenomegaly, and skeletal and soft tissue abnormalities. *Oral Surg* 17:339–342, 1964.

Zimmermann: Über Anomalien des Ektoderms. *Vjschr Zahnheilkd* 44:419–434, 1928.

4.12 Gingival Fibromatosis with Hypertrichosis, Epilepsy, and Mental Retardation

The syndrome is characterized by (1) epilepsy, (2) mental retardation, (3) gingival hyperplasia, and (4) hypertrichosis. The mental retardation and epilepsy are inconsistent features. The syndrome is inherited in an autosomal dominant manner.

Facies. The facies is characterized by protrusion of the lips secondary to gingival enlargement, and hypertrichosis, especially of the eyebrows (Fig. 4.19).

Oral Structures. Gingival enlargement is marked and may completely cover the clinical crowns of the teeth (Fig. 4.20). Gingival hyperplasia usually appears before age 5.

Systemic Features. Mental retardation and epilepsy may be present in

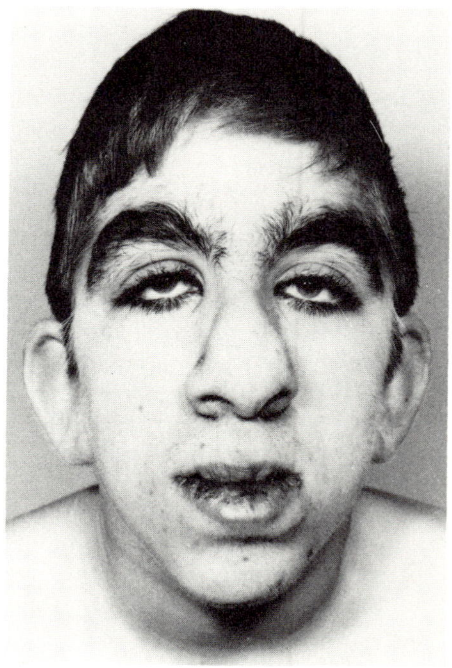

Fig. 4.19. Note marked hypertrichosis in patient with gingival fibromatosis.

rare instances; however, this may represent genetic heterogeneity in the syndrome. Apart from facial involvement, hypertrichosis may be present over the extremities, genitals, and sacral regions.

Differential Diagnosis. Isolated gingival fibromatosis and gingival fibromatosis secondary to Dilantin therapy should be considered in establishing the diagnosis.

Laboratory Aids. None known.

References

Anderson J, et al: Gingival fibromatosis. *Br Med J* 3:218–219, 1969.

Jorgensen RJ, and Cocker ME: Variation in the inheritance and expression of gingival fibromatosis. *J Periodontol* 45:472–477, 1974.

Winter GB, and Simpkiss MJ: Hypertrichosis with hereditary gingival hyperplasia. *Arch Dis Child* 49:394–399, 1974.

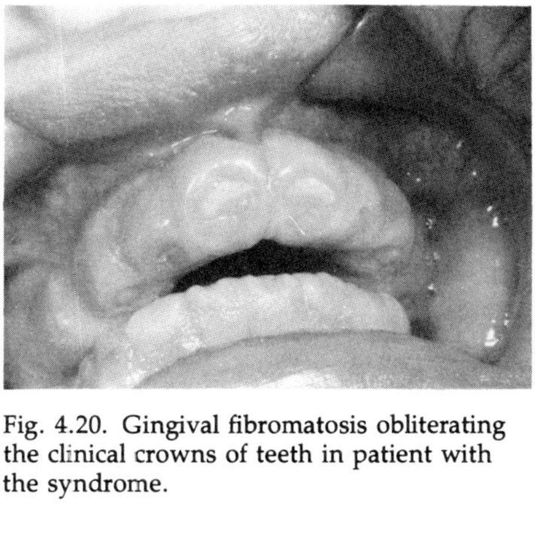

Fig. 4.20. Gingival fibromatosis obliterating the clinical crowns of teeth in patient with the syndrome.

4.13 Gingival Fibromatosis with Multiple Hyaline Fibromas

Murray in 1873 was the first to describe the syndrome. The condition is characterized by (1) hypertrophy of the gingiva, (2) hypertrophy of the nail beds, and (3) fibrotic tumors of the nose, chin, head, and palmar and digital surfaces of the hands. The condition is inherited in an autosomal recessive manner.

Facies. Fibrotic hyaline tumors appear on the nose, chin, and head usually after the age of 2 (Fig. 4.21).

Oral Structures. Gingival enlargement begins at 6 months of age and eventually covers a major portion of the clinical crowns of the teeth by age 2 (Fig. 4.22).

Systemic Features. Mental development is normal; however, height is reduced and sexual maturation retarded. Multiple fibrous tumors resembling those on the face appear on the back, fingers, thighs, and legs, often producing flexion contractures at the knees, elbows, shoulders, and hips.

Differential Diagnosis. The differential diagnosis should include neurofibromatosis, Gardner syndrome, and fibromatosis hyalinica multiplex juvenilis.

Laboratory Aids. Biopsy of the skin tumors reveals a highly vascular pseudocartilage matrix and a ground substance which is homogenous, amorphous, acidophilic, PAS-positive, and contains spindle-shaped cells.

Synonym. Murray-Puretic-Drescher syndrome.

References

Drescher E, et al: Juvenile fibromatosis in siblings (fibromatosis hyalinica multiplex juvenilis). *J Pediatr Surg* 2:427–430, 1967.

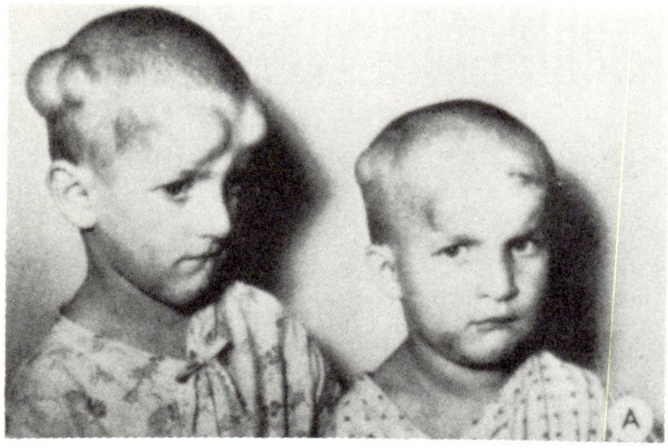

Fig. 4.21. Tumors of the head in 5-year-old male and 4-year-old female sibs, present since age 2 in each.

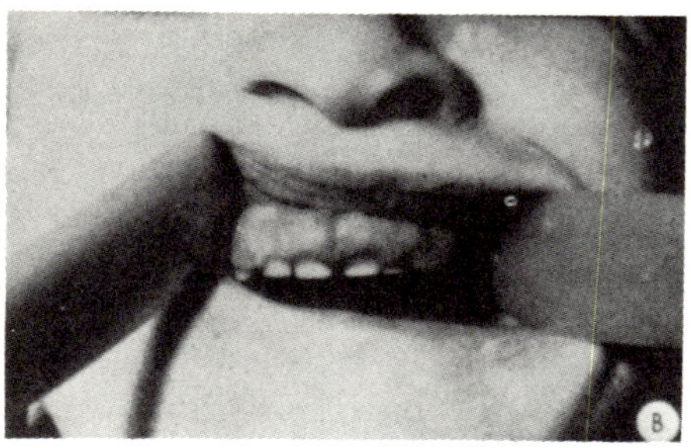

Fig. 4.22. Marked gingival fibromatosis in one of the sibs of Fig. 4.21.

Ishikawa H, Mori S: Systemic hyalinosis or fibromatosis multiplex as a congenital syndrome. *Acta Derm Venereol* (Stockholm) 53:185–191, 1973.

Kitano Y, et al: Two cases of juvenile hyaline fibromatosis: Some histological, electro microscopic and tissue culture observations. *Arch Dermatol* 106:877–883, 1972.

Witkop CJ: Heterogeneity in gingival fibromatosis. *Birth Def* 7(7):215–216, 1971.

4.14 Hereditary Benign Intraepithelial Dyskeratosis

Witkop (1960) and von Sallmann and Paton (1960) concurrently described a syndrome in a North Carolina triracial isolate consisting of (1) plaques of the bulbar conjunctiva and (2) oral mucosal thickenings. The syndrome has autosomal dominant inheritance with a high degree of penetrance.

Facies. The eyes are usually affected within the first year of life. The limbus, both nasally and temporally, reveals foamy gelatinous plaques which are more superficial than pterygia. The bulbar conjunctiva is usually hyperemic. The dyskeratosis may involve the cornea and produces blindness after shedding, with resultant corneal vascularization. Photophobia is especially common in these children.

Oral Structures. Oral mucous membranes exhibit soft white plaques or folds (Fig. 4.23). These lesions are apparent at birth but progressively increase in severity through the first decade. In general, the mucosal lesions are asymptomatic.

Systemic Features. Somatic and mental development are within normal limits. Apart from the ophthalmologic and oral mucosal findings, other mucous membranes do not appear to be affected.

Differential Diagnosis. White sponge nevus, Darier-White disease, and oral lesions of pachyonychia congenita should be included in the differential diagnosis.

Laboratory Aids. Histology of conjunctiva and oral mucous membranes reveals vacuolization of the stratum spinosum, acanthosis, and a waxy eosinophilic dyskeratosis with a "cell-within-a-cell" pattern (Fig. 4.24).

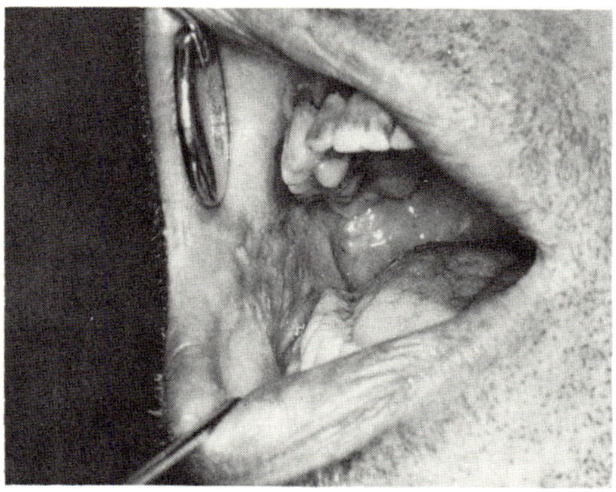

Fig. 4.23. Note prominent leukokeratosis of the buccal mucosa.

Synonym. Witkop-von Sallmann syndrome.

References

Pollitzer WS, et al: Hereditary benign intraepithelial dyskeratosis—a linkage study. *Am J Hum Genet* 17:104–108, 1965.

Sallmann L von, Paton D: Hereditary benign intraepithelial dyskeratosis I; ocular manifestations. *Arch Ophthalmol* 63:421–429, 1960.

Witkop CJ, et al: Hereditary benign intraepithelial dyskeratosis II; oral manifestations and hereditary transmission. *Arch Path* 70:696–711, 1960.

Witkop CJ, Gorlin RJ: Four hereditary mucosal syndromes. *Arch Dermatol* 84:762–771, 1961.

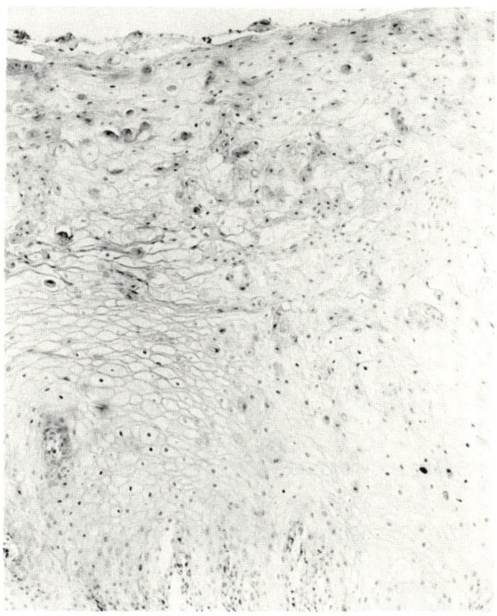

Fig. 4.24. Biopsy of the buccal mucosa shows an acanthotic epithelium with dyskeratotic cells.

4.15 Hereditary Hemorrhagic Telangiectasia

Rendu in 1896 reported a patient suffering from recurrent epistaxis and numerous dilated vessels on the face and oral mucosa. Osler (1901) provided a full account of the syndrome, while Hanes in 1909 first used the term "hereditary hemorrhagic telangiectasia" to describe the condition. The syndrome is characterized by multiple capillary and venous dilations of the skin and mucous membranes with repeated hemorrhage. The condition has an autosomal dominant inheritance pattern. Onset is usually in the second or third decade.

Facies. Pinpoint, spider-like, and nodular telangiectases are observed on the face, nasal orifices, ears, scalp, eyelids, and lips (Fig. 4.25). Lesions on the nasal mucosa produce frequent and at times severe epistaxis that may persist for several days. Generally, nosebleed precedes the appearance of cutaneous telangiectases.

Oral Structures. Telangiectases affect the lips, mucocutaneous junction of the lips, anterior dorsum and tip of the tongue, and occasionally the palate, gingiva, and buccal mucosa (Fig. 4.26). Bleeding from the oral cavity, especially from the lips and tongue, succeeds epistaxis.

Systemic Features. Somatic development is within normal limits. Mucous membranes in the gastrointestinal tract, conjunctiva, vagina, uterus, and bladder may also be affected with telangiectases that hemorrhage. Any organ may be affected (ie, liver, lungs, brain, spinal cord), resulting in cirrhosis of the liver, pulmonary arteriovenous fistulae, and encephalopathies.

Differential Diagnosis. The syndrome should be differentiated from angiokeratoma corporis diffusum (Fabry syndrome), CRST syndrome, Raynaud phenomenon, scleroderma, and isolated telangiectasia.

Syndrome. Osler-Rendu disease.

References

Garland HG, Anning ST: Hereditary hemorrhagic telangiectasia: a genetic and bibliographic study. *Br J Derm* 62:289, 1950.

Lele MV: Oral manifestations of hereditary hemorrhagic telangiectasia. *J All-India Dent Ass* 37:317, 1965.

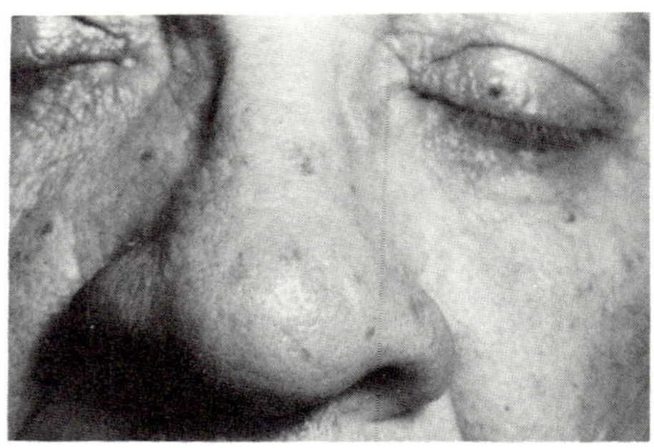

Fig. 4.25. Note telangiectasia over the skin of the nose, face, and eyelid.

Mirra JM, Arnold WD: Skeletal hemangiomatosis in association with hereditary hemorrhagic telangiectasia. *J Bone Joint Surg* 55A:850–854, 1973.

Trell, et al: Familial pulmonary hypertension and multiple abnormalities of large systemic arteries in Osler's disease. *Am J Med* 53:50–63, 1972.

4.16 Hermansky-Pudlak Syndrome

Hermansky and Pudlak (1959) initially described the syndrome of (1) oculocutaneous albinism, (2) hemorrhagic symptoms, especially after the use of aspirin, (3) storage-pool deficiency in platelets, and (4) accumulation of "ceroid-like" pigment in reticuloendothelial and mucosal cells. The condition exhibits autosomal recessive inheritance.

Facies. Clinically, these patients resemble tyrosinase-negative albinos, having scant white hair, white-pink skin, marked nystagmus, and a prominent red reflex. Patients living in tropical areas who are exposed to bright sunlight will often have reddish brown hair, numerous pigmented nevi, and freckles (Fig. 4.27).

Oral Structures. Patients with this disorder may have spontaneous gingival hemorrhage, epistaxis, and prolonged bleeding following tooth extraction, delivery, and surgical procedures. Aspirin administered to such patients may enhance the bleeding diathesis. Examination of oral mucosal scrapings from patients with Hermansky-Pudlak syndrome demonstrates a ceroid-like pigment accumulation.

Systemic Features. Somatic and mental development are within normal limits. Analysis of the pigment defect shows that tyrosinase activity is present and pheomelanin pigment accumulates in melanocytes. A ceroid-like pigment accumulates in reticuloendothelial cells, urinary sediment, and buccal mucosa. Platelets from normal patients examined

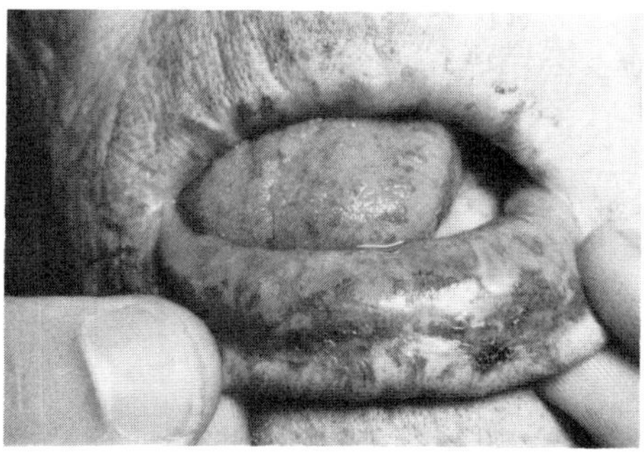

Fig. 4.26. Same patient as Fig. 4.25 with marked telangiectasia of labial and lingual mucosae.

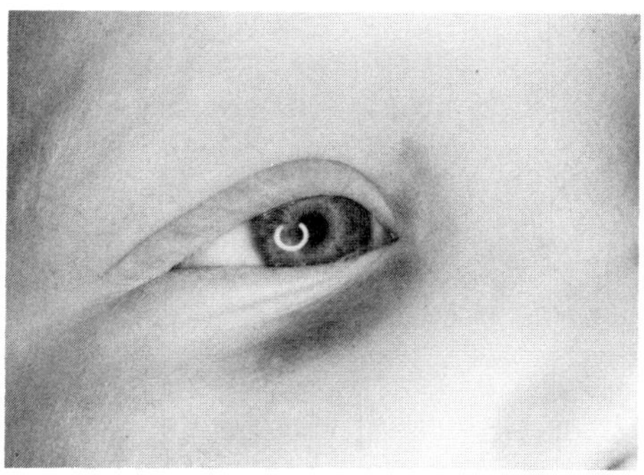

Fig. 4.27. Note marked infraorbital ecchymosis following minor trauma.

under an electron microscope contain dense bodies which are the storage organelles for serotonin and the nonmetabolic nucleotides ADP and ATP, which are released during platelet aggregation. Platelets from patients with this syndrome are markedly deficient in dense bodies, contain reduced amounts of serotonin, ADP, and ATP, and demonstrate single-phase aggregometry curves with platelet-aggregating agents such as epinephrine, collagen, or ADP.

Differential Diagnosis. Tyrosinase-positive albinism, yellow mutant albinism, and platelet storage pool deficiency syndromes without accompanying albinism should be included in the differential diagnosis.

Laboratory Aids. King-tyrosinase hairbulb assay, platelet aggregometry, and electron microscopy of platelets revealing a deficiency of dense bodies are all useful in diagnosis of the syndrome.

Synonyms. Albinism with hemorrhagic diathesis and pigmented reticuloendothelial cells.

References

Hermansky F, Pudlak P: Albinism associated with hemorrhagic diathesis and unusual pigmented reticular cells in bone marrow. *Blood* 14:162–169, 1959.

Witkop CJ Jr, et al: Oculocutaneous albinism. In Nyhan WL (ed), *Heritable Disorders of Amino Acid Metabolism.* New York, John Wiley, 1974.

4.17 Hyperkeratosis Palmoplantaris and Attached Gingival Hyperkeratosis

Raphael and coworkers in 1968 first described the syndrome which is inherited in an autosomal dominant manner.

Facies. There is no characteristic facies for the condition.

Oral Structures. The attached labial and lingual gingiva is covered by a thick layer of keratin. The keratinization follows the normal contour of the attached gingiva, being sharply delineated from the rest of the oral mucosa (Fig. 4.28). The changes appear in childhood and increase in severity with age.

Systemic Features. The only other

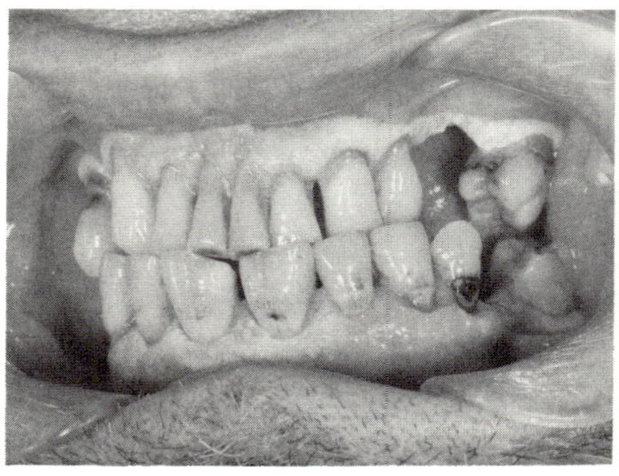

Fig. 4.28. Note marked hyperkeratosis of attached gingiva in a male patient who has a similarly affected brother.

component of the syndrome is palmoplantar hyperkeratosis, which is focal and generally appears at puberty, especially in weight- or trauma-related areas. Hyperhidrosis may also be present. Hyperkeratosis of the distal ends of fingers and toes, as well as subungual keratinization, becomes evident before puberty (Fig. 4.29).

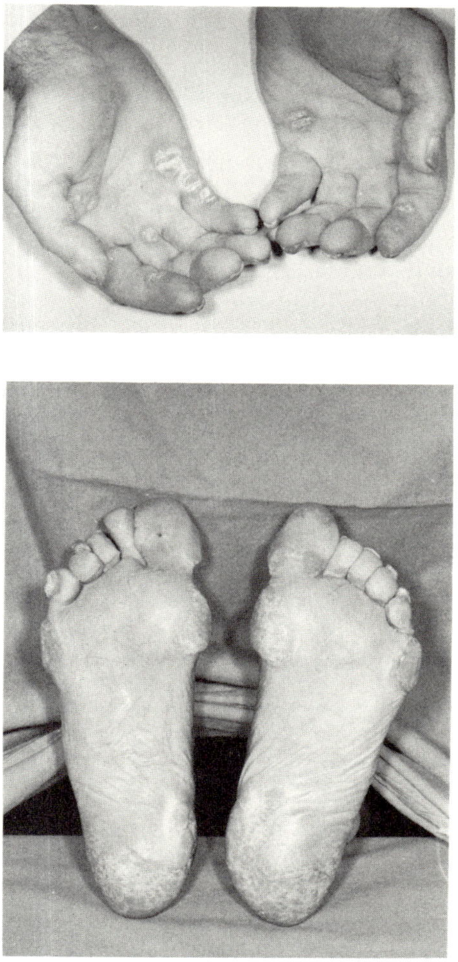

Fig. 4.29. Hyperkeratosis of palms and soles in same patient as Fig. 4.28.

Differential Diagnosis. The Papillon-Lefèvre syndrome, as well as other conditions associated with palmoplantar hyperkeratosis, need to be considered. Intraoral leukoplakia should also be ruled out.

Laboratory Aids. None known.

References

Fred HL, et al: Keratosis palmaris et plantaris. *Arch Intern Med* 113:866–871, 1974.

Gorlin RJ: Hyperkeratosis palmoplantaris and attached gingival hyperkeratosis. *Birth Def*, in press.

Raphael AL, et al: Hyperkeratosis of gingival and plantar surfaces. *Periodontics* 6:118–120, 1968.

4.18 Lesch-Nyhan Syndrome

Lesch and Nyhan in 1964 were the first to recognize this condition as a syndrome composed of (1) hyperuricemia, (2) choreoathetosis, (3) mental and growth retardation, and (4) destructive behavior with self-mutilation. The syndrome is inherited in an X-linked recessive manner and is characterized by the absence of the enzyme hypoxanthine-guanine phosphoribosyltransferase (HGPRTase) in brain, liver, fibroblasts, and erythrocytes, which results in increased purine synthesis with excessive formation of uric acid.

Facies. Affected children exhibit compulsive destructive behavior that leads to self-mutilation. The facies is markedly distorted, due to chewing of the lips (Fig. 4.30). Multiple scars may be seen on the ears, face, and head, due to self-inflicted trauma. Choreoathetosis of the face is also a constant finding.

Oral Structures. As mentioned above, the lips are markedly mutilated due to self-chewing, especially the lower one. Occasionally, destruction of the upper lip mimics clefting. Speech is dysarthric, accentuated by the destruction of the lips.

Systemic Features. There is marked somatic and mental retardation. Amputation by chewing of the distal phalanges of the fingers has been reported. Violent head banging is a constant feature. Apparently there is no sensory anesthesia, since patients scream as if in pain during the process of self-biting. Choreoathetosis of the extremities and neck, from early infancy, is another constant finding.

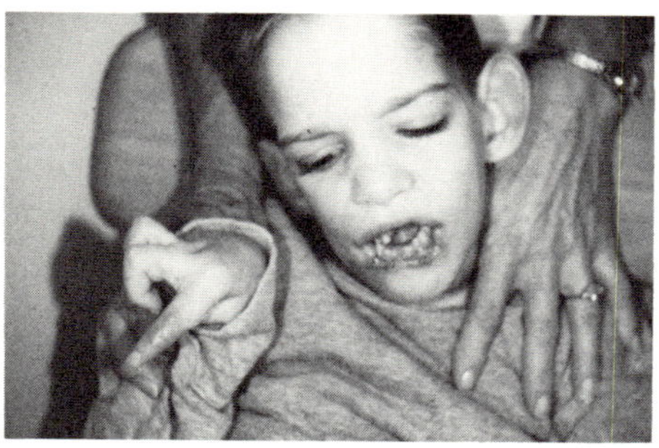

Fig. 4.30. Extensive destruction of lower lip due to self-inflicted trauma.

Opisthotonic spasm, dysphagia, and hyperreflexia are frequently noted. Mild diplegia also can be observed and, less frequently, severe spastic quadriparesis. The central nervous system manifestations seem to be related to dysfunction of the basal ganglia, which in postmortem examination show a complete absence of HGPRTase activity. In normal individuals, HGPRTase shows its maximum activity in the basal ganglia. Hematuria and the passing of uric acid stones are always present.

Differential Diagnosis. All conditions associated with indifference to pain and self-destructive behavior should be included in the differential diagnosis.

Laboratory Aids. Laboratory findings include markedly increased urinary excretion of uric acid and absence of hypoxanthine-guanine phosphoribosyltransferase activity in culture fibroblasts. Identical procedures are used for the determination of carriers and for prenatal diagnosis.

Synonym. HGPRTase deficiency.

References

Boyle JA, et al: Lesch-Nyhan syndrome: Preventive control by prenatal diagnosis. *Science* 169:688–689, 1970.

Emmerson BT, Thompson L: The spectrum of hypoxanthine guanine phosphoribosyltransferase deficiency. *Q J Med* 166:423–440, 1973.

Lesch M, Nyhan WL: A familial disorder of uric acid metabolism and central nervous system function. *Am J Med* 36:561–570, 1964.

Nyhan WL: Clinical features of the Lesch-Nyhan syndrome. *Arch Intern Med* 130:186–192, 1972.

4.19 Moebius Syndrome

The syndrome was described in the early 1880s. The complex consists of (1) congenital, usually bilateral, facial paralysis, (2) unilateral or bilateral loss of the abductors of the eye, (3) anomalies of the extremities, (4) hypoplasia of branchial and thoracic muscles, and (5) involvement of other cranial nerves, especially the hypoglossal. A few cases have been reported in two generations. Rarely there has been consanguinity among parents of affected patients. The majority of cases do not have a familial history and therefore represent isolated examples. The syndrome likely has multifactorial inheritance. Although the etiology of the syndrome is unknown, Moebius indicated that the cause was nuclear agenesis; others have suggested that nuclear atrophy was secondary to failure of muscle formation.

Facies. The face is mask-like due to bilateral facial paralysis (Fig. 4.31). A distinctive facial appearance is noted during crying or laughing. Generally the facial paralysis is partial and does not include the lower face. The eyes can not be abducted beyond the midline; however, convergence can be observed. Other eye anomalies include ptosis of eyelids, epicanthus, nystagmus, and microphthalmia.

Oral Structures. Paralysis of the lips results in downward droop of the angle of the mouth with consequent sialorrhea and defective speech. One-third of affected patients may also present atrophy and tongue paralysis due to hypoglossal involvement. Occasional oral manifestations include bifid uvula, micrognathia, paralysis of masticatory muscles, and dysphagia.

Systemic Features. Somatic growth is within normal limits. Mild mental retardation is seen in about 10% of patients with Moebius syndrome.

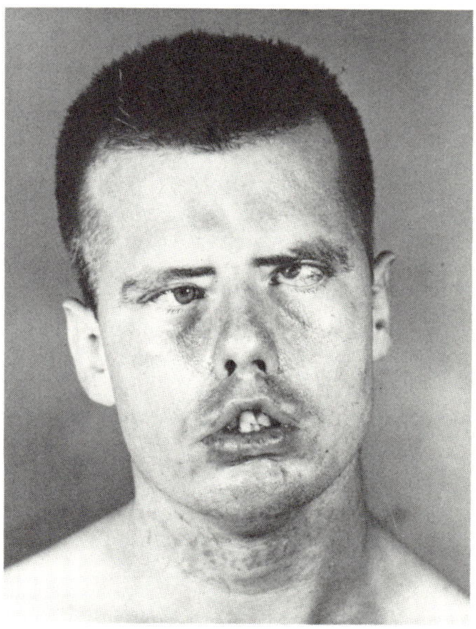

Fig. 4.31. Mask-like face with open mouth and bilateral facial paralysis.

Skeletal anomalies include unilateral or bilateral clubfoot, syndactyly, adactyly, polydactyly, brachydactyly, and congenital dislocation of the hip. Apart from facial musculature, other affected muscular groups include pectoralis, trapezius, quadriceps, serratus magnus and semimembranosus.

Differential Diagnosis. Differential diagnosis should include facial paralysis due to trauma during delivery. The facies should not be confused with that seen in Trisomy 21.

Laboratory Aids. None.

Synonym. Congenital facial diplegia.

References

Hanissian AS, et al: Moebius syndrome in twins. *Am J Dis Child* 120:472–475, 1970.

Olson WH, et al: Moebius syndrome: Lower motor neuron involvement and hypogonadotropic hypogonadism. *Neurology* (Minneap.) 20:1002–1008, 1970.

4.20 Multiple Hamartoma and Neoplasia Syndrome

This syndrome is incompletely defined; however hamartomatous involvement of the breasts, thyroid, and skin appear as characteristics. The syndrome is inherited as a dominant disorder, but whether autosomal or X-linked, has not yet been determined.

Facies. Lichenoid and papillomatous lesions of the pinnae, lateral neck, nasal, periorbital, glabellar, and perioral areas are frequently encountered (Fig. 4.32). Histologic examination of these lesions suggests that they are of hair follicle origin and manifest as hamartomas.

Oral Structures. The lips and gingiva may demonstrate papular lesions; less frequently the palate may also be involved. The buccal, faucial, and oropharyngeal mucosae also are, in most patients, affected with papillomatous lesions (Fig. 4.33). The tongue is pebbly-fissured, while the lesions at the angles of the mouth simulate those of acanthosis nigricans.

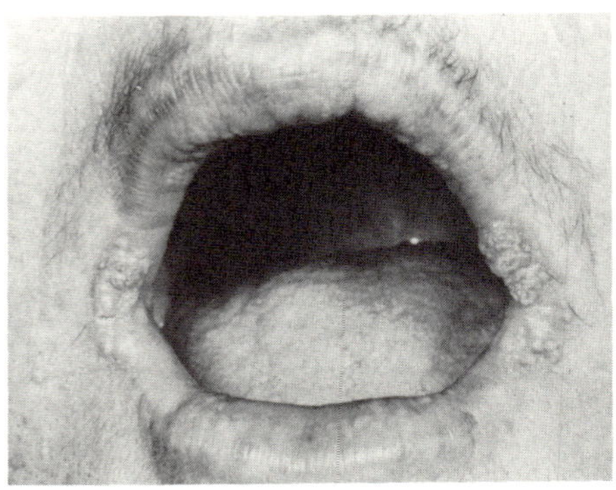

Fig. 4.32. Papillomatous lesions on lip commissures.

Systemic Features. Somatic growth and mental development are within normal limits. The cutaneous lesions in the multiple hamartoma syndrome clinically resemble to some degree those of Darier disease and tuberous sclerosis. The breasts may reveal fibroadenomatosis, virginal hypertrophy, and occasional breast carcinoma. Thyroid alteration has included "goiter," fetal adenoma, and follicular adenocarcinoma (Fig. 4.34). A wide variety of neoplasms has been noted: colonic polyposis or diverticulosis or both, ganglioneuromatosis of the colon, meningoma of ear canal, and angiomatous lesions of soft and hard tissues.

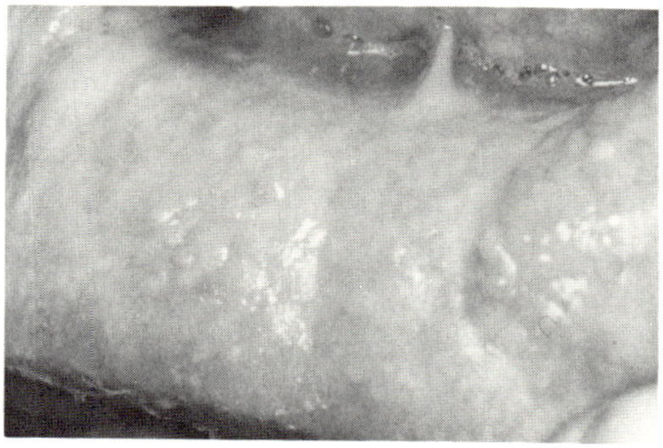

Fig. 4.33. Note papillomatous lesions on labial mucosa in patient with Cowden syndrome.

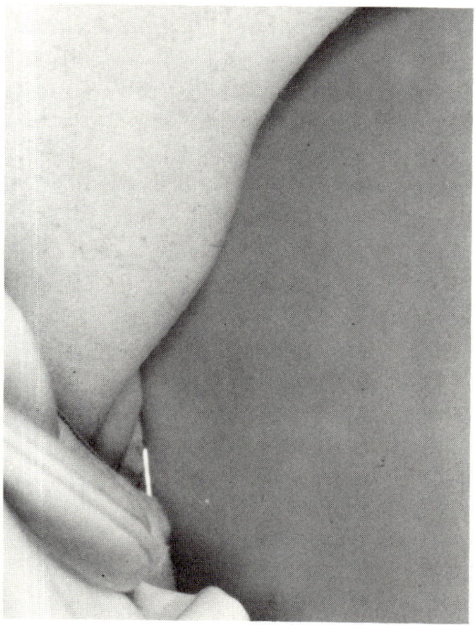

Fig. 4.34. Patient with Cowden syndrome demonstrating thyroid enlargement.

Differential Diagnosis. The differential diagnosis should include (1) Darier disease, (2) tuberous sclerosis, and (3) acanthosis nigricans.

Laboratory Aids. Biopsy of cutaneous lesions limits the differential diagnosis.

Synonym. Cowden syndrome.

References

Gentry WC Jr, et al: Multiple hamartoma syndrome (Cowden's disease). *Arch Dermatol* 109:521–525, 1974.

Gentry WC, et al: Cowden syndrome. *Birth Def* 11(4):137–141, 1975.

Wary PE, et al: Multiple hamartoma syndrome (Cowden's disease). *Arch Dermatol* 106:682–690, 1972.

4.21 Multiple Mucosal Neuromas, Medullary Carcinoma of the Thyroid, Pheochromocytoma, and Marfanoid Body Build with Muscle Wasting

The syndrome described by Wagenmann in 1922 and Froboese in 1923 is characterized by (1) multiple mucosal neuromas, (2) medullary carcinoma of the thyroid, (3) pheochromocytoma, and (4) marfanoid body build with muscle wasting of the extremities. The syndrome is inherited as an autosomal dominant condition.

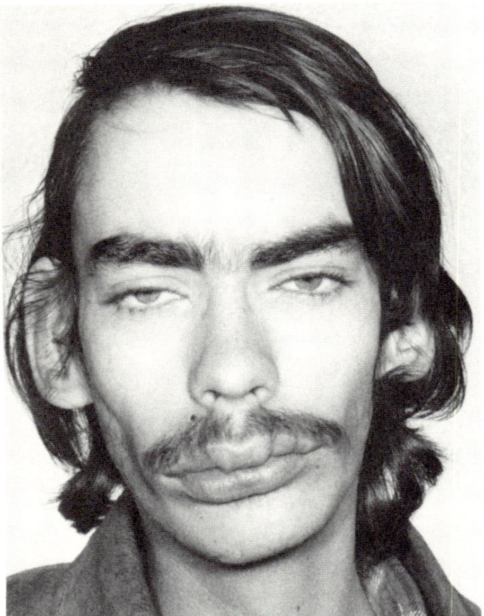

Fig. 4.35. Note coarse facial features and thick, nodular everted lips.

Facies. The large, thick, nodular lips and thick, often everted upper eyelids form a distinct facies (Fig. 4.35).

Oral Structures. The mucosal neuromas usually involve the lips and the anterior dorsal surface of the tongue (Fig. 4.36). Occasionally, the buccal mucosa may also be affected. The mucosal neuromas are microscopically plexiform neuromas without cholinesterase activity. Recently, ganglion cells have been found to be present in the intraoral lesions. These oral and labial neuromas usually appear in the first decade of life.

Systemic Features. The preponderance of affected individuals exhibit a marfanoid or asthenic body build. Muscle wasting of the extremities may resemble a myopathic state. Skeletal changes associated with this syndrome include pes cavus, lordosis, aseptic necrosis, kyphosis, scoliosis, genu valgum, and hyper-

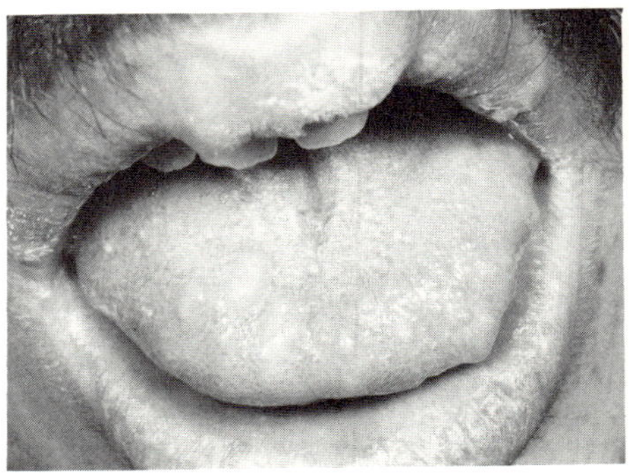

Fig. 4.36. Multiple neuromas are seen on the dorsal surface and lateral borders of the tongue and on the lips.

mobility of joints. In addition to the labial and lingual neuromas, the nasal and laryngeal mucosae may also be affected. Hyperplasia of neurenteric ganglion cells in the entire gastrointestinal tract, bladder, bronchi, and spinal nerve roots have also been described. Diverticulosis and unusual haustral markings with increased mucosal folds and intractable diarrhea or long-standing constipation may also be present.

Another component of the syndrome, medullary carcinoma of the thyroid, has been diagnosed in slightly more than 75% of patients. The thyroid carcinoma usually does not become manifest until the second decade. Approximately 50% of affected patients present metastatic lesions at the time of first diagnosis. Almost 20% of the patients died as a consequence of metastasis from the thyroid carcinoma. The production of ACTH-like peptides by these neoplasms has produced Cushing syndrome in a number of reported cases. In addition, medullary carcinoma of the thyroid can elaborate serotonin, other monoamines, and prostaglandins, all of which may be responsible for the intractable diarrhea. The elaboration of calcitonin by the thyroid carcinoma indicates the presence of primary or metastatic thyroid disease.

Pheochromocytoma has been similarly diagnosed in about half of affected individuals. The pheochromocytoma manifests either in the second or third decades of life and is usually multiple and frequently bilateral. Rare cutaneous findings have included diffuse pigmentation of the hands and feet, café-au-lait pigmentation, and cutaneous neuromas. The eyelid margins or palpebral conjunctiva may exhibit mucosal neuromas, and the corneas demonstrate medullated nerve fibers which extend into the pupil and anastomose.

Differential Diagnosis. Neurofibromatosis, Sipple syndrome (medullary carcinoma with pheochromocytoma), Marfan syndrome, and various myotonic states should be included in the differential diagnosis.

Laboratory Aids. Early endocrine evaluation in patients with the oral manifestations of the syndrome is imperative in view of the high malignant potential of medullary carcinoma of the thyroid. Determination of plasma immunoreactive calcitonin, which is a hormone secreted by the thyroid carcinoma, will demonstrate the presence of even minute thyroid lesions. The presence of pheochromocytoma can be determined by evaluation of urinary levels of epinephrine, vanillylmandelic acid, and metanephrines. Histamine skin tests are also of diagnostic value.

Synonyms. Froboese syndrome; mucosal ganglioneuromatosis, medullary thyroid carcinoma, and pheochromocytoma; multiple endocrine neoplasia, type 2b.

References

Carney JA, et al: Mucosal ganglioneuromatosis, medullary thyroid carcinoma, and pheochromocytoma: Multiple endocrine neoplasia, type 2b. *Oral Surg* 41:739–752, 1976.

Froboese C: Das aus Nervenfascern bestehende, gangliezellenlose echte Neurom in Rankenform-zugleich ein Beitrag zu den nervösen Geschwülsten der Zunge und des Augenlides. *Virchow Arch Pathol Anat* 240:312–327, 1923.

Gorlin RJ, and Vickers RA: Multiple mucosal neuromas, pheochromocytoma, medullary carcinoma of the thyroid and marfanoid body build with muscle wasting: Reexamination of a syndrome of neural crest malmigration. *Birth Def* 7(6):69–72, 1971.

Schimke RN, et al: Syndrome of bilateral pheochromocytoma, medullary thyroid carcinoma and multiple neuromas. A possible regulatory defect in the differentiation of chromaffin tissues. *New Engl J Med* 279:1–7, 1968.

Wagenmann A: Multiple Neurome des Auges und der Zunge. *Ber Dtsch Ophthalmol Ges* 43:282–285, 1922.

4.22 Neurofibromatosis

The syndrome, originally described by von Recklinghausen in 1882, is composed of (1) multiple skin tumors and (2) cutaneous pigmentation. The condition is inherited in an autosomal dominant manner. Its occurrence is estimated at 1 in 3,000 live births. No racial preference is known.

Facies. The facial appearance is quite striking when the tumors develop on the skin of the face, especially the eyelids (Fig. 4.37). Café-au-lait spots are also part of the facies. Less severely affected patients will present only a few or no neurofibromas of the facial skin.

Oral Structures. Oral involvement is seen in about 7% of patients presenting single or multiple tumors, which may affect any area of the oral cavity, but usually occur on the tongue, especially the lateral borders. The intraoral tumors are similar to those found on the skin, namely neurofibromas of the plexiform type. Occasionally neurilemomas are seen associated with the condition, especially on the tongue.

Systemic Features. Physical growth is generally not impaired. Accurate data on incidence and degree of men-

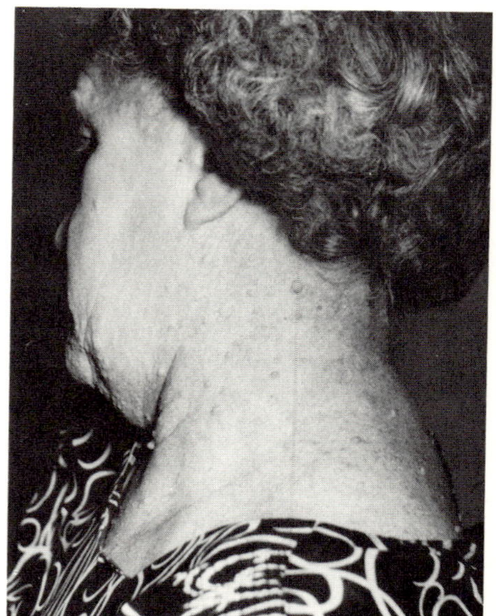

Fig. 4.37. Note numerous neurofibromas scattered over back, neck, and facial skin. The patient had similar intraoral lesions.

tal retardation is lacking. Epilepsy is a frequent finding. Glial proliferations and even large glial brain tumors and neuromas of nearly all cranial nerves may occur, as well as neurinomas of the spinal nerves and fibroblastomas of the meninges. The skin tumors consist of neurinomas, soft fibromas, or most often neurofibromas. They may be present at birth or appear early in life and increase in number and size at puberty. The size varies from that of a pea to a huge, pendulous growth. Malignant transformation of one or more of the neurofibromas occurs in a small percentage of patients.

Multiple café-au-lait pigmentations of the skin usually appear within the first decade and are present in 90 percent of affected individuals. Their color varies from yellowish to chocolate brown. Pigmentation generally precedes the tumors. They occur most often about the axilla (the freckled axilla sign) and the waist, presenting a smooth contour. Neurofibromas can develop in nearly any area of the body, including intraosseous locations. Pheochromocytoma is occasionally found in patients with neurofibromatosis. Phacomas, congenital glaucoma, buphthalmos, corneal opacity, detached retina, and neurofibromatosis of the eyelids are the most frequent ophthalmological findings. Kyphoscoliosis is present in at least 40 percent of affected persons. Other congenital bone anomalies include overgrowth of an extremity or even a digit.

Differential Diagnosis. Multiple lipomatosis and tuberous sclerosis, as well as other phakomatoses, should be included in the differential diagnosis. The multiple mucosal neuroma syndrome and the leopard syndrome also should be considered.

Laboratory Aids. Biopsy of one of the cutaneous or intraoral neurofibromas is of diagnostic value.

Synonym. Von Recklinghausen disease.

References

Freeman MJ, Standish SM: Facial and oral manifestations of familial disseminated neurofibromatosis. *Oral Surg* 19:52–59, 1965.

Kragh LV, et al: Neurofibromatosis of the head and neck. *Plast Reconstr Surg* 25:565–573, 1960.

Saxena K: Endocrine manifestations of neurofibromatosis in children. *Am J Dis Child* 120:265–271, 1970.

4.23 Pachydermoperiostosis

Touraine and collaborators in 1935 first recognized pachydermoperiostosis as a distinct clinical entity. This syndrome is characterized by (1) coarsening of the facial features with thickening and furrowing of the skin of the face, forehead, and scalp, (2) clubbing of the digits, and (3) periosteal new bone formation, especially over the distal ends of the long bones. The disorder usually appears about puberty and slowly progresses for about ten years, when it becomes stationary. The syndrome appears to have autosomal dominant inheritance with marked variability in expressivity, males being more severely affected. Only about 15 percent of reported patients were female, most being sisters of affected males with well-documented pachydermoperiostosis.

Facies. Thickening of the skin occurs over the face, forehead, and scalp (Fig. 4.38). The face is drawn into thick folds, causing a creased or furrowed appearance. This gives the patient a worried or angry look with an appearance of premature aging. The nasolabial folds become deep and sharp. The thickening of the scalp tends to produce a corrugated surface described as "bulldog scalp" or cutis verticis gyrata.

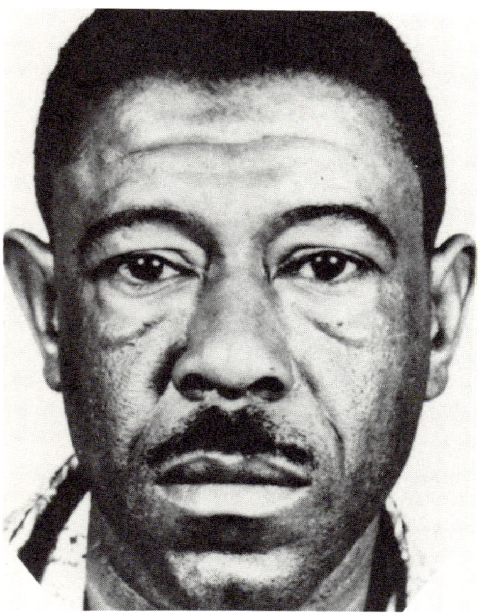

Fig. 4.38. Note cutis gyrata and coarse facial features.

Oral Structure Deepening of the nasolabial folds is exaggerated, thus drawing the lip commissures downward.

Systemic Features. The skin shows widely dilated sebaceous pores filled with plugs of sebum which can be easily expressed. Pseudoptosis, caused by thickening of the eyelids, may be so severe as to obstruct vision. Hyperhidrosis of the hands and feet and, less often, the face is common. The nails may be thickened and curved. The ends of the fingers and toes are bulbous and often grotesque (Fig. 4.39). This clubbing is produced by soft tissue hyperplasia which stops abruptly at the distal interphalangeal joint.

In the early stage of the disease the bony changes tend to be limited to the distal parts of long tubular bones, metacarpals, metatarsals, and proximal phalanges. A diffuse irregular

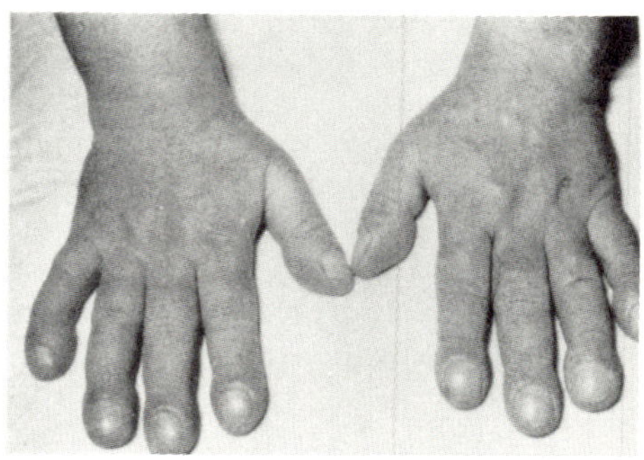

Fig. 4.39. Note clubbing of terminal phalanges.

periosteal ossification increases the circumference of the affected bones without altering their shapes. In the severe and advanced cases, these changes affect virtually all bones of the body except the skull. The bone thickness is greatly increased and the surface is coarse, but they are otherwise not deformed. There is, however, extension of periosteal osteophytic formation into tendinous and membranous insertions. Lastly, joint effusions and ossification of ligaments and tendons occur, leading to ankylosis of the joints and spine.

Differential Diagnosis. Several disorders must be considered before making the diagnosis of pachydermoperiostosis: hypertrophic pulmonary osteoarthropathy, acromegaly, thyroid acropachy, hereditary clubbing, familial idiopathic osteoarthropathy of childhood, and lepromatous leprosy.

Laboratory Aids. None.

Synonym. Touraine-Solente-Golé syndrome.

References

Kerber RE, Vogl A: Pachydermoperiostosis. *Arch Intern Med* 132:245–248, 1973.

Rimoin DL: Pachydermoperiostosis (idiopathic clubbing and periostosis). Genetic and physiologic considerations. *New Engl J Med* 272:923–931, 1965.

Touraine A, et al: Un syndrome ostéodermatopathique: La pachydermie plicaturée avec pachypériostose des extremités. *Presse Méd* 43:1820–1824, 1935.

Vogl A, Goldfischer S: Pachydermoperiostosis: Primary or idiopathic osteoarthropathy. *Am J Med* 33:166–187, 1962.

4.24 Pachyonychia Congenita, Jadassohn-Lewandowski Type

The syndrome consists of (1) pachyonychia congenita, (2) palmoplantar keratosis and hyperhidrosis, (3) follicular keratosis, and (4) oral leukokeratosis. The name "pachyonychia congenita," applied to the thickened nails, was used subsequently to designate the entire syndrome. The condition is inherited in an autosomal dominant manner, though penetrance does not seem to be complete.

Facies. There is no characteristic facies for the condition.

Oral Structures. Oral leukokeratosis is a constant component of the syndrome, the tongue having a marked white to gray coating of parakeratin (Fig. 4.40). Other oral mucosae, especially the buccal, can be similarly affected (Fig. 4.41). Herpetic-like lesions, ie, vesicles and ulcers, are also a frequent finding in the oral mucosa. Natal teeth have been described in several newborns who later developed the syndrome.

Systemic Features. The fingernails and toenails, at birth or shortly thereafter, are thick and hard (Fig. 4.42). The space between nail and nailbed is occupied by a yellowish to brown substance with the consistency of keratin. Therefore, the nails are projected upward and frequently lost on that account. Regrowth occurs, but the process is repeated and generally with increased severity. Periungual inflammation is almost always present. Other dermatologic findings include hyperhidrosis of palms and soles in contrast to a generalized hypohidrosis, keratosis palmo-plantaris, and bullous eruption on the plantar surface of toes and heels, especially during the summer. Small-sized papules, with central keratinized plugging, appear during infancy on elbows, knees, popliteal areas and buttocks (Fig. 4.43). Verruca-like lesions can be seen with a similar distribution.

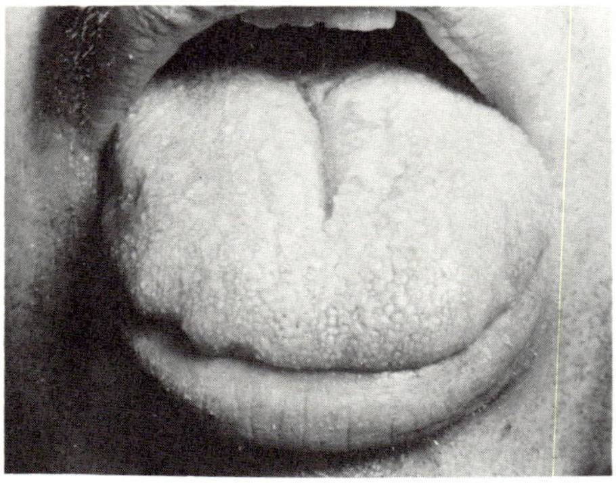

Fig. 4.40. Note marked thickening of lingual mucosa.

Differential Diagnosis. The Jackson-Lawler type of pachyonychia congenita is essentially similar to the Jadassohn-Lewandowski type, but the following differences are recognized in the Jackson-Lawler syn-

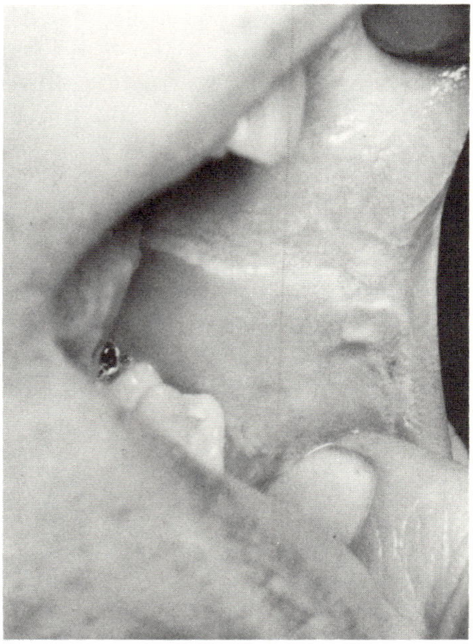

Fig. 4.41. Moderate keratinization of the buccal mucosa in patient with the syndrome.

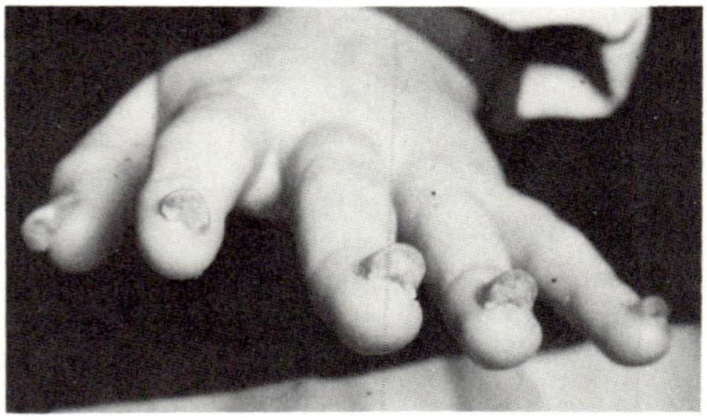

Fig. 4.42. Thickening and elevation of free edge of fingernails.

drome: (1) absence of oral keratosis, (2) presence of neonatal teeth with hypoplastic enamel, and (3) presence of cutaneous epidermoid cysts. The rest of the clinical manifestations are identical. Other conditions to be included in the differential diagnosis are white sponge nevus of Cannon, hereditary benign intraepithelial dyskeratosis, and dyskeratosis congenita.

Laboratory Aids. None known.

Synonym. Jadassohn-Lewandowski syndrome.

References

Anneroth G, et al: Pachyonychia congenita. A clinical, histological and microradiographic study with special reference to oral manifestations. *Acta Derm Vener* 55:387–394, 1975.

Besser FS, Moynahan EJ: Pachyonychia congenita with epidermal cysts and teeth at birth: 4th generation. *Br J Dermatol* 84:95–96, 1971.

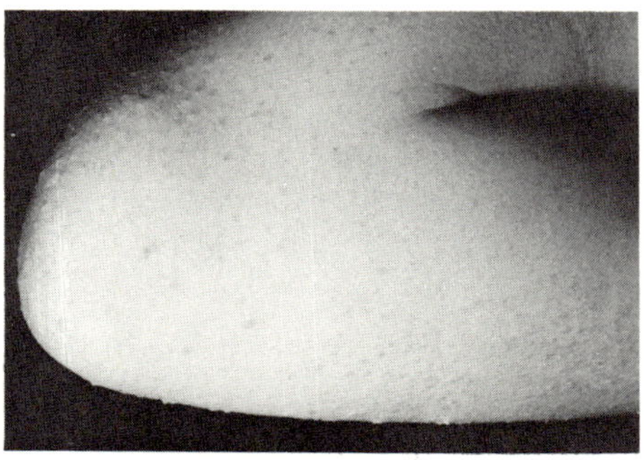

Fig. 4.43. Note follicular papules over the elbows.

Gorlin RJ, Chaudry AP: Oral lesions accompanying pachyonychia congenita. *Oral Surg* 11:541–544, 1958.

Lang CR, et al: Pachyonychia congenita. *Am J Dis Child* 111:649–652, 1966.

4.25 Peutz-Jeghers Syndrome

The syndrome of (1) mucocutaneous melanotic pigmentation and (2) gastrointestinal polyposis was probably first described by Hutchinson in 1896. Peutz, in 1921, reported the condition in several generations of a family, and Jeghers, in 1949, published an exhaustive description of several cases of the syndrome. The condition is clearly inherited in an autosomal dominant manner with high penetrance.

Facies. The typical facial finding is the presence of discrete, brown to bluish black macules on the skin, chiefly around the oral, nasal, and orbital orifices in over half of the affected individuals. The pigmented macules generally are not more than a few millimeters in diameter, and they vary in number and degree of pigmentation, especially with age. The older the patient, the less the number of macules and the degree of pigmentation. Occasionally, macules occur on the dorsum of the nose and other facial skin areas.

Oral Structures. The lips, especially the lower, and the oral mucosa are involved with pigmented macules in about 98% of the patients (Fig. 4.44); less frequently the gingiva and palate and rarely the tongue and oral floor are involved. The melanotic spots are larger than those on the skin, up to 12 mm in diameter. The cutaneous pigmented macules tend to fade after puberty, but the intraoral pigmentation is more stable (Fig. 4.45).

Systemic Features. Mental and physical development are within normal limits. Pigmentation of the extremities, conjunctiva, and nasal mucosa also can be found, with the number of pigmented spots varying in different patients. The most important component of the syndrome is the polyposis of the gastrointestinal tract. The polyps are hamartomatous in origin. The following sites, in order of frequency, are involved: jejunum, ileum, large bowel, rectum, stomach, duodenum, and appendix.

Polyps may produce intussusception and occasionally lead to severe intestinal obstruction and death. The age of onset cannot be precisely determined, but generally there is a history of gastrointestinal problems before the third decade of life. There is no evidence that the polyps are premalignant. Some patients have had polyps of the bladder, nose, cervix, and bronchi, but this is unusual. Theca cell tumors of the ovary are found with increased frequency.

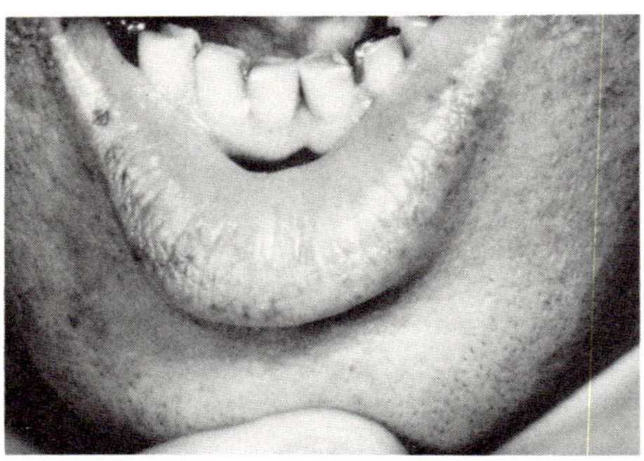

Fig. 4.44. Note small areas of pigmentation on the vermilion border of lower lip.

Differential Diagnosis. Intestinal polyposis I (colonic polyposis), Gardner syndrome, and Addison disease should be considered in the differential diagnosis.

Laboratory Aids. Roentgenographic survey of the gastrointestinal tract is helpful in establishing the diagnosis.

Synonym. Intestinal polyposis II.

References

Bartholomew LG, et al: Intestinal polyposis associated with mucocutaneous melanin pigmentation: Peutz-Jeghers syndrome; review of literature and re-

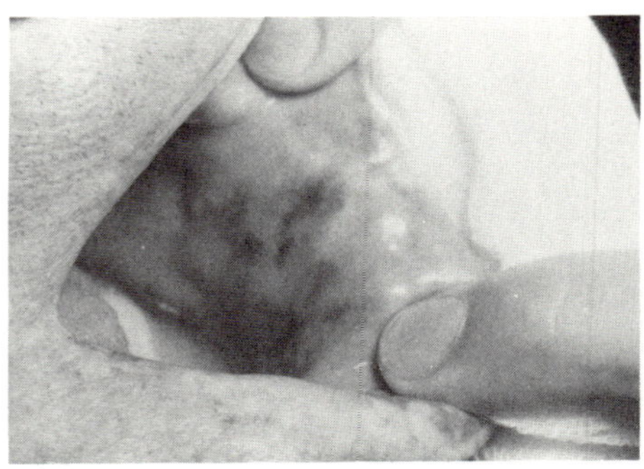

Fig. 4.45. Intraoral areas of pigmentation in the buccal mucosa of patient with the syndrome.

port of six cases with special reference to pathologic findings. *Gastroenterology* 32:434–451, 1957.

Dozis RR, et al: The Peutz-Jeghers syndrome. *Arch Surg* 98:509–517, 1969.

Jeghers H, et al: Generalized intestinal polyposis and melanin spots of the oral mucosa, lips and digits. *N Engl J Med* 241:993–1005, 1031–1036, 1949.

Lowe NJ: Peutz-Jeghers syndrome with pigmented oral papillomas. *Arch Dermatol* 111:503–505, 1975.

Utsonomiya J, et al: Peutz-Jeghers syndrome: Its natural course and management. *Johns Hopkins Med J* 136:71–82, 1975.

4.26 Pseudoxanthoma Elasticum

The syndrome comprises (1) dermatologic changes, (2) angioid streaks, (3) recurrent hemorrhagic episodes of the gastrointestinal tract, (4) weak pulse, and (5) failing vision. Pseudoxanthoma elasticum exhibits genetic heterogeneity, with the majority of cases being inherited in an autosomal recessive manner. Two dominant and two recessive forms are recognized. The basic defect in the syndrome is calcification of elastic fibers. For simplicity, only a summary of the general clinical findings in the various forms will be presented here. For further details the interested reader is referred to the excellent review by Pope (1975).

Facies. The facial skin is the site of dermatologic changes as described below. Failing vision is seen in older patients. Around puberty, but occasionally earlier, the perioral skin becomes redundant, accentuating the skin creases and folds with a resultant "hound dog" appearance.

Oral Structures. In addition to the perioral changes, yellowish nodules formed by heavily packed and whorly collagen fibers can be seen in the labial, buccal, soft and hard palatal, and tonsilar mucosae (Fig. 4.46).

Systemic Features. Physical development is within normal limits. Between infancy and the beginning of the second decade, the dermatologic changes take place. Thickening of the skin with accumulation of flat yellowish papules slightly elevated from the skin surface occurs in almost any area of the body (Fig. 4.47). Most fa-

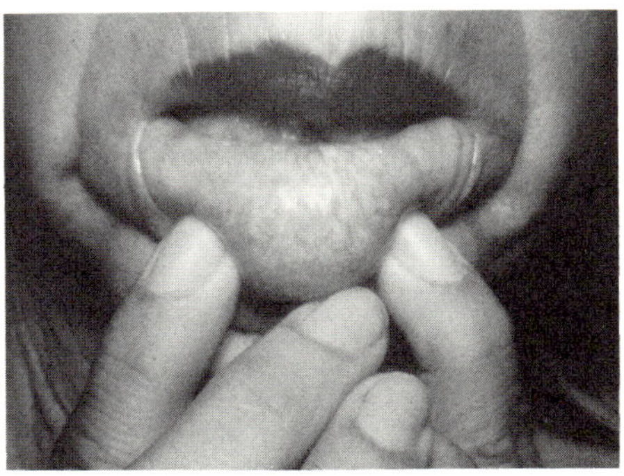

Fig. 4.46. Inner surface of lower lip showing yellowish papules simulating Fordyce granules.

vored locations are perioral skin, neck, axilla, groin, and elbows. The skin loses its elasticity and acquires a leathery appearance.

Angioid streaks seen on fundoscopic examination in almost all patients represent involvement of the Bruch membrane and are usually found around the optic discs. Other ocular findings include retinal hemorrhage with failing vision, central chorioretinitis, and macular degeneration. Calcification of peripheral arteries generally occurs in the late twenties with consequent diminished or absent pulse in both arms and legs. Hypertension, angina pectoris, and abdominal angina are common complications. Hemorrhagic episodes can occur in the gastrointestinal tract, kidneys, bladder, uterus, nasal mucosa, joints, and cranium.

Differential Diagnosis. A variety of conditions associated with angioid streaks should be differentiated, as well as senile elastosis.

Laboratory Aids. Biopsy of skin or mucous membrane will demonstrate calcification of elastic fibers. Increased levels of collagenic lysine and hydroxylysine as well as elevated amounts of glutamine in the elastin have been reported.

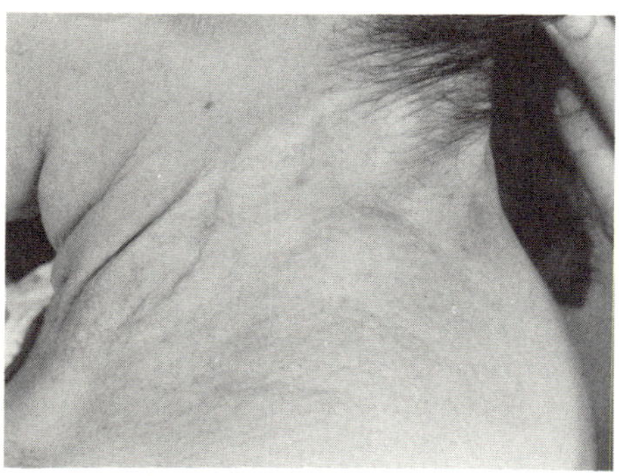

Fig. 4.47. Left side of neck, in patient of Fig. 4.46, showing accentuation of transverse folds and yellowish plaques in confluent and reticular arrangement.

Synonym. Grönblad-Strandberg syndrome.

References

Altman LK, et al: Pseudoxanthoma elasticum. *Arch Intern Med* 134:1048–1054, 1974.

Martinez-Hernandez A, Huffer WE: Pseudoxanthoma elasticum: dermal polyanions and mineralization of elastic fibers. *Lab Invest* 31:181–186, 1974.

Pope FM: Two types of autosomal recessive pseudoxanthoma elasticum. *Arch Dermatol* 110:209–212, 1974.

Pope FM: Historical evidence for the genetic heterogeneity of pseudoxanthoma elasticum. *Br J Dermatol* 92:493–510, 1975.

4.27 Xerodermic Idiocy

Although described as early as 1870 by Hebra and Kaposi, the association of (1) xeroderma pigmentosum, (2) mental deficiency, (3) microcephaly, (4) dwarfism, (5) gonadal hypoplasia, and (6) various neurologic complications was first pointed out by De

Sanctis and Cacchione in 1932. The frequent occurrence of the syndrome in siblings and the increased rate of parental consanguinity indicate autosomal recessive inheritance. The mothers of affected individuals often present a history of increased incidence of spontaneous abortions. The syndrome appears to have a higher frequency in Arab countries.

Facies. The skin of the face is severely sensitive to sunlight, with consequent sunburn effects and freckling (Fig. 4.48). Malignant neoplasms of the skin, as explained below, are part of the facies.

Oral Structures. Squamous cell carcinomas of the lips, developing as early as age 17, as well as other malignant neoplasms, are frequent oral findings.

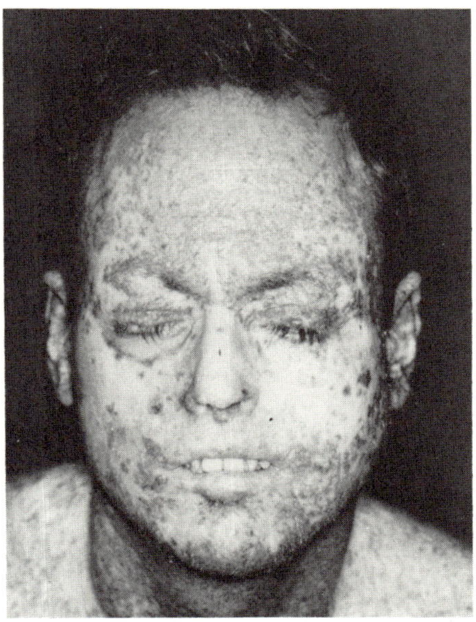

Fig. 4.48. Typical appearance of patient with xerodermic idiocy. Several areas exhibit early malignant transformation.

Systemic Features. Mental retardation is marked. Physical development and bone age are retarded. Mental retardation usually becomes evident within the first year of life and is progressive. Microcephaly, premature closure of cranial sutures, retarded sexual development, choreoathetosis, cerebellar ataxia, and other signs of spinocerebellar disease are frequent. Necropsy has revealed cerebral and olivopontocerebellar atrophy.

Marked sensitivity to sunlight (especially wavelengths from 2,800 to 3,100 Ångstroms) is noted early in life. Many of these children experience severe sunburn reactions, and subsequent freckling of exposed skin areas, between the sixth month and the first birthday. Within the first few years, the condition rapidly progresses to a development of cutaneous malignancies in areas of both ectodermal and mesodermal origins. Keratoacanthoma, squamous cell carcinoma, basal cell carcinoma, melanoma, and fibrosarcoma often appear on the facial skin and other sun-exposed areas. Leukemia has also been noted. Early death, resulting from malignancy or from poor resistance to infection, is common. The acute sensitivity to sunlight tends to disappear in adulthood. Ocular manifestations include photophobia with consequent conjunctivitis and profuse lacrimation, malignancy of the eye, ulceration of the cornea, iritis, ectropion, and symblepharon.

Differential Diagnosis. Other forms of xeroderma pigmentosum are recognized; one is similar to the present syndrome but lacks mental retardation and dwarfism, and another form is milder and is inherited as an autosomal dominant condition. Still other photodermatoses associated with malignancies or neurologic involvement should be considered. Bloom syndrome and Cockayne syndrome also should be included in the differential diagnosis.

Laboratory Aids. The repair mechanism of DNA following visible and ultraviolet light exposure appears to be defective in this disorder. Fibroblasts from patients with the xeroderma pigmentosum syndrome have 10% to 20% of the normal ability to repair. Increased chromosomal breakage has been found in fibroblasts from these patients but has not been found in lymphocyte culture.

Synonyms. De Sanctis-Cacchione syndrome, xeroderma pigmentosum with mental retardation syndrome.

References

Botsma D, et al: Different inherited levels of DNA repair replication in xeroderma pigmentosum cell strains, after exposure to ultraviolet irradiation. *Mutat Res* 9:507–516, 1970.

Cleaver JE: Xeroderma pigmentosum—progress and regress. *J Invest Dermatol* 60:374–380, 1973.

De Sanctis C, Cacchione A: L'idiozia xerodermica. *Riv Sper Freniatr* 56:269, 1932.

Friedman A, et al: Xerodermic idiocy or De Sanctis-Cacchione syndrome. *Clin Pediatr* 12:56–58, 1973.

Robbins JH, et al: Xeroderma pigmentosum: An inherited disease with sun sensitivity, multiple cutaneous neoplasms, and abnormal DNA repair. *Ann Intern Med* 80:221–248, 1974.

4.28 White Sponge Nevus

This disorder may be present at birth or may appear at puberty. It is characterized by white spongy

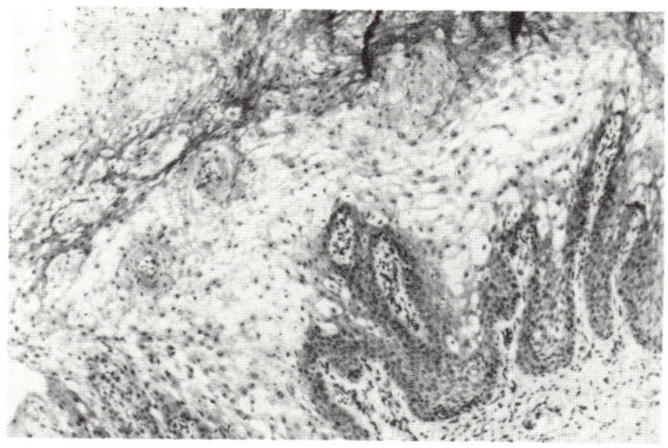

Fig. 4.50. Biopsy of the buccal mucosa showing prominent spongiosis of all epithelial cell layers.

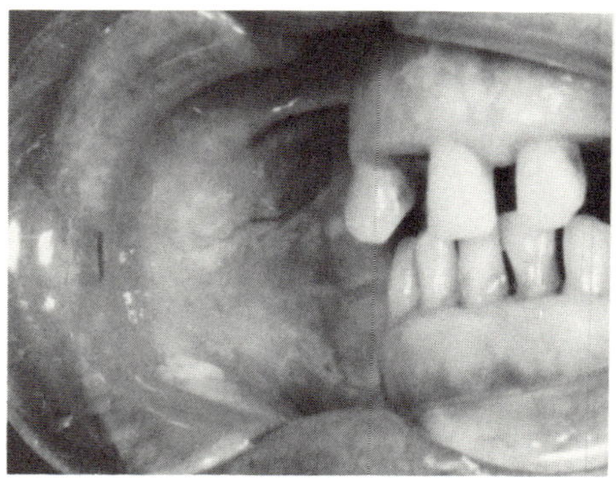

Fig. 4.49. Thickening of buccal mucosa in a 65-year-old male with white sponge nevus.

plaques on nearly any part of the oral mucosa, with variable involvement of other mucous membranes. The sexes are equally affected and the condition is inherited in an autosomal dominant manner.

Facies. No characteristic facies.

Oral Structures. The mucosa is thickened, corrugated, or folded and soft (Fig. 4.49). The superficial keratin has a tendency to desquamate at times, leaving a raw surface. The free gingival margin appears to be spared. Buccal mucosal involvement is constant and nearly always symmetrical; in rare instances, it is unilateral. The white plaques are symptomless; hence, the disorder is often discovered by accident.

Systemic Features. Somatic and mental development are normal. There may be variable thickening of the nasal, laryngeal, esophageal, anal, and vaginal mucosae.

Differential Diagnosis. Pachyonychia congenita, hereditary benign intraepithelial dyskeratosis, and leuko-edema should be included in the differential diagnosis.

Laboratory Aids. Histologic alterations are characterized by marked spongiosis of all epithelial layers (Fig. 4.50).

Synonyms. White sponge of nevus of Cannon, Cannon disease.

References

Cohen L, Young AH: The white sponge naevus. *Brit J Oral Surg* 5:206–210, 1968.

Cooke BED: Keratinizing lesions affecting the oral mucosa. *Proc R Soc Med* 60:819–822, 1967.

Kamalamma MK, et al: The white sponge nevus. *Oral Surg* 30:51–54, 1970.

Witkop CJ, Gorlin RJ: Four hereditary mucosal syndromes. *Arch Derm* 84:762–771, 1961.

CHAPTER 5

Systemic Inherited Disorders with Involvement of Jaw Bones

5.1 Apert Syndrome

Apert syndrome is a form of craniosynostosis consisting of (1) turribrachycephaly and (2) syndactyly of hands and feet. The syndrome was mentioned as early as 1842 by Baumgartner, though eponymic credit is given to Apert for his presentation of the syndrome in 1906. In 1938, Valentin thoroughly reviewed 93 cases from the literature, and in 1960 Blank established distinct criteria for the syndrome and estimated the incidence to be 1 in 160,000 live births with an equal distribution between sexes. Because of the high infant mortality, he found the frequency decreased to about 1 in 2 million in the general population. The majority of cases of acrocephalosyndactyly are sporadic. The syndrome is transmitted as an autosomal dominant condition. An advanced paternal age effect has been demonstrated.

Facies. The middle third of the face appears flat and underdeveloped, producing a relative mandibular prognathism. The nose is sometimes small and somewhat parrot-shaped. Hypertelorism and strabismus are often noted (Fig. 5.1). The orbits are flattened, and the eyes tend to be proptosed. A horizontal groove extends across the forehead just above the supraorbital ridges in some infants.

Oral Structures. A high-arched palate, occasionally with a marked median furrow, is frequently observed (Fig. 5.2). Cleft palate or bifid uvula is found in at least 25% of these patients. Associated with

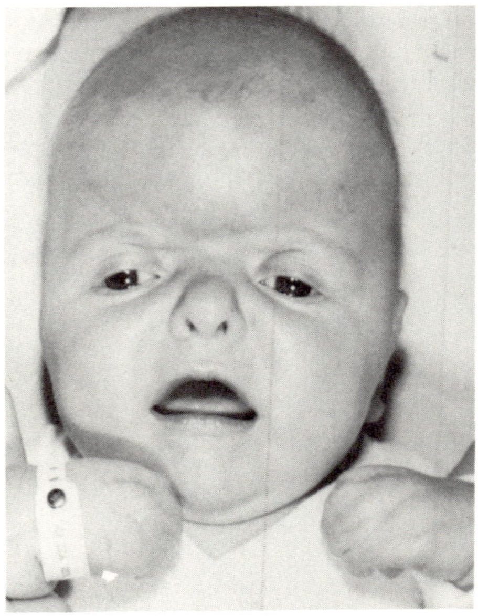

Fig. 5.1. Marked frontal bulging, ocular hypertelorism, and fusion of fingers.

hypoplastic maxilla is relative mandibular prognathism and compression of the upper arcade, which becomes V-shaped, leading to an irregular positioning of the teeth. Crowding of the teeth leads to a marked thickening of the alveolar process. The pointed palate causes protrusion of the middle portion of the upper lip.

Systemic Features. Physical development is within normal limits. Most patients have an intelligence below normal. The cranium has a characteristic oxycephalic appearance. It is ovoid and brachycephalic, with a high, prominent, steep forehead. The frontal and temporal areas bulge. The apex of the cranium is located near or anterior to the bregma, the occipital region being flat and in the same vertical place as the neck. A number of patients possess an open anterior fontanel, which at times continues to an open frontal suture. There is irregular early obliteration of cranial sutures. Roentgenographically, the fusion of the coronal suture is found most often, alone or together with fusion of the sagittal suture.

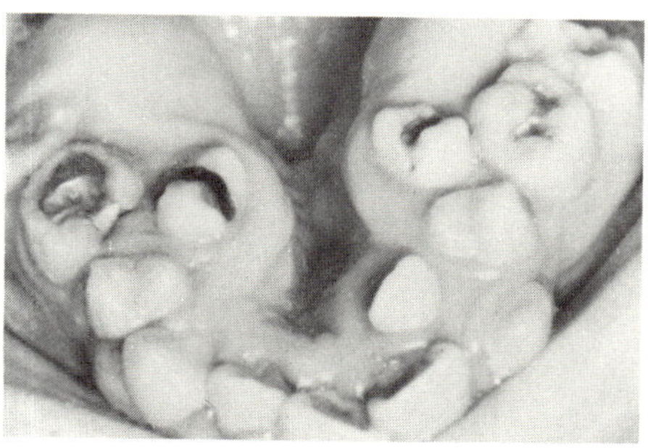

Fig. 5.2. Bizarre formation of palate—"Byzantine arch palate"—and unusual crowding of teeth.

Marked accentuation of digital markings is usually observed. The symmetrical syndactyly of both hands and feet varies in degree from partial fusion of the skin to a true progressive osseous syndactyly of metacarpals, metartarsals, and phalanges. When the three middle fingers are completely fused, there is often a common nail that gives the hand the appearance of a mitten ("mid-digital hand mass"). Miscellaneous abnormalities have included aplasia or ankylosis of several joints, especially elbow, shoulder, and hip; ankylosis of vertebrae, spina bifida, and fixed stapes with consequent hearing loss.

Differential Diagnosis. The other types of acrocephalosyndactyly, Saethre-Chotzen syndrome, and Crouzon syndrome should be considered in the differential diagnosis.

Laboratory Aids. None known.

Synonym. Acrocephalosyndactyly type I.

References

Apert E: De l'acrocephalosyndactylie. *Bull Soc Med (Paris)* 32:1310–1330, 1906.

Blank CE: Apert's syndrome (a type of acrocephalosyndactyly): Observations on a British series of thirty-nine cases. *Ann Hum Genet* 24:151–164, 1960.

Cohen MM Jr, et al: Facial variability in Apert type acrocephalosyndactyly. *Birth Def* 7(7):143–152, 1971.

Hoover GH, et al: The hand in Apert's syndrome. *J Bone Joint Surg* 52A:878–895, 1970.

Valentin B: Die Korrelation (Koppelung) von Missbildungen, erläutert am Biespiel der Akrocephalosyndactylie. *Acta Orthop Scand* 9:235–316, 1938.

5.2 Carpenter Syndrome

The syndrome originally described by Carpenter (1901) consists of (1) acrocephaly, (2) soft tissue syndactyly, especially involving the third and fourth fingers, and brachymesophalangy, (3) preaxial polydactyly and syndactyly of the toes, (4) coxa valga and pes varus, (5) congenital heart disease, (6) mental retardation, (7) hypogenitalism, (8) mild obesity, and (9) hernia. The syndrome is inherited as an autosomal recessive condition.

Facies. Dystopia canthorum is a constant feature and is generally associated with epicanthal folds and depressed nasal bridge (Fig. 5.3). Maldeveloped cornea, microcornea, slight optic atrophy, corneal opacity, and blurring of disc margins have also been described associated with the syndrome. Low-set ears and short neck are constant findings.

Oral Structures. The mandible is quite hypoplastic and consequently retrognathic. The palate is high-arched.

Systemic Features. A low level of intelligence is generally observed in those patients who do not die of congenital heart disease. Height is usually below the 25th percentile, but weight is above average. The obesity mainly involves the trunk, proximal portion of the limbs, face, and back of neck. Premature synostosis of all cranial sutures often occurs asymmetrically, producing distorted calvaria and a tower-shaped skull. The sagittal and lambdoidal sutures fuse first, the coronal last. The anterior fontanel occasionally exhibits Wormian bones.

The hands are short with stubby fingers. Soft tissue syndactyly can be seen between the third and fourth fingers; a minor degree of syndactyly is also present between the other fingers. The proximal phalanges of the thumb and hallux have two

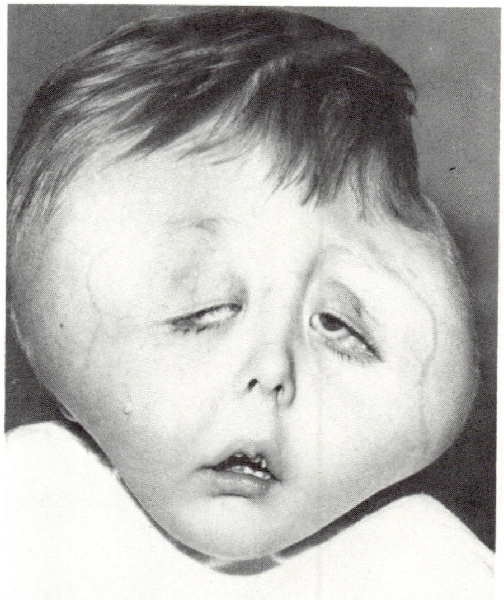

Fig. 5.3. Child with Carpenter syndrome presenting acrocephaly, asymmetric cloverleaf skull, dystopia canthorum, and depressed nasal bridge.

round ossification centers; in addition the hallux presents a distal triangular center. A tongue-shaped projection may extend from the radial side of the epiphysis of the proximal phalanx of the index finger. Often there is brachymesophalangy of all digits or agenesis of some middle phalanges of the second to fifth digits.

Usually there are bilateral varus deformities of the feet and preaxial polydactyly with duplication of the second toes. In many cases, toes exhibit soft tissue syndactyly. Radiographically, there are metatarsus varus and replication of the second toe and, to a lesser extent, the second metatarsal. The first metatarsals are broad and short. The toes are formed by only two phalanges. Genua valga with lateral displacement of the patellae is a constant finding. Mobility of the hip is reduced. Congenital heart disease, such as ventricular septal defect, atrial septal defect, patent ductus arteriosus, pulmonary stenosis, and tetralogy of Fallot, has been reported in several cases.

Differential Diagnosis. Noack syndrome, Laurence-Moon syndrome and the acrocephalosyndactylies should be included in the differential diagnosis.

Laboratory Aids. None known.

Synonyms. Acrocephalopolysyndactyly, ACPS type II.

References

Carpenter G: Two sisters showing malformations of the skull and other congenital abnormalities. *Rep Soc Study Dis Child (London)* 1:110, 1901.

Der Kaloustian et al: Carpenter's syndrome. Acrocephalopolysyndactyly type II. *Am J Dis Child* 124:716–718, 1972.

Sakati N, et al: A new syndrome with acrocephalopolysyndactyly, cardiac disease and distinctive defects of the ear, skin and lower limbs. *J Pediatr* 79:104–109, 1971.

Sunderhaus E, Wolter JR: Acrocephalosyndactylism. *J Pediatr Ophthal* 5:118–120, 1968.

Temtamy SA: Carpenter's syndrome: Acrocephalopolysyndactyly. An autosomal recessive syndrome. *J Pediatr* 69:111–120, 1966.

5.3 Cerebrohepatorenal Syndrome

Bowen and associates in 1964 and, independently, Smith and coworkers in 1965 described a syndrome consisting of (1) hypotonia, (2) high forehead and other craniofacial anomalies, (3) flexion contractures, (4) hypoprothrombinemia, (5) hepatomegaly, (6) renal cortical cysts, and (7) developmental abnormalities of the brain. The syndrome has autosomal recessive inheritance, with female predilection. Death generally ensues in the first six months of life.

Facies. The facies and the supraorbital ridges are flat and the forehead is high (Figs. 5.4–5). Ocular manifestations have included hypertelorism, mild mongoloid obliquity of the palpebral fissures, edematous eyelids, epicanthal folds, nystagmus, Brushfield spots, and cataracts. The facial appearance is completed by anteverted nostrils, puffy cheeks, and micrognathia. The skull may be pear-shaped, the skin of the neck is redundant and the ears are generally rotated posteriorly.

Oral Structures. High-arched palate, micrognathia, and protruding tongue are constant findings.

Systemic Features. Birth weight is below 3,000 gm. Severe hypotonia, seizures, abnormal electroencephalographic findings, and dilated ventricles are quite constant findings. Other CNS findings have included macrogyria, absent corpus callosum, and olfactory hypoplasia, among others. Fontanels and sutures are widely open, with occasional Wormian bones. Hypomineralization and retarded bone age are also evident. Calcific stippling of the acetabular cartilages, stippled epiphyses in long bones, calcification of the thyroid cartilage and the hyoid bone, and metaphyseal radiolucencies have also been noted. A plethora of abnormalities have been described as associated with the condition. Also observed are camptodactyly of one or more fingers, cubitus valgus, talipes equinovarus, rocker bottom feet, patent ductus arteriosus, and patent foramen ovale, hepatomegaly, iron pigment deposition, renal cortical cysts, small penis, hypospadias, prominent clitoris, umbilical hernia, splenomegaly, and pancreatic islet cell hyperplasia.

Differential Diagnosis. All other forms of infantile hypotonia should be considered.

Laboratory Aids. Serum iron levels may be of diagnostic value during the neonatal period, although increased iron has not been reported in every case. Decreased immunoglobulins have also been reported.

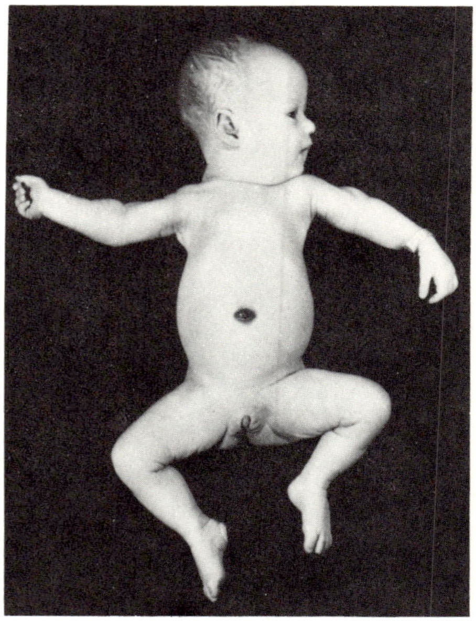

Fig. 5.4. Note high forehead, pear-shaped skull with flattened occiput, and cubitus valgus.

Synonyms. Zellweger syndrome, Bowen syndrome.

References

Bowen P, et al: A familial syndrome of multiple congenital defects. *Johns Hopkins Med J* 114:402–414, 1964.

Danks DM, et al: Cerebrohepatorenal syndrome of Zellweger, *J Pediatr* 86:382–387, 1975.

Gilchrist KW, et al: Immunodeficiency in cerebro-hepato-renal syndrome. *Lancet* 1:164–165, 1974.

Jan JE, et al: Cerebro-hepato-renal syndrome of Zellweger. *Am J Dis Child* 119:274–277, 1970.

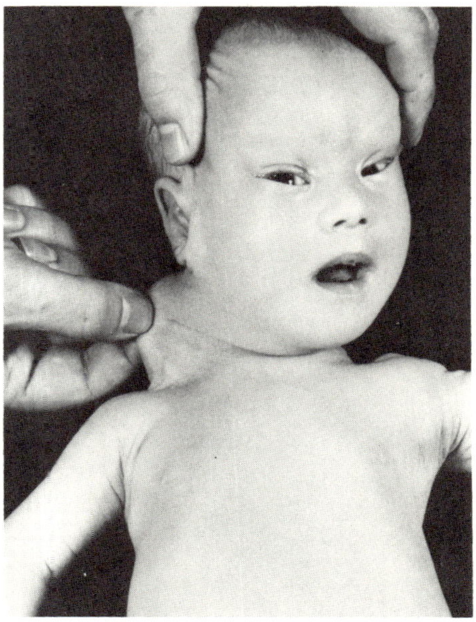

Fig. 5.5. Note redundant skin on the neck and various craniofacial anomalies in this hypotonic infant with the syndrome.

Smith DW, et al: A syndrome of multiple developmental defects including polycystic kidneys and intrahepatic biliary dysgenesis in 2 siblings. *J Pediatr* 67:617–624, 1965.

5.4 Cherubism

This disorder was first described by Jones in 1933 as a familial multilocular bone disease that almost exclusively affects the jaws. The condition is inherited in an autosomal dominant mode with variable expressivity and incomplete penetrance in females. Cherubism is not considered to be a form of fibrous dysplasia of the jaws.

Facies. The syndrome first becomes manifest as a painless swelling between the ages of 18 months and 4 years of age, the affected individual being normal at birth. Generally involvement is bilateral, but occasional unilateral cases have been reported. Maxilla and mandible can be affected at the same time, but the maxilla is less often involved (in about 65% of cases). If the maxilla is affected, involvement of the orbital floor will produce upward displacement of the eye, exposing a characteristic rim of sclera beneath the iris. This, associated with the bilateral swelling, gives the typical cherubic appearance (Fig. 5.6). Ocular hypertelorism is an almost constant feature.

Oral Structures. In involved maxilla or mandible the bone is replaced by fibrous connective tissue with scattered multinucleated giant cells. This produces displacement of primary teeth as well as abortive formation or absence of permanent molar teeth. Radiographically, a "soap bubble" appearance of the bone is observed, generally extending bilaterally from the molar region to the angle and ramus of the mandible (Fig. 5.7). The condyle is never affected. Severe cases may evince total involvement of the mandible. The maxilla is most frequently affected in the area of the antrum and the tuberosity.

The jaws increase rapidly in size until about puberty, when the swelling tends to remain stationary and then progressively disappears (Fig. 5.8). After the age of 20, and in some cases 30, the only remaining radiographic evidence is scattered areas of slightly increased bone density. Severe cases may exhibit a grotesque appearance with complications in mastication, deglutition, respiration, and speech.

Systemic Features. Rarely, extraoral lesions have been reported occurring in the humerus, ribs, femur, etc. Occasionally, submandibular and cervical lymphadenopathy can be observed during the active phase of the condition.

Differential Diagnosis. Odontogenic tumors (ie, ameloblastoma), fibrous dysplasia, primary and metastatic tumors of the jaws, aneurysmal bone cysts, and central giant cell tumor of the jaws should

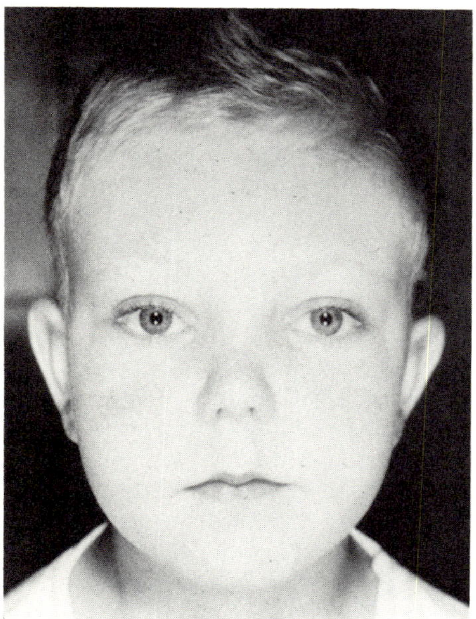

Fig. 5.6. Note rounded face and slight hypertelorism.

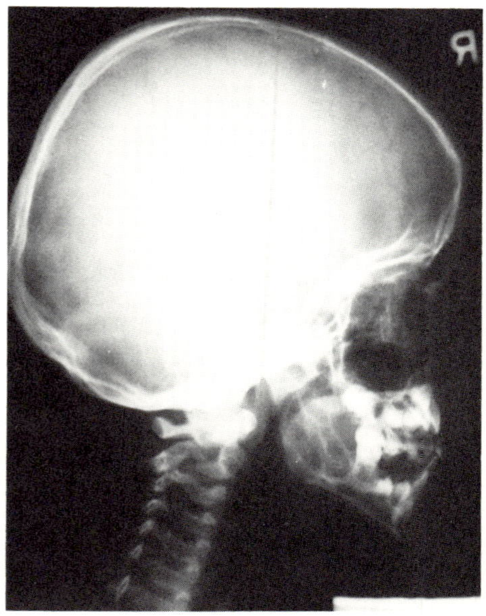

Fig. 5.7. Radiograph showing multilocular cyst-like areas in the ascending ramus of the mandible.

be considered in the differential diagnosis.

Laboratory Aids. Serum alkaline phosphatase levels may occasionally be elevated during the active phase of the disease.

Synonym. Familial fibrous dysplasia.

References

Anderson DE, McClendon JL: Cherubism, hereditary fibrous dysplasia of the jaws. I. Genetic considerations. *Oral Surg* 15(Suppl 2):5–16, 1962.

Cornelius EA, McClendon JL: Cherubism; hereditary fibrous dysplasia of the jaws. *Am J Roentgen* 106:136–143, 1969.

Jones WA: Familial multilocular cystic disease of the jaws. *Amer J Cancer* 17:946–950, 1933.

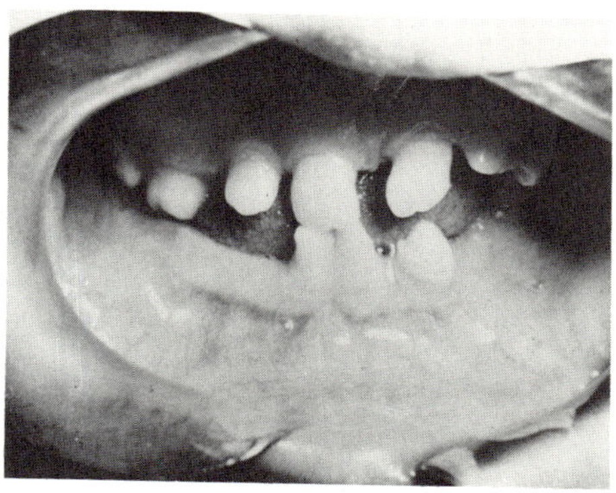

Fig. 5.8. Intraoral view showing lack of tooth eruption due to intrabony retention.

5.5 Chondrodysplasia Punctata

Chondrodysplasia punctata was described by Conradi in 1914. The condition is characterized by (1) punctate or stippled alterations of the epiphyses of the long bones, (2) congenital cataract, and (3) joint contractures and other skeletal changes. The syndrome is inherited in an autosomal dominant mode (Conradi-Hünermann type), or in an autosomal recessive mode (rhizomelic type). The condition is extremely rare, the estimated frequency being about two to three cases per million births. The consanguinity rate is about 8% for the rhizomelic type, and about 50% of these individuals die before the end of the first year of life.

Facies. A severe saddle-nose deformity as a result of nasal bone deficiencies, ocular hypertelorism, optic atrophy and congenital cataracts characterize the facies; however, only about one-half of either type exhibit a typical facies (Fig. 5.9).

Oral Structures. High-arched and cleft palates have been reported in a few patients with the rhizomelic form of the syndrome.

Systemic Features. The Conradi-Hünermann type usually manifests normal psychomotor development. Height is reduced, but head circumference is within normal limits. Punctate calcifications may be present in epiphyses, flat and round bones, and vertebrae. The tubular bones are asymmetrically shortened. Multiple dysplastic alterations in the epiphyses with flattened or irregular outlines have been noted; however, the metaphyses are unaffected. The vertebral bodies reveal punctate calcifications, are deformed, and exhibit scoliosis after the first year of life. Contractures of the large joints are present in about 25% of the cases. Talipes calcaneovalgus is present in 20% of affected individuals.

In contrast, individuals affected with the rhizomelic type of chondrodysplasia punctata usually have retarded mental development, cerebral atrophy, optic atrophy, and spastic diplegia. Skeletal changes include severe congenital rhizomelic shortening of the extremities and small head circumference persisting into infancy and childhood. Epiphyseal and extra epiphyseal calcifications are common and extensive. Contractures have been noted in 60% of affected individuals and foot deformities in 10% of cases. Roentgenologic examination often reveals severe shortening, metaphyseal cupping, splaying and disrupted ossification of the humerus and/or femur. A universal coronal cleft of the vertebral bodies is observed on lateral views of the spine. Congenital cataracts have been described in about 20% of the Conradi-Hünermann form and in 70% of the rhizomelic type. The skin is atrophic, dry, and scaly in 25% of affected individuals. Similar skin

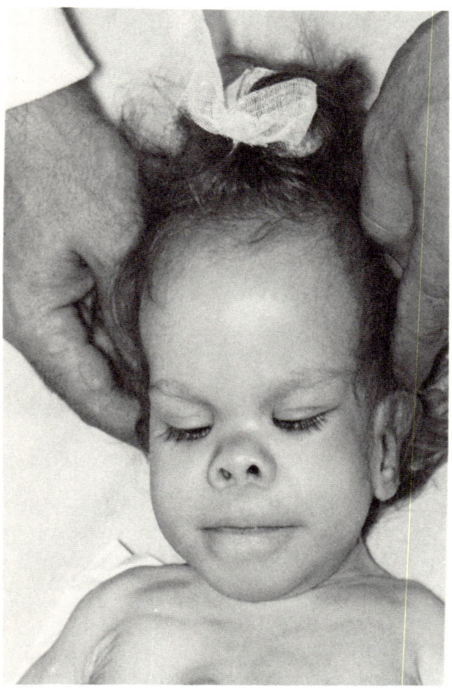

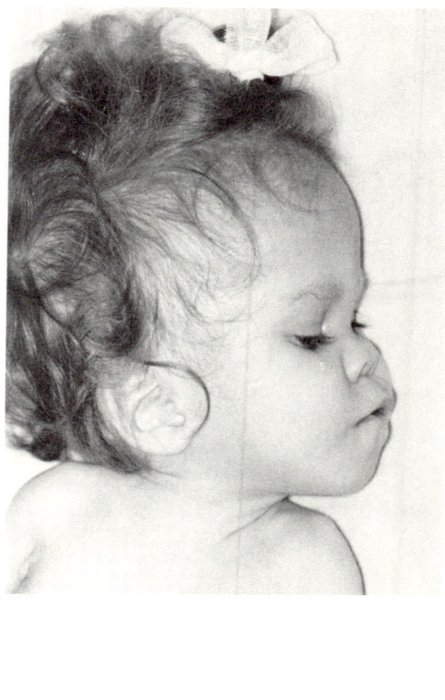

Fig. 5.9a, b. Note severe hypoplasia of nasal bones resulting in saddle deformity.

changes and incidence have been reported for both forms.

Differential Diagnosis. Maternal ingestion of dicoumaral or Warfarin during the first trimester of pregnancy may produce a similar disorder. Punctate intracartilaginous and extracartilaginous calcifications are nonspecific and may be seen in a wide variety of hereditary and nonhereditary conditions.

Laboratory Aids. None.

Synonyms: Conradi-Hünermann syndrome, stippled epiphyses, chondrodystrophia calcificans congenita.

References

Spranger JW, et al: Chondrodysplasia punctata (Chondrodystrophia calcificans). II. Der rhizomelic Typ. *Fortschr Roentgenstr* 114:327–335, 1971.

Spranger JW, et al: Heterogeneity of chondrodysplasia punctata. *Humangenetik* 11:190–212, 1971.

Tasker WG, et al: Chondrodystrophia calcificans congenita (dysplasia epiphysalis punctata). Recognition of the clinical picture. *Am J Dis Child* 119:122–127, 1970.

5.6 Craniofacial Dysostosis

The syndrome of (1) cranial synostosis, (2) bilateral exophthalmus with external strabismus, (3) parrot-beaked nose, and (4) relative mandibular prognathism with drooping lower lip was first described by Crouzon in 1912. The syndrome is inherited as an autosomal dominant condition with almost complete penetrance. Not uncommonly, sporadic cases with a negative family history have been reported, thus representing new mutations.

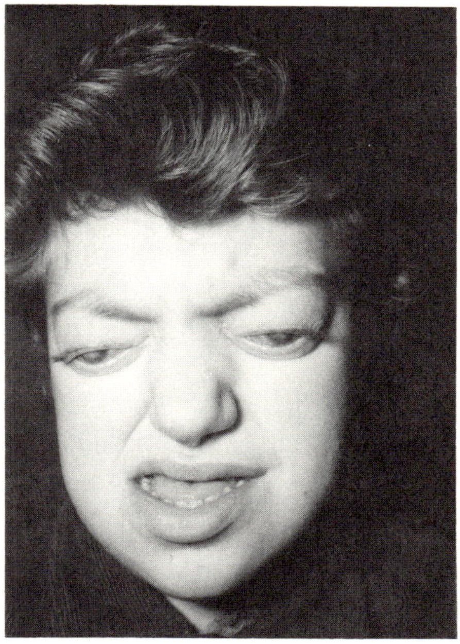

Fig. 5.10. Note marked exophthalmus, hypertelorism, beaked nose, and short upper lip.

Facies. The facies is easily recognized and characterized by marked exophthalmus, probably due to shallow orbits (Figs. 5.10–11). At times there is spontaneous luxation of the eyes. Ocular hypertelorism and hypoplastic maxilla are also constant facial findings. This last feature produces a marked relative mandibular prognathism and short upper lip. The cranium is brachycephalic with frontal bossing and ridging of the sagittal suture.

Oral Structures. Oral manifestations include hypoplastic maxilla, a V-shaped palatal arch in contrast to the normal U-shape, dental malocclusion, open bite, and partial clefting of the palate.

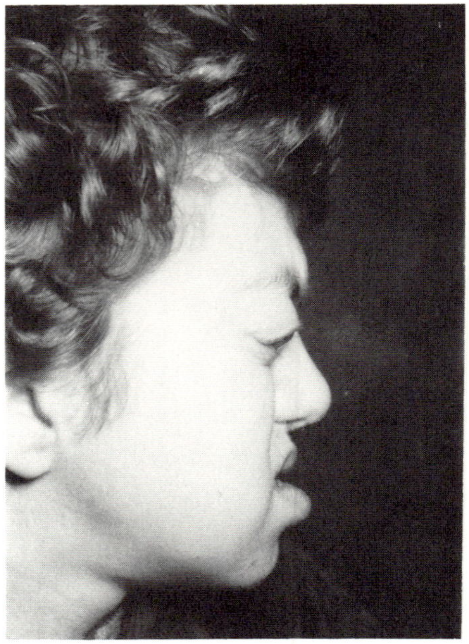

Fig. 5.11. Profile showing exophthalmus and midline hypoplasia.

Systemic Features. Physical development is within normal limits. Roentgenographically, the coronal, sagittal, and lambdoidal sutures are prematurely synostosed (Fig. 5.12). Increased digital markings are almost always present. Other sporadically associated anomalies have included epilepsy and various ear malformations. Eighty percent of affected individuals have optic nerve damage. Nystagmus is seen occasionally.

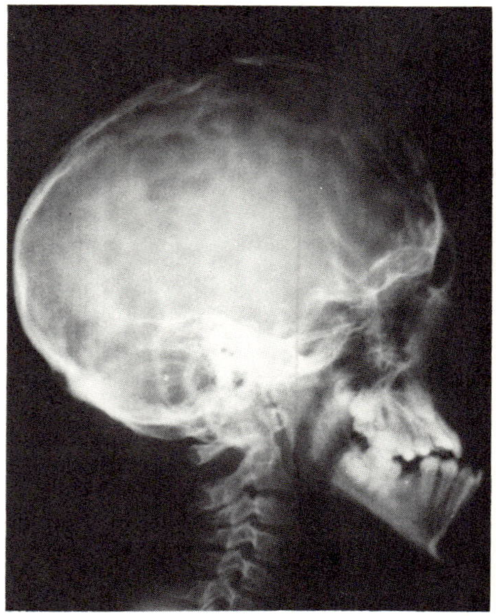

Fig. 5.12. Roentgenogram of patient showing marked digital impressions and mid-facial hypoplasia.

Differential Diagnosis. Cleidocranial dysplasia and the acrocephalosyndactyly syndromes, as well as the craniosynostosis syndrome, should be included.

Laboratory Aids. None known.

Synonym. Crouzon syndrome.

References

Cohen MM Jr: An etiologic and nosologic overview of craniosynostosis syndromes. *Birth Def* 11(2):137–189, 1975.

Kelly EE, et al: Oral manifestations of Crouzon's disease. *Oral Surg* 13:1245–1248, 1960.

5.7 Craniometaphyseal Dysplasia and Craniodiaphyseal Dysplasia

Craniometaphyseal dysplasia consists of (1) alterations in the metaphyses of long bones similar to those seen in metaphyseal dysplasia, increased diaphyseal density, and reduced metaphyseal density; and (2) bony overgrowth of the face and jaws, especially of the paranasal areas. Craniometaphyseal dysplasia may be transmitted in an autosomal dominant manner or in an autosomal recessive manner. Craniodiaphyseal dysplasia has autosomal recessive inheritance.

Facies. A rather large head with an extremely broad and flat nasal bridge, ocular hypertelorism, and an open mouth give the patient a vacuous expression (Fig. 5.13). The open mouth is due to nasal blockage. Soon after birth, the skull exhibits marked thickening and increased density of the vault with elimination of the diploë, especially in the frontal and occipital areas. The paranasal sinuses are similarly obliterated.

The bones of the skull base, maxilla, and mandible also become enlarged, thickened, and increased in density. Blindness resulting from optic atrophy in early infancy is not uncommon, and ocular hypertelorism has been a relatively constant finding (Fig. 5.14). Facial nerve paralysis and deafness have also been common features, presumably due to overgrowth of the foramina.

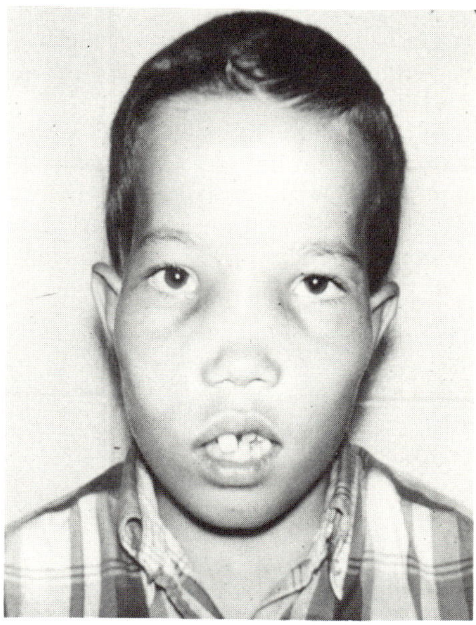

Fig. 5.13. Craniometaphyseal dysplasia, dominant form: bony growth in glabellar area in eight-year-old boy, who also has severe nerve deafness.

Oral Structures. The increased density observed in the skull with obliteration of the paranasal sinuses may extend to involve the maxilla and mandible. Thus, the jaws may appear enlarged and thickened and reveal increased density in roentgenologic examination.

Systemic Features. In craniometaphyseal dysplasia, the long bones, especially the femurs, assume an "Erlenmeyer flask" shape in the metaphyseal area with decreased density. The diaphyseal area is increased in density, the medullary bone being porotic and lacking the usual trabecular pattern. Similar changes are seen in the epiphyseal ends of the metacarpals and phalanges. Generalized late motor development is usual in these syndromes. Several patients with the recessive form show marked mental retardation, headache, vomiting, and irritability.

What appears to be a different disease, yet having several facets in common with craniometaphyseal dysplasia, is craniodiaphyseal dysplasia. It is much more severe, producing marked facial distortion and severe mental retardation (Fig. 5.15). Nasal obstruction and facial alteration are noticeable within the first few years. Vision fails by the seventh or eighth year.

There is marked sclerosis of the calvaria and facial bones, and the paranasal sinuses are overgrown. The ribs are widened and extremely dense, the clavicles being most severely involved and thickened in the midportions. The vertebrae, for the most part, are not involved. The long bones are straight with a thin cortex and a remarkably uniform thickness of the shaft. In the metacarpals, similar changes are seen. There is some degree of ballooning of the midportion of the shaft. The cortex is thinner than normal except for the first metacar-

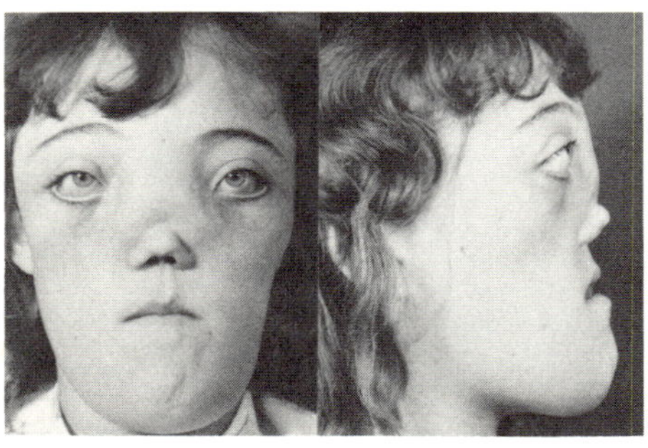

Fig. 5.14. Craniometaphyseal dysplasia, recessive form: note marked frontonasal hyperostosis and hypertelorism.

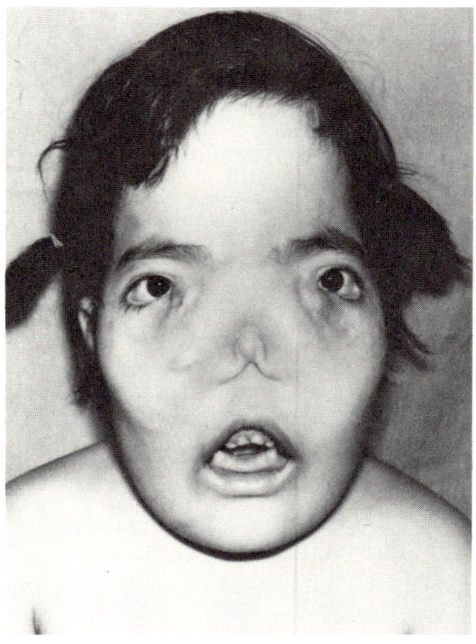

Fig. 5.15. Craniodiaphyseal dysplasia: severe distortion of face and skull. Note marked hypertelorism.

pal, which shows some osteosclerosis.

Differential Diagnosis. Van Buchem disease, metaphyseal dysplasia (Pyle disease), Schwarz-Lelek syndrome, and sclerosteosis should be included in the differential diagnosis.

Laboratory Aids. The blood count, serum calcium, phosphorus, and alkaline phosphatase are normal and may be used to exclude several entities.

References

Gorlin RJ, et al: Genetic craniotubular bone dysplasias and hyperosteosis, a critical analysis. *Birth Def* 5(4):79–95, 1969.

Halliday J: A rare case of bone dysplasia. *Brit J Surg* 37:52–63, 1949–50.

Hermel MB, et al: Familial metaphyseal dysplasia. *Am J Roentgenol* 70:413–421, 1953.

5.8 Infantile Cortical Hyperostosis

Infantile cortical hyperostosis was originally described by Röske in 1930 and later clinically and roentgenographically defined by Caffey and Silverman (1945), and Smyth and coworkers (1946). The syndrome consists of (1) bilateral swelling over the mandible or other bones, (2) new bone formation in these areas, (3) hyperirritability, and (4) mild fever. The condition is manifest before six months of age and may possibly be inherited in an autosomal dominant manner. It seems to be a disappearing disorder. The onset is generally observed between the second to the sixth month of life. Some cases have been reported in utero. Congenital anomaly of the arteries supplying the affected areas and resultant hypoxia have been suggested as etiologic factors.

Facies. Facial swelling usually occurs over the ramus, angle, and body of the mandible bilaterally, giving the face a striking appearance with

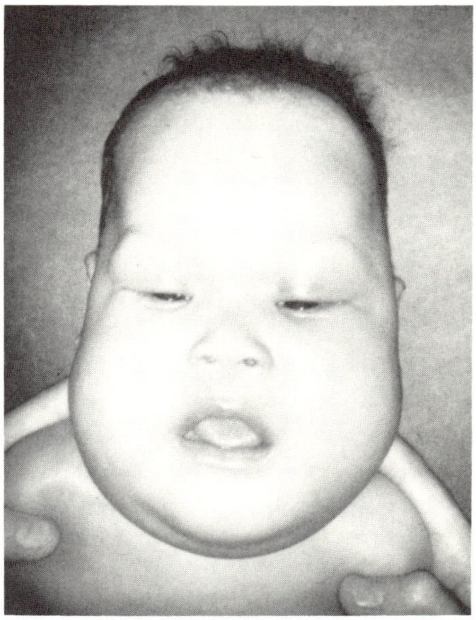

Fig. 5.16. Note marked bilateral swelling over ramus of mandible.

pallor over the involved sites (Fig. 5.16). There is usually roentgenographic evidence of new bone formation in the affected area.

Oral Structures. Seventy-five percent of affected patients will reveal mandibular involvement. Pseudoparalysis of the face may result from intense pain conveyed by the tender, edematous soft tissue involvement. Severe malocclusion has been noted as a consequence of the condition.

Systemic Features. Somatic and mental development are within normal limits. Several bones may be concurrently involved. Most common involvements apart from the mandible are the fifth and sixth ribs. Other bones affected may include ulna, femur, clavicle, tibia, humerus, and fibula. In the latter, only the shaft of the bone is affected. The covering soft tissues are tender and edematous, undergoing mixed stages of exacerbation and remission. In 70% of affected infants, irritability, pain, and fever may precede the bone involvement.

Differential Diagnosis. Differential diagnosis should include osteomyelitis, epidemic parotitis, and parotid tumors.

Laboratory Aids. The finding of anemia, leukocytosis, increased erythrocyte sedimentation rate, and increased serum alkaline phosphatase levels during periods of increased bone formation frequently aids in the diagnosis of the syndrome.

Synonyms. Caffey-Silverman syndrome, Smyth syndrome.

References

Ball MJ, Feingold M: Autosomal dominant inheritance of Caffey's disease. *Birth Def* 10(9):139–146, 1974.

Caffey J, Silverman WA: Infantile cortical hyperostosis: preliminary report of a new syndrome. *Am J Roentgen* 54:1–16, 1945.

Caylor GC, Peterson CA: Infantile cortical hyperostosis; report of 17 cases. *Am J Dis Child* 91:119–125, 1956.

Cochran W: Infantile cortical hyperostosis: a review with illustrative case report. *Acta Paediatr* 51:442–453, 1962.

Röske G: Eine eigenartige Knochenerkrankung im Säuglingsalter. *Monatschr Kinderheilkd* 47:385–400, 1930.

Smyth FS, et al: Periosteal reaction, fever and irritability in young infants: a new syndrome? *Am J Dis Child* 71:333–350, 1946.

5.9 Mandibulofacial Dysostosis

Treacher Collins described the essential components of the syndrome.

Franceschetti published extensive reviews of the syndrome and gave it the name of mandibulofacial dysostosis. It is inherited in an autosomal dominant manner with incomplete penetrance and variable expressivity. About 300 cases have been described to date.

Facies. The facial appearance reveals downward sloping palpebral fissures, hypoplastic malar bones, deformed or malplaced pinnae, and receding chin. A coloboma in the outer third of the lower lid is characteristic (Fig. 5.17). A deficiency of cilia medial to the coloboma is also noted in half of the reported cases. Deafness due to defects in ossicles and absence of the external auditory canal is present in one-third of cases (Fig. 5.18). Ear tags and blind fistulas have been reported from the tragus of the ear to the angle of the mouth. The nose often exhibits obliteration of the nasal-frontal angle with the bridge of the nose raised. Lack of malar development creates the impression of an enlarged nose. Hypoplasia of alar cartilages results in narrowing of the nares.

Oral Structures. The mandible is nearly always hypoplastic. Roentgenographic studies reveal a more obtuse mandibular angle than normal. Also the ramus may be deficient and the body of the mandible may be markedly concave on the under surface (Fig. 5.19). Flat or aplastic coronoid and condyloid processes may be evident. The palate is high or cleft in over 30% of the cases. The

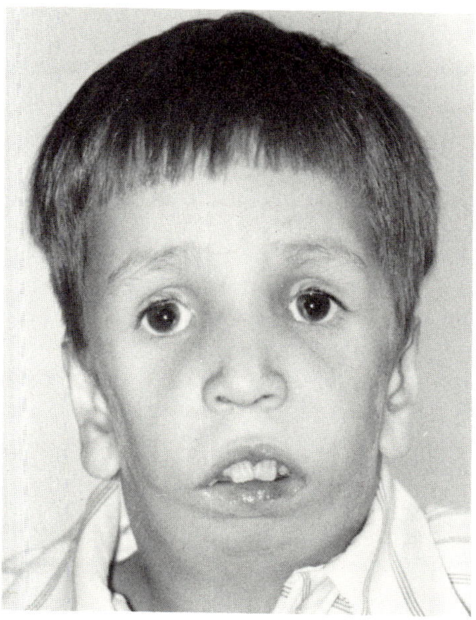

Fig. 5.17. Antimongoloid obliquity of palpebral fissures, poor development of the mandible and malar bones, and coloboma of the outer third of the lower lid.

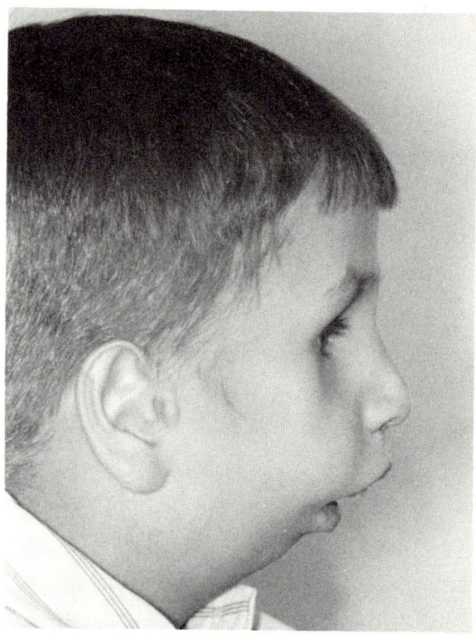

Fig. 5.18. Profile demonstrating unusual development of pinnae and marked retrognathia.

teeth may be maloccluded or associated with open bite.

Systemic Features. Somatic development is within normal limits. Mental development is rarely retarded. However in some cases the "retardation" may be secondary to severe hearing loss.

Differential Diagnosis. Differential diagnosis should include dominantly inherited maxillofacial dysostosis, oculoauriculovertebral syndrome, and Nager acrofacial dysostosis.

Laboratory Aids. None.

Synonyms. Treacher Collins syndrome, Franceschetti-Zwahlen-Klein syndrome.

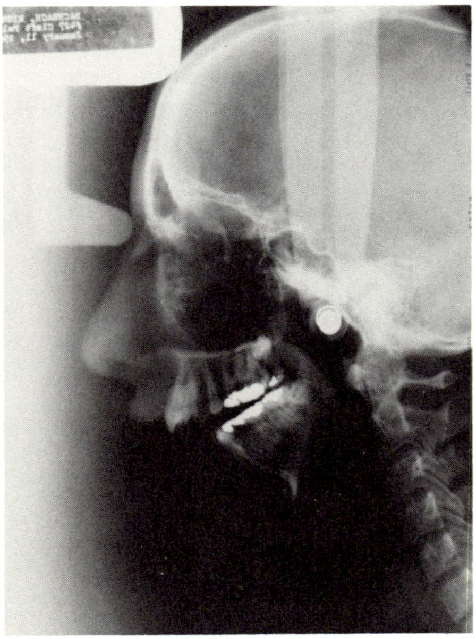

Fig. 5.19. Cephalometric radiography showing marked retrognathia.

References

Klein D, et al: Sur une forme extensive de dysostose mandibulo-faciale (Franceschetti) accompagnée de malformations des extrémités. *Rev Oto-Neuro-Ophthal* 42:422–440, 1970.

Rovin S, et al: Mandibulofacial Dysostosis: A familial study of five generations. *J Pediatr* 65:215–221, 1964.

Vatre J: Etude génétique et classification clinique de 154 cas de dysostose mandibulo-faciale (syndrome de Franceschetti) avec description de leurs associations malformatives. *J Génét Hum* 19:17–100, 1971.

5.10 Marfan Syndrome

The syndrome named for Marfan consists of (1) arachnodactyly, disproportionate skeletal growth and other skeletal anomalies; (2) extopia lentis; and (3) fusiform and dissecting aneurysms of the aorta and aortic insufficiency. The syndrome is inherited in an autosomal dominant manner. The condition appears with a frequency of about 3 per 200,000 population.

Facies. A dolichocephalic head with prominent supraorbital ridges and a long, thin face are characteristic. Bilateral ectopia lentis as a result of weakened or broken suspensory ligaments is present in about half of the patients; as a result, the lenses often dislocate upward. The lens may be small and spherical, or completely dislocated into the anterior or, occasionally, posterior chamber. Myopia is usually present. Blue sclerae and spontaneous retinal detachment have been reported.

Oral Structures. A high palatal vault is a constant finding. Malocclusion is common. Temporomandibular dysarthrosis has been reported as a presenting symptom.

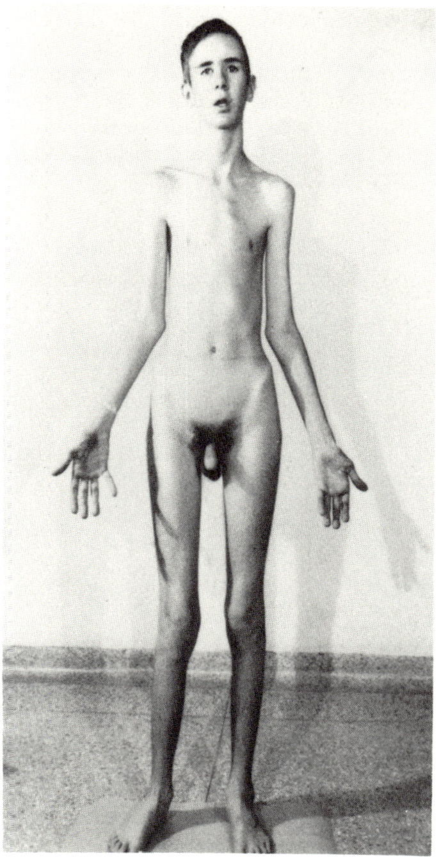

Fig. 5.20. Tall thin patient with pectus excavatum and arachnodactyly.

Systemic Features. The extremities are disproportionately long, and the pubis to sole segment is greater than the vertex to pubis segment (Figs. 5.20–21). Normally the upper to lower segment ratio is 0.93 in white adults, while the corresponding ratio in Marfan syndrome is about 0.85 for white adults. The hand-to-height and foot-to-height ratios are usually in excess of 11% and 15%, respectively. The metacarpal index ranges from 8.5 to 10.5 (normal values are 5.5 to 8.0). The length of the middle finger usually exceeds 1.5 times the length of its metacarpal.

Late-developing kyphoscoliosis, pectus excavatum and carinatum, weakness of joint capsules manifested by flat foot, and hyperextensibility of joints with habitual dislocations are usual findings. Hernias and deficiency of subcutaneous fat are common. Stria distensae of the pectoral and anterior deltoid areas are often noted. Many patients exhibit diffuse dilatation of the ascending aorta and/or dissecting

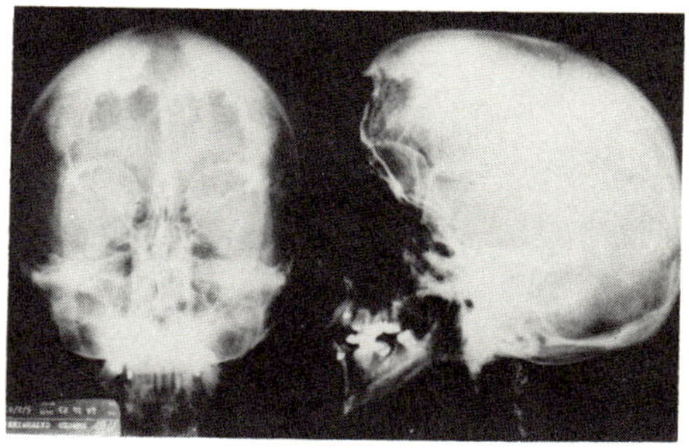

Fig. 5.21. Skull radiograph in a case of Marfan syndrome, showing enlarged maxillary sinuses and mandibular prognathism.

aneurysm, which may be preceded by aortic regurgitation. The pulmonary artery occasionally is similarly involved.

Differential Diagnosis. Disproportionate upper and lower segments may also be present in sickle cell anemia, the eunuchoid state, Klinefelter syndrome, and homocystinuria. Pectus excavatum, hyperextensible joints, and hernia may be seen in several other heritable disorders of connective tissue.

Laboratory Aids. Determination of upper to lower segment ratio and the metacarpal index are useful diagnostic aids.

Synonyms. Dolichostenomelia, arachnodactyly.

References

Bowers D: Marfan's syndrome: The S family re-visited. *Canad Med Assoc J* 89:337, 1963.

McKusick VA: *Heritable Disorders of Connective Tissue.* 4th Ed., 1972, St. Louis, CV Mosby Co.

Massumi RA, et al: Multiple aortic aneurysms (thoracic and abdominal) in twins with Marfan's syndrome: Fatal rupture during pregnancy. *J Thorac Cardiovasc Surg* 53:223–230, 1967.

Matalon R, Dorfman A: The accumulation of hyaluronic acid in cultured fibroblasts of the Marfan syndrome. *Biochem Biophys Res Commun* 32:150–154, 1968.

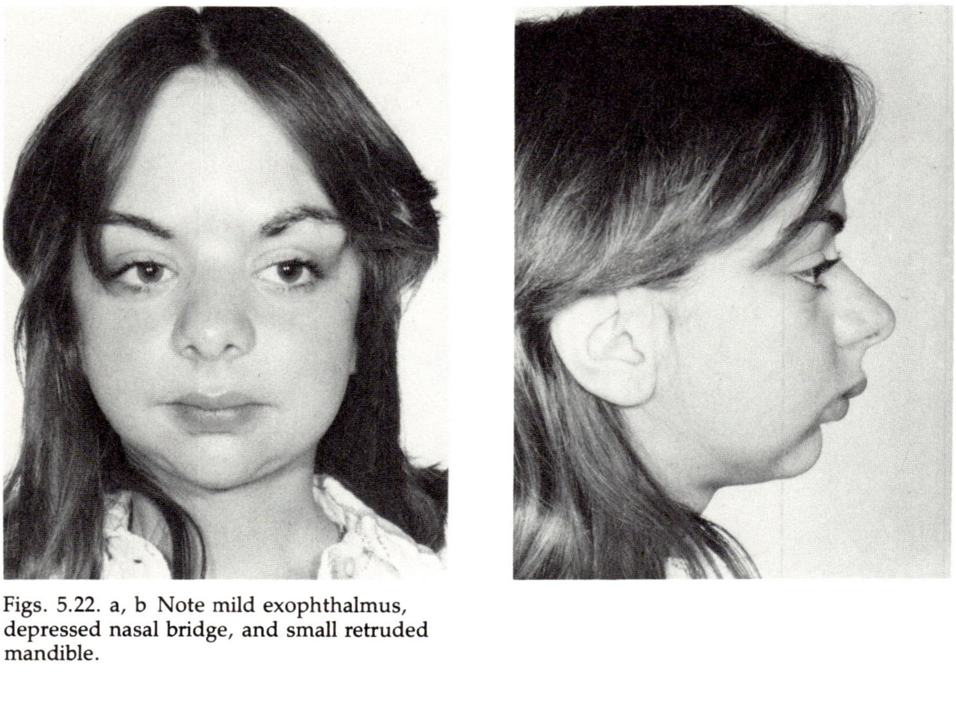

Figs. 5.22. a, b Note mild exophthalmus, depressed nasal bridge, and small retruded mandible.

5.11 Melnick-Needles Syndrome

Melnick and Needles in 1966 described a syndrome characterized by (1) generalized bone dysplasia and (2) abnormal facies. The condition has autosomal dominant inheritance. The diagnosis is essentially made on roentgenograms, but the typical facies should suggest the bony abnormalities.

Facies. The facies is so typical that unrelated patients look like siblings. Marked exophthalmus, full cheeks, large ears, micrognathia, and a transversally long mouth form the characteristic facial features (Fig. 5.22).

Oral Structures. Micrognathia, marked malocclusion, and the aforementioned mouth shape are constant features.

Systemic Features. Mental development is not impaired. There is slow development in height and weight. Adult patients are generally slightly shorter than the normal mean. The neck is long, the shoulders narrow, and the upper arms are short. Delayed closure of the anterior fontanel and sclerosis of the skull base and mastoid processes are seen radiographically. The paranasal sinuses are generally not well developed. The clavicles have cortical irregularity with flaring. The vertebral bodies are higher than normal; this is best seen in the axis, atlas, and occipital condyles. The thoracic vertebrae have an anterior concavity with double beaking.

The radius and tibia have an S-shaped appearance, due to marked bowing. Both metaphyseal areas of the humerus, fibula, and tibia are markedly flared. Coxa valga is evident. The iliac bones are also flared at the crest, but flat at the acetabular area. The ribs are thin and ribbon-like.

Differential Diagnosis. The Weissman-Netter syndrome should be considered.

Laboratory Aids. Serum chemistry is within normal limits with the exception of serum alkaline phosphatase, which is generally slightly elevated.

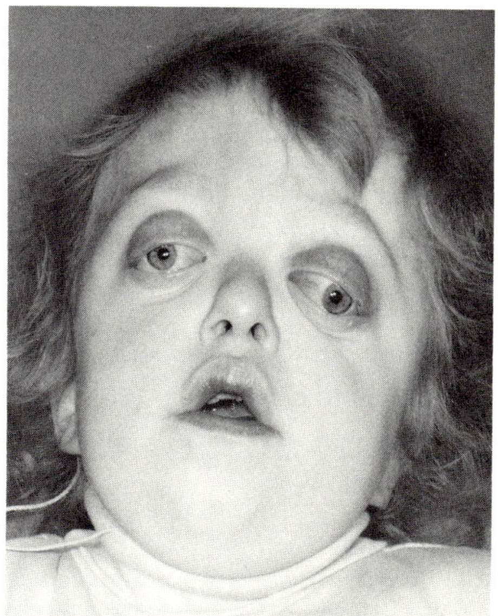

Fig. 5.23. Note hypertelorism, antimongoloid obliquity of palpebral fissures, and midfacial hypoplasia.

Synonym. Osteodysplasty.

References

Coste F, et al: Osteodysplasty (Melnick and Needles syndrome). *Ann Rheum Dis* 27:360–366, 1968.

Melnick JC, Needles CF: An undiagnosed bone dysplasia. A 2-family study of 4 generations and 3 generations. *Am J Roentgenol* 97:39–48, 1966.

5.12 Mucopolysaccharidosis VII

Sly and colleagues in 1973 reported and defined MPS VII. The condition is manifest clinically by (1) short stature, (2) progressive skeletal deformities, (3) hepatosplenomegaly, and (4) mental retardation after the first few years of life. MPS VII is inherited as an autosomal recessive condition. The absence of β-glucoronidase appears to be the etiology of the condition. The intracellular accumulation of acid mucopolysaccharides (AMPS) is responsible for the phenotype.

Facies. The depressed nasal bridge, hypertelorism, and anteverted nostrils resemble in part MPS I-H; however, in MPS VII the corneas are clear. The head is large and exhibits frontal prominence. Radiographically, premature closure of sagittal and lambdoidal sutures can be noted.

Oral Structures. Thickening and widening of the alveolar processes appear to be the only oral manifestation of the condition.

Systemic Features. After age 2 the diminished stature becomes apparent and there is progressive mental retardation. In addition, thoracolumbar gibbus and pigeon-breast deformity may be noted from birth. Roentgenologic examination reveals hook-like deformities of lower thoracic and upper lumbar vertebrae, shortening of tubular bones, and prominent proximal tapering of metacarpals II-V. Inguinal and umbilical hernias, hepatosplenomegaly, and lax skin are prominent findings.

Differential Diagnosis. MPS I and MPS VI should be specifically included in the differential diagnosis.

Laboratory Aids. Bone and peripheral granulocytes reveal coarse metachromatic intracellular inclusions. The absence of β-glucuronidase activity in fibroblasts and white cells in pathognomic for MPS VII. Diminished β-glucuronidase activity is present in heterozygotes.

Synonym. β-glucuronidase deficiency.

References

Sly WS, et al: β-glucuronidase deficiency: A report of clinical, radiologic and biochemical features of a new mucopolysaccharidosis. *J Pediatr* 82:249–257, 1973.

5.13 Pfeiffer Syndrome

Pfeiffer in 1964, using the name of dominant hereditary acrocephalosyndactyly, described a syndrome characterized by (1) craniosynostosis with turribrachycephaly and (2) broad thumbs and halluces. The condition is inherited in an autosomal dominant manner with variable expressivity.

Facies. The condition is characterized by mid-face hypoplasia with consequently shallow orbits, depressed nasal bridge, mildly prominent supraorbital ridges, and relative mandibular prognathism. Hypertelorism and occasionally strabismus, proptosis, and antimongoloid obliquity can be seen (Fig. 5.23). The turribrachycephalic skull, due to early closure of sutures (especially the coronal suture), contributes to the facial appearance.

Oral Structures. There is marked maxillary hypoplasia with resultant narrow and high-arched palate. The mandible is within normal limits. Therefore, the relationship between these two bones is altered: there is maxillary hypoplasia with resultant relative mandibular prognathism and class III malocclusion (Fig. 5.24). Bifid uvula and malposition of teeth have also been described in patients with the syndrome.

Systemic Features. Mild mental retardation has been reported occasionally, but the majority of affected individuals are of normal intelligence. Thumbs and halluces are broad and generally have varus deformity. Partial soft tissue syndactyly is a variable component of the syndrome; when present, it is generally mild and involves either digits 2 and 3, or 3 and 4, of both hands and

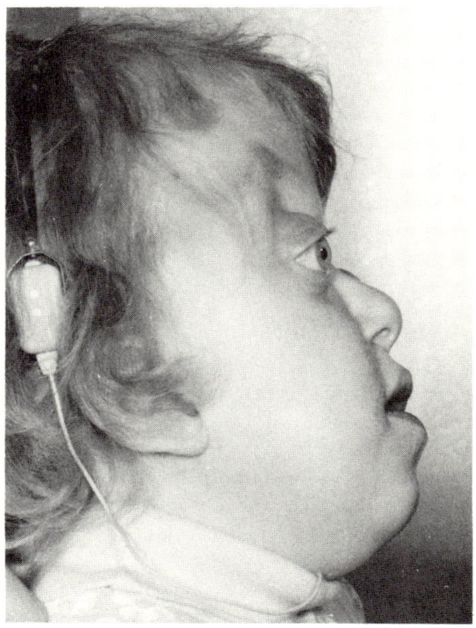

Fig. 5.24. Profile view showing exophthalmus, depressed nasal bridge, and pseudoprognathism due to maxillary hypoplasia.

feet. A variety of skeletal abnormalities of hands and feet have been observed, such as brachymesophalangy, absent phalanges, pollex varus, abnormal phalangeal shape, broad metatarsals with accessory epiphyses, and multiple phalangeal ossification centers. Synostosis of the following bones can also be seen: carpals, tarsals, metacarpals, metatarsals, cervical vertebrae, radiohumeral, and radioulnar.

Differential Diagnosis. Apert-type acrocephalosyndactyly is clinically almost indistinguishable from Pfeiffer syndrome. Some investigators believe that the latter is a mild form of the Apert syndrome. Comparison of family pedigrees of both conditions has shown that there are no transition forms from one syndrome to the other. The differential diagnosis is based on the mode of inheritance and the milder clinical manifestations in the Pfeiffer syndrome, especially hand and foot anomalies. The majority of cases of Apert syndrome are sporadic. Other types of craniosynostosis as well as the Saethre-Chotzen syndrome should be considered in the differential diagnosis.

Laboratory Aids. None known.

References

Asnes RS, Morehead CD: Pfeiffer syndrome. *Birth Def* 5(3):198–203, 1969.

Martsolf JT, et al: Pfeiffer syndrome. *Am J Dis Child* 121:257–262, 1971.

Pfeiffer RA: Dominant erbliche Akrocephalosyndaktylie. *Z Kinderheilkd* 90:301–320, 1964.

Saldino RM, et al: Familial acrocephalosyndactyly (Pfeiffer syndrome). *Am J Roentgenol* 116:609–622, 1972.

5.14 Smith-Lemli-Opitz Syndrome

Smith, Lemli, and Opitz in 1964 described a syndrome having multiple skeletal and urogenital anomalies and a characteristic facies. The syndrome comprises (1) fetal hypoactivity and (2) intrauterine growth retardation. Thus, at birth, affected infants are moderately small and hypotonic. Failure to thrive, observed during the first years of life, progressively changes to spasticity in later years. The syndrome is inherited in an autosomal recessive manner.

Facies. The patient often reveals microcephaly, bilateral blepharoptosis, short nose with broad bridge, anteverted nostrils and micrognathia (Fig. 5.25).

Oral Structures. Intraorally, a broad maxillary anterior alveolar ridge has been reported to be associated with the syndrome.

Systemic Features. Patients are of short stature with narrow shoulders and short neck. Mild to severe mental retardation is a constant finding. Irritable behavior with typical shrill screaming, as if in constant pain, is also observed. Frequent vomiting with inhalation may result in secondary pneumonia. Urogenital anomalies are present only in affected males, comprising hypospadias, cryptorchidism, and cleft scrotum (Fig. 5.26). Marked soft tissue syndactyly of second and third toes is a constant finding. Affected individuals present abnormal dermatoglyphics characterized by palmar simian creases, a high number of digital whorls, and arch tibial pattern.

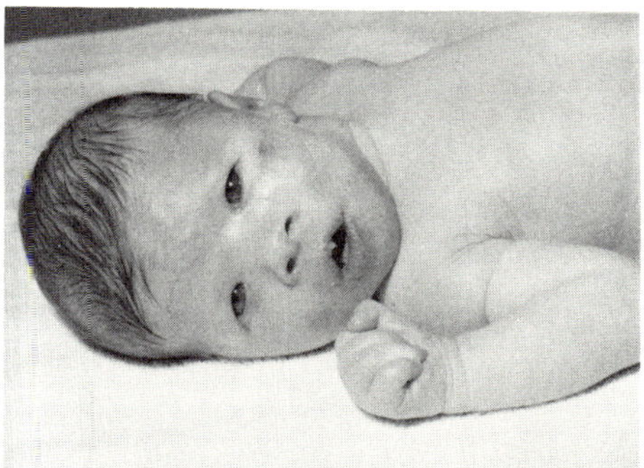

Fig. 5.25. Newborn child presenting ptosis of eyelids, broad nasal tip, and micrognathia.

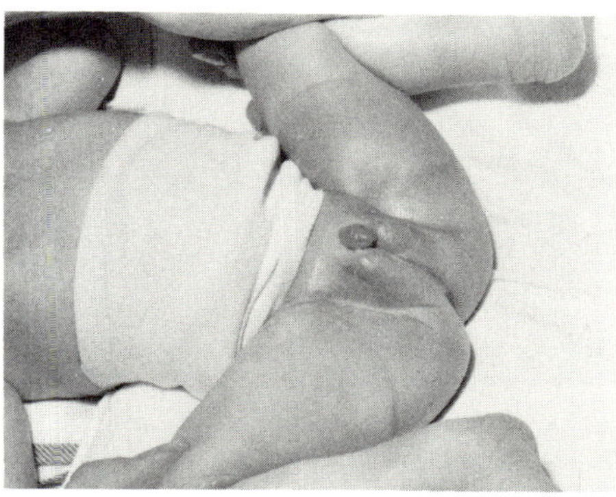

Fig. 5.26. Same child as Fig. 5.25, with hypospadias and hypoplastic scrotum.

Other less frequent findings have included stippled epiphyses, cleft palate, polydactyly, sacral dimples, lowset ears, strabismus, epicanthal folds, cataracts, pyloric stenosis, and abnormal EEG and EKG.

Differential Diagnosis. Meckel syndrome and trisomy 13 may be confused with the S-L-O syndrome and should be differentiated.

Laboratory Aids. None.

References

Cherstroy ED, et al: The pathological anatomy of the Smith-Lemli-Opitz syndrome. *Clin Genet* 7:382–387, 1975.

Dallaire L: Syndrome of retardation with urogenital and skeletal anomalies (Smith-Lemli-Opitz syndrome): Clinical features and mode of inheritance. *J Med Genet* 6:113–120, 1969.

Dallaire L, Fraser FC: The syndrome of retardation with urogenital and skeletal anomalies in siblings. *J Pediatr* 69:459–460, 1966.

Smith DW, et al: A newly recognized syndrome of multiple congenital anomalies. *J Pediatr* 64:210–217, 1964.

5.15 Waardenburg Syndrome

The syndrome described by Waardenburg in 1948 consists essentially of (1) congenital sensorineural deafness, (2) lateral displacement of the medial canthi and lacrimal punctae with broad nasal root, (3) white forelock or poliosis, (4) heterochromia irides, and (5) hyperplasia of the medial portion of the eyebrows. The condition is inherited in an autosomal dominant manner. Estimates of incidence have suggested that Waardenburg syndrome is seen in about 2% of all congenitally deaf persons.

Facies. The facies is quite characteristic; a broad nasal root and hypoplastic alar cartilages result in narrow nostrils and a slightly protruding mandible. The tip of the nose tends to be rounded and slightly upturned, revealing the columella. Although the interpupillary and outer canthal distances are normal, there is an increased distance between the inner canthi (dystopia canthorum), resulting in blepharophimosis. This appears to be the most constant facial finding. A white forelock is present in fewer than one of five affected persons, but when present, its effect is dramatic (Fig. 5.27). Detection of this trait in females may be difficult, because of their tendency to mask it by coloring the hair. Premature graying of the eyebrows and lashes may also occur. The eyebrows in about half of the patients are confluent at the midline, only the medial ends being hyperplastic. This characteristic may be less evident in women, who tend to pluck these hairs.

Vitiligo is infrequent, but may occur in this syndrome. Heterochromia irides, or more accurately hypoplasia of the irides, is seen in about 25% of persons with the syndrome. It may be partial or total, both irides being completely blue. Especially striking is the presence of one blue and one brown eye, or two pale blue eyes in an Afro-American. Commonly there is a peculiar pig-

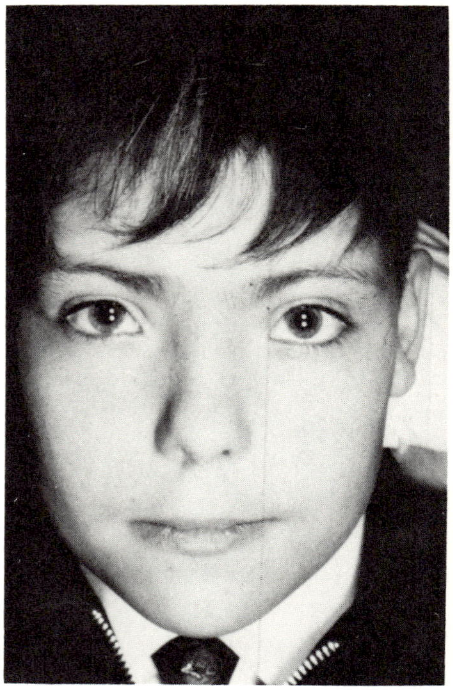

Fig. 5.27. Note small white forelock, synophrys, pale lavender irises, dystopia canthorum, lateral displacement of lacrimal points, and hypoplasia of nasal alae. Patient had high-tone deafness.

mentary mottling at the periphery of the fundi. Little or no sclera may be visible on the medial side, giving the impression of convergent squint. The inferior lacrimal points are displaced laterally even as far as the cornea.

Oral Structures. Prognathism, with protruding lower lip and high-arched palate, has been reported in a number of cases. Additional oral findings have included cleft lip-palate and lateral displacement of the mandibular angle.

Systemic Features. Congenital sensorineural deafness is present in about 20% of affected individuals. The degree is variable, ranging from mild to moderate bilaterally. Some patients have profound unilateral impairment. The deafness has been shown to be due to absence of the organ of Corti.

Differential Diagnosis. When the syndrome presents all or most of the facial characteristics, it is almost impossible to confuse it with other conditions. Nevertheless, some disorders associated with heterochromia irides, such as the Romberg syndrome, should be included. Vitiligo also should be included in the differential diagnosis.

Laboratory Aids. None known.

Synonym. Congenital deafness, white forelock, dystopia canthorum, and heterochromia irides.

References

Arias S: Genetic heterogeneity in the Waardenburg syndrome. *Birth Def* 7(4):87–101, 1971.

Pantke OA, Cohen MM Jr: The Waardenburg syndrome. *Birth Def* 7(7):147–152, 1971.

Waardenburg PJ: Dystopia punctorum lacrimalium, blepharophimosis, en partiele irisatrophia bij een doofstomme. *Nederl tijdschr geneesk* 92:3463–3466, 1948.

CHAPTER 6

Systemic Inherited Disorders Associated with Facial Clefting

6.1 Cleft Lip-Palate and Congenital Lip Pits

The syndrome of (1) cleft lip-palate and (2) congenital lip pits has been recognized for over 100 years. The condition is transmitted as an autosomal dominant condition with 80% penetrance of any component of the syndrome. The syndrome is seen with a frequency of about 1 in 75,000–100,000 live births and affects both sexes equally.

Facies. Cleft lip or the repaired cleft scar, together with the paramedian pits of the lower lip, are characteristic. Occasionally, adhesions between the eyelids (ankyloblepharon filiforme adnatum) are present.

Oral Structures. Bilateral, symmetrical pits are located on the vermilion portion of the lower lip (Fig. 6.1). These fistulas may be 3 mm or more in diameter, or so small as barely to allow the introduction of a thin probe. The dimple may be circular or may present as a transverse slit. Rarely, they may be located at the apex of a nipple-like elevation. These depressions often exude saliva, spontaneously or upon pressure, because of their association with minor salivary glands. On microscopic sections, the pits have proven to be blind sinuses, descending through the orbicularis oris muscles.

The pits may be an isolated finding (ca. 33%) or associated with cleft lip-palate (ca. 76%). When associated with cleft lip-palate, the clefts are bilateral in over 80% of patients. A few cases have been reported in which there has been but a single pit. Adhesions between maxilla and mandible have also been noted. In those cases of the syndrome in which cleft lip is absent, the maxillary lateral incisors are missing or are hypoplastic (peg lateral). Miscellaneous oral findings have included ankyloglossia and cleft uvula.

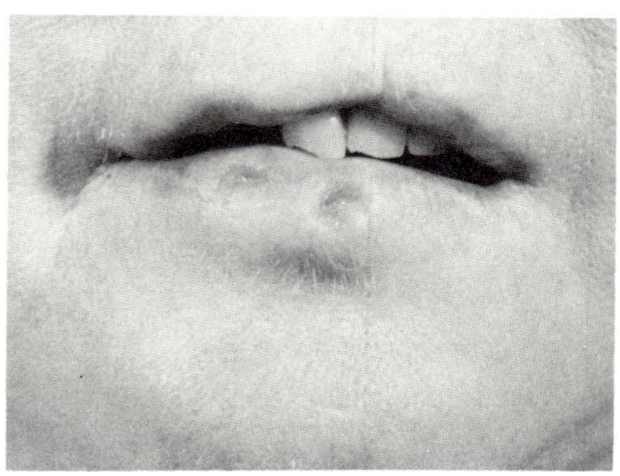

Fig. 6.1. Note pits of the lower lip and corrected cleft lip.

Systemic Features. Mental and physical development are within normal limits. Rarely, there is an associated syndactyly of hands.

Differential Diagnosis. All the clefting syndromes should be included as well as the OFD I and popliteal pterygium syndromes.

Laboratory Aids. None known.

Synonym. Van der Woude syndrome.

References

Cervenka J, et al: The syndrome of pits of the lower lip and cleft lip and/or palate: Genetic considerations. *Am J Hum Genet* 19:416–432, 1967.

Schneider EL: Lip pits and congenital absence of second premolars. Varied expression of the lip pits syndrome. *J Med Genet* 10:346–349, 1973.

Taylor WB, Lane DK: Congenital fistulas of the lower lip: Associations with cleft lip-palate and anomalies of the extremities. *Arch Dermatol* 94:421–424, 1966.

6.2 Cleft Lip-Palate and Tetraphocomelia

The syndrome consists of (1) cleft lip-palate, (2) tetraphocomelia with a reduction in digit number, (3) exophthalmus and ocular hypertelorism, and (4) deficient growth. Parental consanguinity and occurrence in sibs have been reported in this syndrome, which is clearly inherited in an autosomal recessive manner. The condition is usually lethal, and most affected infants die within the first few months of life of unknown causes.

Facies. The facies is characterized by ocular hypertelorism, exophthalmus and usually bilateral cleft lip-palate (Fig. 6.2). The pinnae are generally underdeveloped. Other eye anomalies, such as colobomas and cataracts, can also be present.

Oral Structures. Oral manifestations are essentially confined to bilateral cleft lip with or without cleft palate, or isolated cleft palate.

Systemic Features. Mental retardation is most likely to be present. Physical development is obviously retarded. Usually there is reduction in size, of variable degree, in the bones of all four extremities. Reduc-

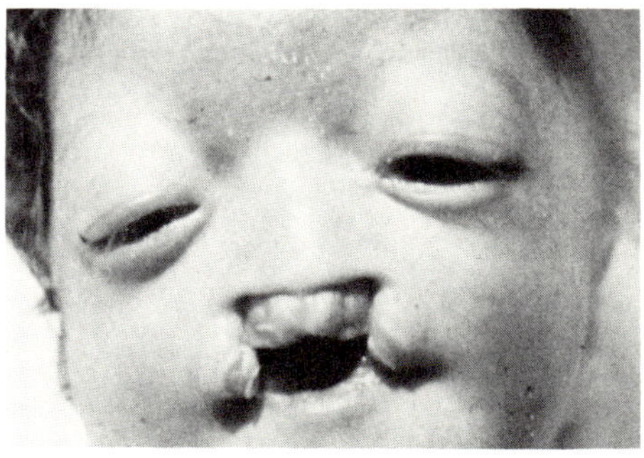

Fig. 6.2. Note bilateral cleft lip, hypertelorism and exophthalmus; the infant also had cleft palate.

tion in the number of digits, with soft tissue syndactyly of the hands, is almost always present. Feet are less frequently affected in such a manner. Genital anomalies include enlarged and cleft labia minora, inguinal hernia, and cryptorchidism (Fig. 6.3). The clitoris or penis appears enlarged due to the marked reduction in size of the lower extremities.

Differential Diagnosis. The differential diagnosis should include tetraphocomelia due to thalidomide, pseudothalidomide syndrome, and the clefting syndromes. It has recently been suggested that this syndrome is identical to the pseudothalidomide syndrome (Gorlin and collaborators, 1976).

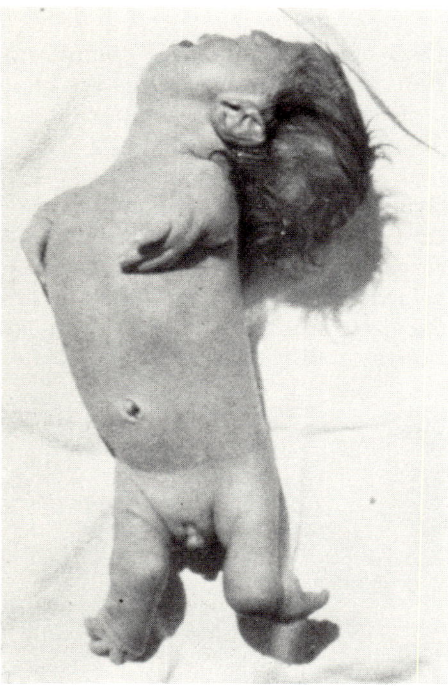

Fig. 6.3. Same patient as in Fig. 6.2. Note shortened extremities, tetraphocomelia, and missing digits. The infant had marked clitoral enlargement.

Laboratory Aids. None known.

Synonyms. Roberts syndrome; Appelt-Gerken-Lenz syndrome; tetraphocomelia, cleft lip-palate, and penile or clitoral enlargement.

References

Freeman MVR, et al: The Roberts syndrome. *Clin Genet* 5:1–16, 1974.

Gorlin RJ, et al: *Syndromes of the Head and Neck.* 2d Ed. New York, McGraw-Hill, 1976.

Grosse FR, et al: The tetraphocomelia-cleft palate syndrome. *Humangenetik* 28:353–356, 1975.

Roberts JB: A child with double cleft of lip and palate, protrusion of the intermaxillary portion of the upper jaw and imperfect development of the bones of the four extremities. *Ann Surg* 70:252, 1919.

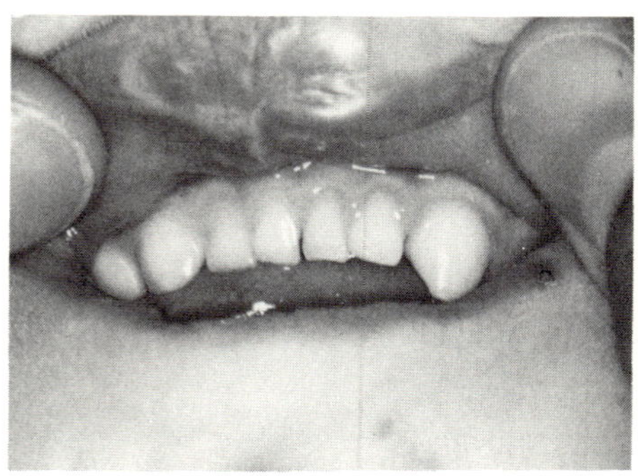

Fig. 6.4. Bilateral congenital lower lip pits present in a patient with the syndrome.

Temtamy SA, Loutfy AH: Some genetic and surgical aspects of cleft lip/cleft palate problem in Egypt. *Cleft Palate J* 7:578–594, 1970.

6.3 Cleft Lip-Palate, Popliteal Pterygium, Digital and Genital Anomalies Syndrome

This syndrome was probably first reported by Trélat in 1869. Several examples are found in the German literature. Gorlin, Sedano, and Cervenka in 1968 proposed the name popliteal pterygium syndrome. A thorough review of published cases reveals the following basic components: (1) popliteal and intercrural pterygia, (2) cleft lip-palate, (3) lower-lip pits, (4) digital anomalies, and (5) genital anomalies. The syndrome is inherited in an autosomal dominant manner, with incomplete penetrance and variable expressivity.

Facies. The most striking facial finding is clefting of the upper lip. Also of note, but less obvious, are pits or fistulas of the lower lip (Fig. 6.4). Ankyloblepharon, when present, adds to the facial appearance, especially in newborns with the syndrome. Some cases present a short upper lip and flattened facies, due to absence of the premaxillary bones.

Oral Structures. Relative prognathism may be present due to absence of the premaxilla. The most frequent oral finding is cleft lip-palate, usually unilateral. Some cases have shown only cleft palate or even clefting confined to the soft palate. Fibrous bands extending from the maxillary alveolar processes to the floor of the mouth have been observed in several cases. Syngnathia and pits and fistulas of the lower lip are also commonly seen. Teeth are within normal limits. Agenesis of central and lateral incisors is seen in those cases presenting absence of the premaxilla.

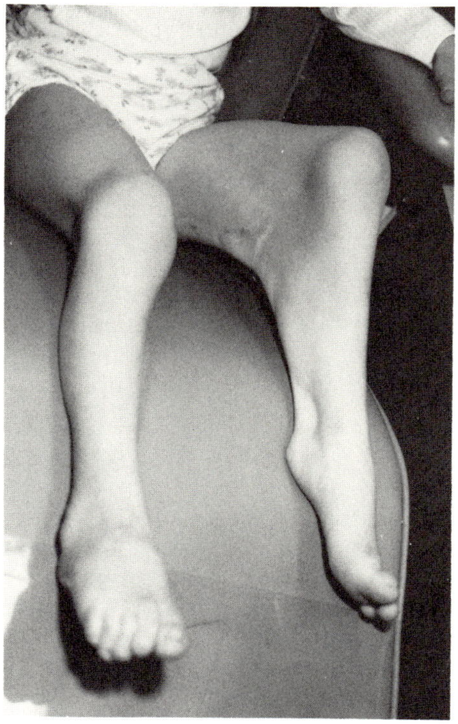

Fig. 6.5. Same patient as in Fig. 6.4. Note popliteal pterygium extending from the heel to the ischial tuberosity, present in both legs. Beneath the free margin lies the sciatic nerve.

Systemic Features. Mental status is within normal limits. The most striking feature is a pterygium or skin web, nearly always bilateral, which extends from the heel to the ischial tuberosity (Fig. 6.5). This limits extension and abduction, as well as rotation of the leg, and interferes with walking. Along its free edge is a hard, inelastic fibrous band. Beneath this is the sciatic nerve. Awareness of this is important to the surgeon correcting the defect.

Often associated are hypoplasia or agenesis of digits, talipes equinovarus and valgus, syndactyly of hands and feet, spina bifida occulta, and scoliosis or lordosis. A pyramidal skin fold is often present on the hallux, extending over the nail. Filiform adhesions (ankyloblepharon filiforme adnatum) may join the eyelids. Cryptorchidism, absent or cleft scrotum, inguinal hernia, absence of labia majora, infantile uterus, and intercrural pterygium are frequently part of the clinical picture. These genital abnormalities limit the capability of these patients to procreate, which explains the relatively small number of cases observed.

Differential Diagnosis. The popliteal pterygium is so evident and distinctive as to make this syndrome easily recognizable. Nevertheless, multiple pterygium syndrome and arthromyodysplasia congenita should be considered in the differential diagnosis.

Laboratory Aids. None known.

Synonyms. Congenital webbing of lower limbs, congenital popliteal webbing, popliteal pterygium syndrome.

References

Bixler D, et al: Phenotypic variation in the popliteal pterygium syndrome. *Clin Genet* 4:220–228, 1973.

Gorlin RJ, et al: Popliteal pterygium syndrome: A syndrome comprising cleft lip-palate, popliteal and intercrural pterygia, digital and genital anomalies. *Pediatrics* 41:503–509, 1968.

Rintala A, Lahti A: The facio-genito-popliteal syndrome. *Scand J Plast Reconstr Surg* 4:67–71, 1970.

6.4 Cleft Palate, Flattened Facies, and Multiple Congenital Dislocations

The components of the syndrome, first recognized as an entity by Larsen in 1950, include (1) peculiar facies, (2) multiple congenital dislocations, (3) foot deformities, and (4) cleft palate. The syndrome is apparently inherited both as an autosomal recessive and autosomal dominant condition. Occurrence in siblings and a predilection for females have been observed.

Facies. The face is markedly flattened with depressed nasal bridge and frontal bossing (Fig. 6.6). Interocular distance is normal; the eyes appear widely spaced due to the depressed nasal bridge.

Oral Structures. Cleft palate is the only oral component of the syndrome. In some cases, cleft of the soft palate or cleft uvula have been noted.

Systemic Features. Mental and physical development are within normal limits. Impairment of variable degree is due to speech difficulties, as a consequence of cleft palate, and abnormal gait due to multiple dislocations. The skeletal anomalies are bilateral and include anterior dislocation of the tibia on the femur, antenatal elbow and hip dislocations, and talipes equinovarus or equinovalgus (Fig. 6.7). The fingers are long and cylindrical, with extra finger creases. The thumb is spatulate, without normal taper, and the metacarpals are slightly shorter than normal. Abnormal segmentation of vertebrae or multiple vertebrae and a juxtacalcaneal accessory bone or bifid calcaneous have also been seen. Interventricular septal defect has been described in a few cases.

Differential Diagnosis. The otopalatodigital syndrome and the clefting syndromes should be included in the differential diagnosis.

Laboratory Aids. None known.

Synonym. Larsen syndrome.

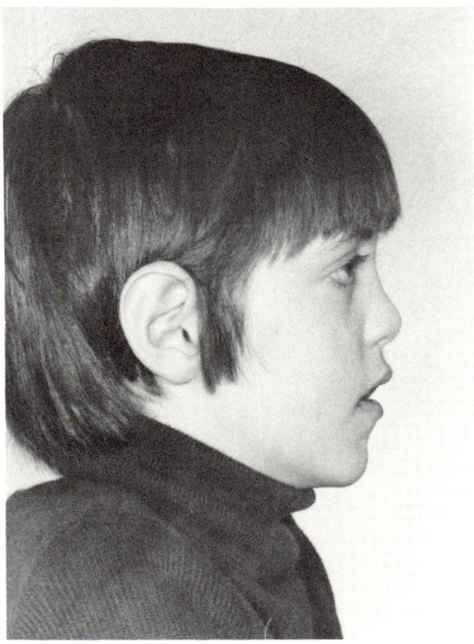

Fig. 6.6 Note depressed nasal bridge. The patient also had cleft palate.

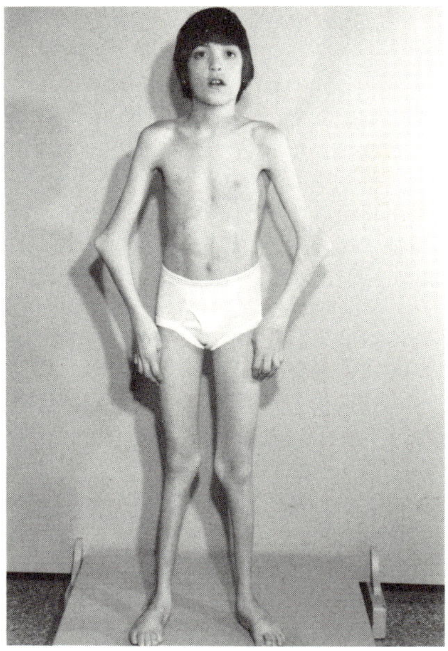

Fig. 6.7. Dislocations at elbows and knees, talipes equinovarus, and flattened face.

References

Harris R, Cullen CH: Autosomal dominant inheritance in Larsen's syndrome. *Clin Genet* 2:87–90, 1971.

Larsen LJ, et al: Multiple congenital dislocations associated with characteristic facial abnormality. *J Pediatr* 37:574–581, 1950.

Robertson FW, et al: Larsen's syndrome. *Clin Pediatr* 14:53–60, 1975.

6.5 Diastrophic Dwarfism

In 1960, Lamy and Maroteaux defined a new syndrome which they named "diastrophic dwarfism" to emphasize the progressive kyphoscoliosis which is usually evident at birth. The syndrome consists of (1) micromelic dwarfism, (2) talipes equinovarus, with limited dorsiflexion, (3) anomalies of the pinna, (4) restricted joint motion, (5) progressive kyphoscoliosis, (6) adduction of thumbs and halluces, (7) severe epimetaphyseal ossification defects, and (8) cleft palate. Diastrophic dwarfism is clearly inherited as an autosomal recessive condition.

Facies. The facies is not especially remarkable, although the cystic ears, if viewed in the florid hemorrhagic stage, are quite striking (Figs. 6.8–9). This process soon resolves and plates of calcium can then be felt in the helices. Some patients have a mildly depressed nasal bridge.

Oral Structures. At least 50% of affected individuals have cleft palate. Additional findings are mandibular hypoplasia and protruding lower lip.

Systemic Features. Mental development is within normal limits, but dwarfism is the outstanding feature of the syndrome. The limbs are severely shortened. The trunk is also foreshortened but less so, proportionately, as a result of the severe kyphoscoliosis. The latter is absent at birth but may appear during infancy, and then progresses. The feet are usually supinated and adducted. Attempts at correction have failed. The hallux and thumb are often widely

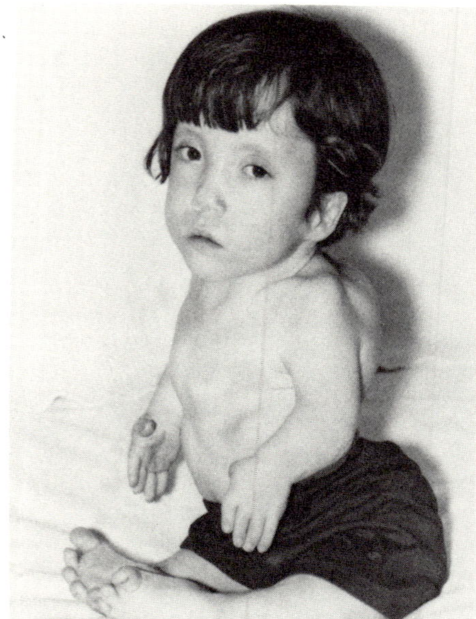

Fig. 6.8. Note characteristic abbreviation of limbs, kyphoscoliosis, and talipes equinovarus. Child also has cleft palate.

opposed and hypermobile ("hitch-hiker's thumb"). The fingers are short with extension contractures of the interphalangeal joints. The hands may be ulnarly deviated at the wrists. Most peripheral joints are markedly restricted in motion, and posterior dislocation of the ulna and subluxation of the knees are common. Progressive degeneration of the hips is a frequent finding, and ambulation becomes difficult.

Roentgenographically, there are several alterations in the metaphyses of long tubular bones. The epiphyses appear late and are severely flattened or deformed. The phalanges, metacarpals, and metatarsals are plump, their metaphyses are broad, and their epiphyses are deformed. The first metacarpals are broad with widened distal ends. The second, third, and fourth cervical vertebrae often are keel-shaped and produce a severe cervical kyphosis and subluxation, the cervical spine appearing to slide under the bone of the skull. The thoracic and lumbar vertebrae are of normal height. The interpediculate distance in the lumbar area is essentially normal, a finding which clearly distinguishes this condition from achondroplasia.

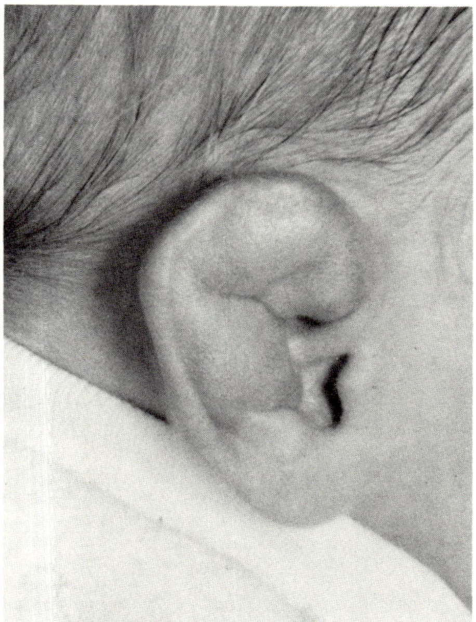

Fig. 6.9. Cystic ear during hemorrhagic phase from another patient with diastrophic dwarfism.

Differential Diagnosis. Most commonly the disorder is erroneously considered to be atypical achondroplasia, a grievous mistake if genetic counseling is to be given. Arthrogryposis congenita should also be considered in the differential diagnosis.

Laboratory Aids. None known.

References

Lamy M, Maroteaux P: Le nanisme diastrophique. *Presse Méd* 68:1977–1980, 1960.

Walker BA, et al: Diastrophic dwarfism. *Medicine* 51:41–59, 1972.

Wilson DW, et al: Diastrophic dwarfism. *Arch Dis Child* 44:48–59, 1969.

6.6 Ectrodactyly-Ectodermal Dysplasia-Clefting (EEC) Syndrome

The syndrome, originally described in 1804 by Eckoldt and Martens, consists of (1) ectrodactyly (lobster-claw deformity) of the hands and feet, (2) obliteration of nasolacrimal ducts, and (3) cleft-lip palate. The condition is most likely inherited in an autosomal dominant manner with incomplete penetrance and variable expressivity. In several families the EEC syndrome appears to be inherited as an autosomal recessive condition; therefore, genetic heterogeneity is suggested.

Facies. The most typical facial finding is the presence of cleft lip, generally bilateral (Fig. 6.10). Obliteration of the nasolacrimal duct results in tearing, keratoconjunctivitis, dacrocystitis, blepharitis, and photophobia. The facial features are accentuated by diminished scalp hair, eyebrows, and lashes. Albino-like appearance of the facial skin has been seen in some cases.

Oral Structures. Bilateral cleft lip-palate is present in around 50% of affected individuals. Other orodental findings include oligodontia, hypoplasia of enamel, xerostomia, and markedly fissured tongue.

Systemic Features. Mental retardation associated with microcephaly is occasionally seen. Physical development is within normal limits. The main component of the syndrome is ectrodactyly, generally present in both hands and feet. A few patients have only soft tissue syndactyly. Other less frequently associated anomalies have included conduction deafness, hypoplastic nails, pigmented nevi, and urethral and kidney malformations.

Differential Diagnosis. Isolated ectrodactyly, various clefting syndromes, and some of the ectodermal dysplasias should be excluded.

Laboratory Aids. None known. Skin biopsy has shown diminished numbers of sebaceous glands.

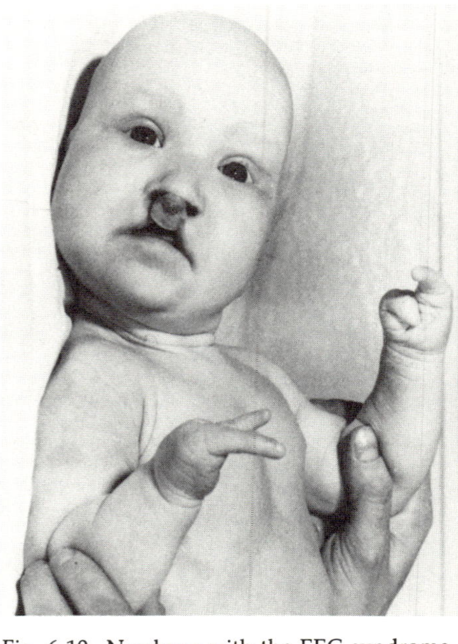

Fig. 6.10. Newborn with the EEC syndrome demonstrating bilateral cleft lip and ectrodactyly of hands. The palate was also cleft.

Synonyms. Cleft lip-palate, lobster-claw deformity, and nasolacrimal duct obstruction.

References

Pries C, et al: The EEC syndrome. *Am J Dis Child* 127:840–844, 1974.

Preus M, Fraser FC: The lobster-claw defect with ectodermal defects, cleft lip-palate, tear duct anomaly and renal anomalies. *Clin Genet* 4:369–375, 1973.

Reed WB, et al: The REEDS syndrome. *Birth Def* 10(8):61–73, 1974.

Rosenmann AT, et al: Ectrodactyly, ectodermal dysplasia and cleft palate (EEC syndrome). Report of a family and review of the literature. *Clin Genet* 9:347–353, 1976.

6.7 Hereditary Progressive Arthroophthalmopathy

Stickler and colleagues in 1965 first described five generations of a family with a syndrome composed of (1) progressive myopia and (2) arthropathy. The condition is inherited in an autosomal dominant manner with complete penetrance and variable expressivity.

Facies. Affected individuals present a characteristic facies with depressed nasal bridge, maxillary hypoplasia, and long philtrum (Fig. 6.11). Progressive myopia (to minus 18 diopters) is associated frequently with lattice degeneration and retinal detachment, especially in childhood, accompanied by glaucoma and amblyopia.

Oral Structures. Cleft palate or submucous cleft palate and bifid uvula are common findings.

Systemic Features. Mental and physical development are within normal limits. Joint involvement is characterized by irregularly shaped articular surfaces and enlargement of the joints, with marked stiffness, progressive impairment of locomo-

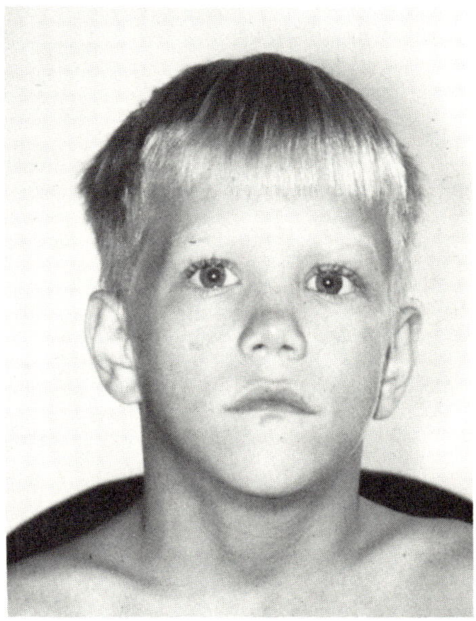

Fig. 6.11. Mild maxillary hypoplasia, long philtrum, and depressed nasal bridge. The patient also had cleft uvula.

tion, and pain. In some patients, joint hypermobility is observed. The spine shows narrow intervertebral spaces and flattened vertebral bodies, which may lead to kyphosis and sometimes to scoliosis. Thoracic kyphosis and mild flexion in the hips, knees, and ankles is the typical body posture of affected individuals. Causally related to the skeletal defects is the abnormal development of the epiphyseal plates in the vertebrae and long bones. Rarely, progressive sensorineural hearing loss has been seen in association with the syndrome.

Differential Diagnosis. None.

Laboratory Aids. None known.

Synonym. Stickler syndrome, arthroophthalmopathy.

References

Herrmann J, et al: The Stickler syndrome (hereditary ophthalmopathy). *Birth Def* 11(2):76–103, 1975.

Stickler GB, et al: Hereditary progressive arthroophthalmopathy. *Mayo Clin Proc* 40:433–455, 1965.

Stickler SB, Pugh DG: Hereditary progressive arthroophthalmopathy. II. Additional observations on vertebral abnormalities, a hearing defect, and a report of a similar case. *Mayo Clin Proc* 42:495, 1967.

6.8 Meckel Syndrome

The syndrome was probably first reported by Meckel in 1822 and consists of (1) microcephaly, (2) posterior exencephalocele, (3) microphthalmia, (4) congenital heart defects, (5) polydactyly, (6) polycystic kidneys, liver, and pancreas, and (7) cleft palate. The syndrome, which is inherited in an autosomal recessive manner, is lethal. Death usually occurs during the first month of life, generally due to renal insufficiency.

Facies. Even though not part of the facies, the posterior exencephalocele is the most salient feature. The head is microcephalic with a sloping forehead. Hypertelorism and microphthalmia complete the facial appearance.

Oral Structures. Cleft palate is present in the majority of affected newborns. Cleft lip is less frequently seen. Natal teeth have been noted in several cases. Tongue abnormalities, which are less frequent, include multiple papillomas and clefting. Occasionally a thick buccal frenulum has been described, fixing the lip mucosa to the attached gingiva. Micrognathia is also evident.

Systemic Features. Holoprosencephaly, internal hydrocephalus, and meningoencephaloceles are frequent features (Fig. 6.12). Cysts of the kidneys are seen in around 90% of cases, and less frequently cysts of the liver or pancreas. Skeletal anomalies such as polydactyly involving all four extremities with hexadactyly, heptodactyly or an even greater number of postaxial digits, and talipes equinovarus have been noted. Genital anomalies such as hypoplastic penis, undescended testes, septate vagina, bicornuate uterus, and hypoplastic urinary bladder have been observed in about 20% of cases.

Differential Diagnosis. Trisomy 13 and Smith-Lemli-Opitz syndrome should be considered in the differential diagnosis.

Laboratory Aids. None known.

Synonyms. Dysencephalia splanchnocystica, Gruber syndrome.

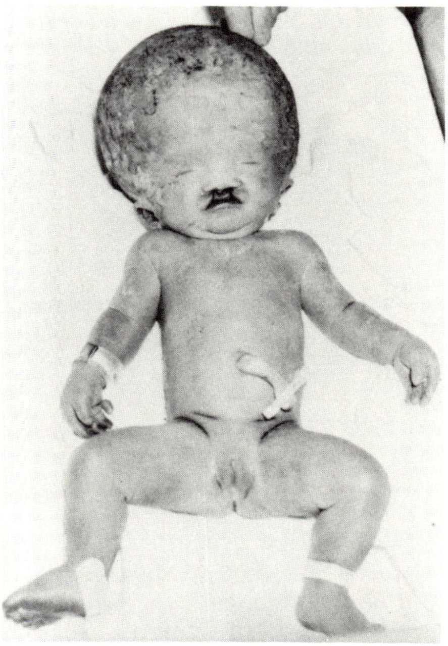

Fig. 6.12. Newborn with Meckel syndrome presenting hydrocephalus, microphthalmia, ocular hypertelorism and premaxillary agenesis with cleft lip-palate.

References

Fried K, et al: Polycystic kidneys associated with malformations of brain, polydactyly, and other birth defects in newborn sibs. *J Med Genet* 8:285–290, 1971.

Hsia YE, et al: Genetics of the Meckel syndrome (dysencephalia splanchnocystica). *Pediatrics* 48:237–247, 1971.

Opitz J, Howe JJ: Meckel's syndrome. Dysencephalia, splanchnocystica, Gruber's syndrome. *Birth Def* 5(2):167–179, 1969.

6.9 Multiple Pterygium Syndrome

The syndrome consists of (1) growth retardation, (2) multiple pterygia involving the neck, fingers, antecubital, popliteal, and intercrural areas, and (3) cleft palate. Parental consanguinity and affected sibs have been described. The syndrome is inherited as an autosomal recessive condition.

Facies. Characteristically, the palpebral fissures have mild antimongoloid obliquity; mild ptosis of the eyelids is also seen.

Oral Structures. Cleft palate, present in the majority of affected patients, is the only oral manifestation of the syndrome.

Systemic Features. Growth is usually below the third percentile; adult height does not exceed 135 cm. Mental development is within normal limits. The popliteal pterygia, even if only mild, interferes with walking and produces an abnormal stance. Pterygium colli rarely may surround the neck (Fig. 6.13). Soft tissue syndactyly between the fingers and flexion deformity of the digits are occasionally present.

Unilateral or bilateral talipes equinovarus and rocker bottom feet have been noted. Scoliosis and rib and vertebral anomalies have also been seen associated with the syndrome. When intercrural web is present in males, the penis and scrotum are retropositioned. This finding can be associated with cryptorchism and inguinal hernia. The labia majora may be absent in female patients with intercrural web.

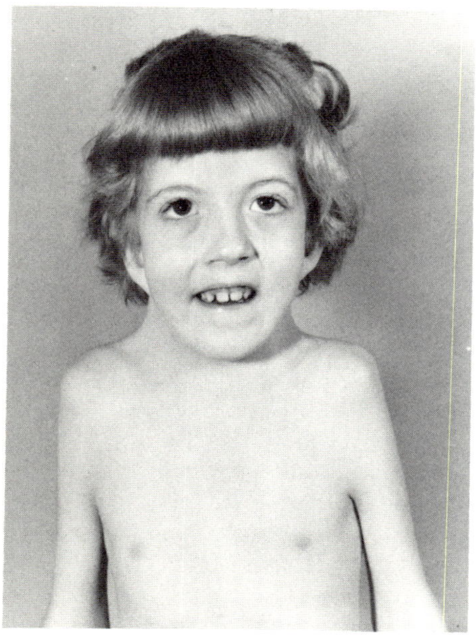

Fig. 6.13. Note pterygia of the neck and cubital area. The child also had popliteal pterygium and cleft palate.

Differential Diagnosis. The following conditions should be included: popliteal pterygium syndrome, arthrogryposis congenita, Turner syndrome, and Noonan syndrome.

Laboratory Aids. None known.

References

Aarskog D: Pterygium syndrome. *Birth Def* 7(6):232–234, 1971.

Gillin ME, Pryse-Davis J: Pterygium syndrome. *J Med Genet* 13:249–251, 1976.

Norum RA, et al: Pterygium syndrome in three children in a recessive pattern. *Birth Def* 5(2):233–235, 1969.

Scott C: Pterygium syndrome. *Birth Def* 5(2):231–232, 1969.

6.10 Otopalatodigital Syndrome

Taybi, in 1962, reported a case of "generalized skeletal dysplasia with multiple anomalies," suggesting that this possibly represented a new entity. Dudding, Gorlin, and Langer in 1967 presented three new cases, collected data from unreported cases, and proposed the name otopalatodigital (OPD) syndrome. The disorder comprises (1) deafness, (2) cleft palate, (3) generalized bone dysplasia, and (4) characteristic facies. The condition is inherited in an X-linked recessive manner. Only males have the full-blown syndrome. Carrier females present less severe manifestations in accordance with the Lyon hypothesis.

Facies. The facies of the affected male has a characteristic pugilistic appearance, with prominent supraorbital ridges, frontal bossing, apparent ocular hypertelorism, and antimongoloid obliquity of the palpebral fissures (Fig. 6.14). The nose is flat with a broad and flat nasal bridge. The mouth is generally small and open. The facies of the female carrier exhibits prominence of the lateral supraorbital ridges.

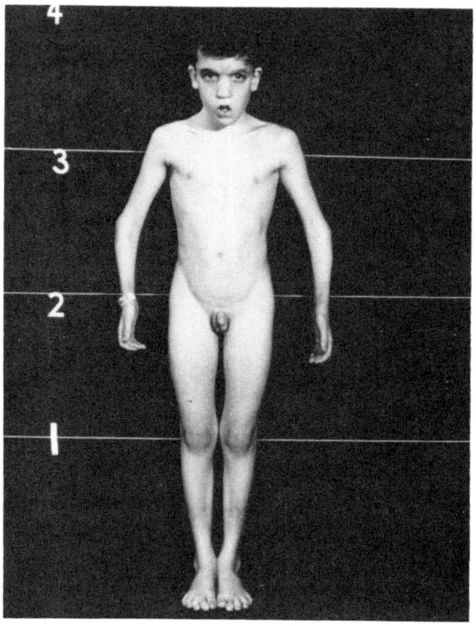

Fig. 6.14. Patient with OPD syndrome. Note pugilistic appearance of face; also note toes resembling those of a tree frog. The patient had cleft palate.

Oral Structures. Cleft palate has been reported in all affected males, but never in female heterozygotes. Small mandible with an obtuse angle is another constant finding.

Systemic Features. In general, skeletal growth is retarded below the 10th percentile. All patients are mildly mentally retarded with slow speech development, but this may be related to the hearing loss and palatal clefting. Skeletal findings include a large variety of malformations, such as coxa valga and hypoplasia of proximal radius with posterior dislocation. The hands show clinodactyly, short broad distal phalanges of all fingers, shortening of the thumb, second ossification center at proximal of second metacarpal, and teardrop-shaped lesser multangular. The feet also show distinctive anomalies, such as short phalanges and metatarsal of great toe, long abnormally shaped second and third metatarsals, and absence of normal modeling in metaphyseal regions of tubular bones. The feet have a marked resemblance to those of a tree frog. Bilateral conductive hearing loss is noted early in life. Abnormally shaped ossicles have been reported.

Differential Diagnosis. Larsen syndrome should be differentiated.

Laboratory Aids. None known.

Synonym. OPD syndrome.

References

Gall JC Jr, et al: Oto-palato-digital syndrome: Comparison of clinical and radiographic manifestations in males and females. *Am J Hum Genet* 24:24–36, 1972.

Gorlin RJ, et al: The oto-palato-digital (OPD) syndrome in females. Heterozygotic expression of an X-linked trait. *Oral Surg* 35:218–224, 1973.

Langer LO: The roentgenologic features of the otopalatodigital syndrome. *Am J Roentgenol* 100:63–70, 1967.

Podoshin L, et al: The oto-palato-digital syndrome. *J Laryngol Otol* 90:407–411, 1976.

Taybi H: Generalized skeletal dysplasia with multiple anomalies. *Am J Roentgenol* 88:450–457, 1962.

CHAPTER 7

Systemic Inherited Disorders with Involvement of Multiple Oral Structures

Jaw Bones and Teeth

7.1 Bird-Headed Dwarfism

The condition, recognized as an entity by Seckel in 1960, comprises (1) dwarfism, (2) low birth weight, (3) microcephaly, (4) mental retardation, and (5) beak-like appearance of the mid-face. The syndrome is inherited as an autosomal recessive condition.

Facies. The face is narrow with a receding mandible. The eyes are large with mild antimongoloid obliquity of the palpebral fissures, strabismus, and ocular hypertelorism. The most characteristic finding is the beak-like protrusion of the mid-face. The facial features are so typical as to make unrelated patients look like siblings. Zygomatic hypoplasia produces an "Aztec-like" facial appearance in affected individuals (Fig. 7.1).

Oral Structures. Patients have a receding chin due to mandibular hypoplasia; consequently the teeth are in malposition and are maloccluded. Other oral and dental

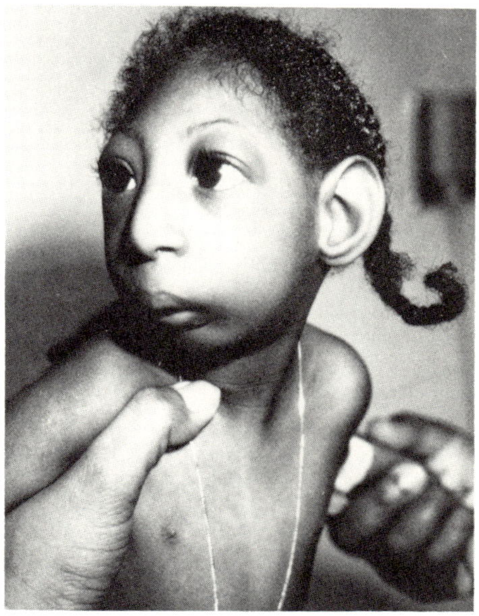

Fig. 7.1. Characteristic facies with small head circumference, micrognathia, and typical "Aztec-like" appearance.

findings have included enamel hypoplasia, cleft lip or palate or both, and high-arched palate.

Systemic Features. Physical growth is retarded, adults rarely reaching 120 cm in height. Mental retardation is evident and worsens with age. An IQ of 50 at around 6 to 8 years of age has been reported. Other abnormalities include dislocation of joints, kyphoscoliosis, clubbing of fingers, absence of patellae, proximal shortening of the fibula, and hypotonicity. Several patients have been reported with hypertrichosis, abnormal pigmentation of the skin, lobeless ears, bilateral cryptorchidism, and pancytopenia.

Differential Diagnosis. The facies is so distinctive as to make the differential diagnosis almost unnecessary; nevertheless all those conditions associated with dwarfism in conjunction with mental retardation and microcephaly should be considered.

Laboratory Aids. None known.

Synonyms. Seckel syndrome, nanocephalic dwarfism.

References

McKusick VA, et al: Seckel's bird-headed dwarfism. *New Engl J Med* 277:279–286, 1967.

Sauk JJ, et al: Familial bird-headed dwarfism (Seckel's syndrome). *J Med Genet* 10:196–198, 1973.

Seckel HPG: *Bird-headed Dwarfs*. Springfield, Ill, CC Thomas, 1960.

7.2 Cleidocranial Dysplasia

The first accurate descriptions of this condition were made by Scheuthauer in 1871 and by Marie and Sainton in 1897. The syndrome consists of (1) aplasia or hypoplasia of one or both clavicles, (2) exaggerated development of the transverse diameter of the cranium, and (3) delayed ossification of the fontanels. Cleidocranial dysplasia is transmitted in an autosomal dominant manner, although in less than half the cases it arises spontaneously, caused either by mutation or a gene with poor penetrance.

Facies. The face appears small, the nasal bridge is depressed, and the nose is broad at the base. The skull is brachycephalic with marked frontal, parietal, and occipital bossing. Fontanels and sutures remain open, often for life. Wormian bones are formed through secondary centers of ossification in the suture lines. The paranasal sinuses are often underdeveloped or absent. The mastoids may not be pneumatized because of functional alteration of the sternocleidomastoid muscles.

Oral Structures. Oral manifestations in the syndrome include supernumerary teeth and submucous or complete cleft palate. The so-called pseudoanodontia is due to delayed eruption and impaction of deciduous, permanent, and supernumerary teeth (Fig. 7.2). Cyst formation around these impacted teeth has been described by a number of investigators. In addition, the impacted teeth appear to lack a layer of cellular cementum. Probably the most prominent oral manifestation is the number of supernumerary teeth present, which at times simulate a third dentition (Fig. 7.3). Nonunion at the mandibular symphysis has been described. Development of the premaxilla is poor, resulting in a false or relative prognathism.

Systemic Features. Individuals with the syndrome are short in stature with long necks and narrow shoulders. The clavicles may be unilaterally or bilaterally aplastic or hypoplastic, generally at the acromial end. Due to this bony defect, patients with the condition are able to approximate their shoulders in front of the chest (Fig. 7.4). Other anomalies include congenital dislocation of hip, underdevelopment of pelvis, coxa vara or coxa valga, genu valgum, scoliosis, kyphosis, and cervical ribs.

Differential Diagnosis. Pyknodysostosis, mandibuloacral dysplasia, and cleidofacial dysplasia should be included in the differential diagnosis.

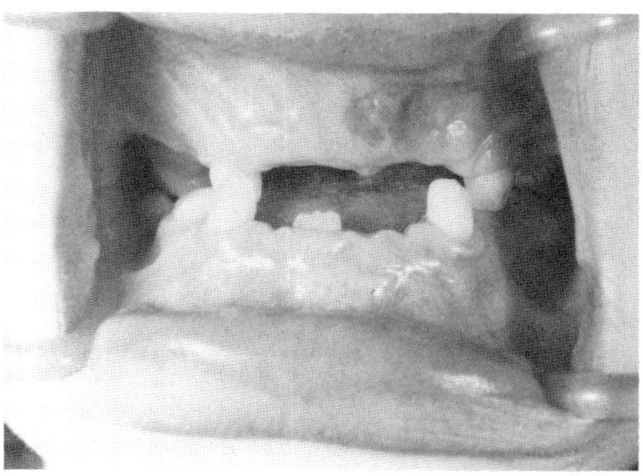

Fig. 7.2. Intraoral view showing lack of teeth eruption due to retention.

Laboratory Aids. None known.

Synonyms. Scheuthauer-Marie-Sainton syndrome, cleidocranial dysostosis.

References

Jarvis JL, Keats TE: Cleidocranial dysostosis: A review of 40 new cases. *Am J Roentgenol* 121:5–16, 1974.

Keats TE: Cleidocranial dysostosis; some atypical roentgen manifestations. *Am J Roentgenol* 100:71–74, 1967.

Skokeir, MHK: Complete failure of eruption of all permanent teeth: An autosomal dominant disorder. *Clin Genet* 5:322–326, 1974.

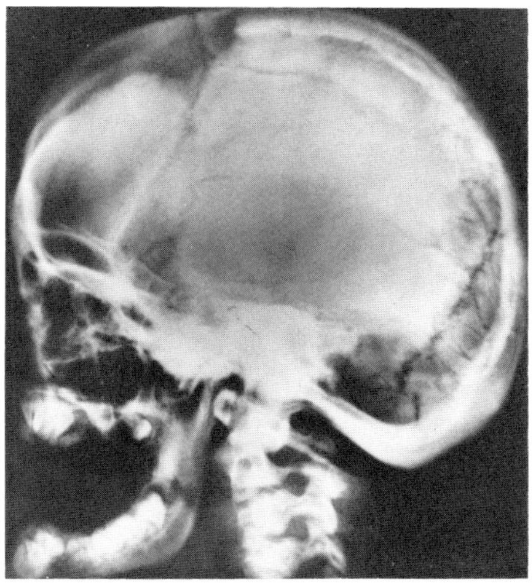

Fig. 7.3. Skull radiograph in patient showing open sutures, numerous Wormian bones, and multiple retention of teeth.

Witkop-Oostenrijk GA: Contribution to the study of the inheritance of dysostosis cleidocranialis. *Acta Genet* (Basel) 7:223–228, 1957.

7.3 Cockayne Syndrome

The syndrome is characterized by (1) cachectic dwarfism, (2) premature aging, (3) mental deficiency, (4) microcephaly, (5) intracranial calcifications, (6) neurological deficits, (7) retinal pigmentary abnormalities, (8) sensorineural deafness, and (9) photosensitivity. The condition was first described by Cockayne in 1936. It is inherited in an autosomal recessive manner.

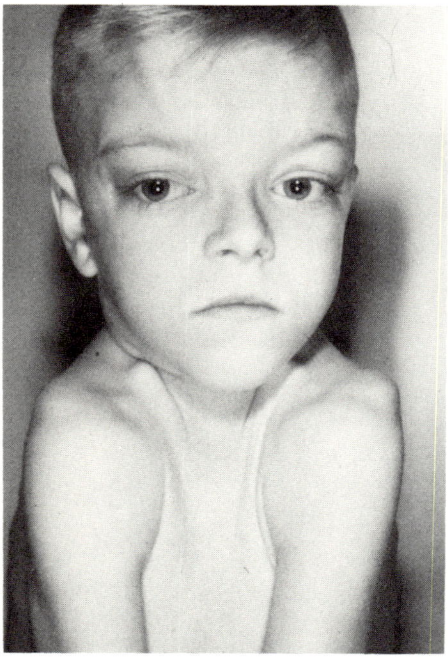

Fig. 7.4. Child with cleidocranial dysplasia demonstrating ability to approximate shoulder to the midline due to absent clavicles.

Facies. The facies has a typical bird-like appearance, accentuated by a beak-like nose, sunken eyes, and prominent cheek bones (Fig. 7.5). The superficial facial veins are readily seen because of absence of subcutaneous fat. Microcephaly and large ears add to the facial appearance.

Oral Structures. Oral findings include marked prognathism, which adds to the facial characteristics, and extensive dental caries, which most likely is not related to the condition itself. Condylar hypoplasia and partial congenital anodontia have also been reported.

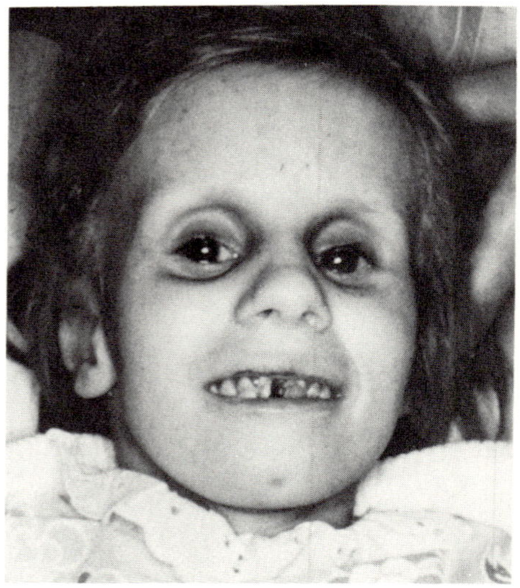

Fig. 7.5. Note birdlike appearance with sunken eyes and prominent cheek bones. The patient had an ataxic gait, microcephaly, and mental retardation.

Systemic Features. Birth weight is within normal limits, but growth retardation becomes apparent around the second year of life, with resultant dwarfism. Advanced mental retardation is evident. CNS findings include microcephaly; widespread mineralization in the cortex, basal ganglia, and cerebellum; patchy demyelinization, often severe, in the subcortical white matter; cerebellar ataxia; choreoathetosis; sensorineural deafness; and blindness. Skeletal findings include kyphosis, ankylosis, long limbs, large hands and feet, flexion contractures involving the ankles, knees, and elbows, and occasionally periarticular thickening of the interphalangeal joints of the hands and feet. Over 50 percent of affected males present cryptorchidism.

Photosensitivity is marked, especially in the sun-exposed areas of the skin. The forehead is generally spared, but the butterfly area of the face is severely involved. The photodermatitis is responsible for scarring and pigmentation in older patients. Enophthalmos, optic atrophy, and ocular arteriolar narrowing are usually present. The macula shows numerous fine speckles of pigment apposition. Cataracts may develop around puberty.

Differential Diagnosis. Progeria, bird-headed dwarfism, Rothmund-Thomson syndrome, Bloom syndrome, and the photodermatoses should be included in the differential diagnosis.

Laboratory Aids. Hyperinsulinemia and hyperlipoproteinemia have been noted in some patients with the syndrome.

References

Cockayne EA: Dwarfism with retinal atrophy and deafness. *Arch Dis Child* 11:1–8, 1936.

Conly PW, et al: Hyperinsulinemia in Cockayne's syndrome. *S Med J* 63:1491, 1970.

Crome L, Kanjilal GC: Cockayne's syndrome. *J Neurol Neurosurg Psychiatr* 34:171–178, 1971.

Riggs W Jr, Seibert J: Cockayne's syndrome. Roentgen findings. *Am J Roentgenol* 116:623–633, 1972.

7.4 Frontometaphyseal Dysplasia

Frontometaphyseal dysplasia was recognized as an independent entity by Gorlin and Cohen in 1969. The syndrome consists of (1) deafness, (2) pronounced supraorbital ridge, and (3) other skeletal alterations. It is a rare syndrome of unknown etiology. An autosomal dominant mode of inheritance has been suggested by Weiss and coworkers (1975); however, an X-linked form may also exist according to Jarvis and Jenkins (1975).

Facies. The facies is quite striking, presenting a pronounced supraorbital ridge, mild facial asymmetry, wide nasal bridge, slight antimongoloid obliquity of palpebral fissures, hirsutism above the eyebrows, and a small, pointed chin (Fig. 7.6). Roentgenographic alterations include thick frontal ridge, absence of frontal sinuses, and "Hershey kiss" defects of the supraorbital rims.

Oral Structures. Malocclusion appears with antegonial notching of the lower mandibular border and hypoplasia of the angle and condyloid processes. Absence of permanent dentition and retained primary teeth has been reported (Fig. 7.7).

Systemic Features. Somatic development is diminished and mental development may be retarded, although in most cases it appears to be within normal limits. The long bones present an increased density in the diaphyseal region with lack of modeling of the metaphyseal region, producing an Erlenmeyer-flask-type deformity. Carpal bones, with the exception of the pisiform, become fused into a conglomerate mass. Marked flaring of the iliac bones and coxa valga are also present. The occiput has an abnormal relationship to the first cervical vertebra, with the foramen magnum distally placed.

Conductive deafness due to bony changes appears to be part of the syndrome. Associated anomalies may include pectus carinatum, generalized body hirsutism, arachnodactyly and camptodactyly of the fingers, clinodactyly of the toes, ankylosis and diminished motion of the elbows, wrists, knees, and ankles, and keloid formation. Fibroblast metachromasia has also been reported.

Differential diagnosis. Pyle disease, craniometaphyseal dysplasia, craniodiaphyseal dysplasia, and osteopetrosis should be included in the differential diagnosis.

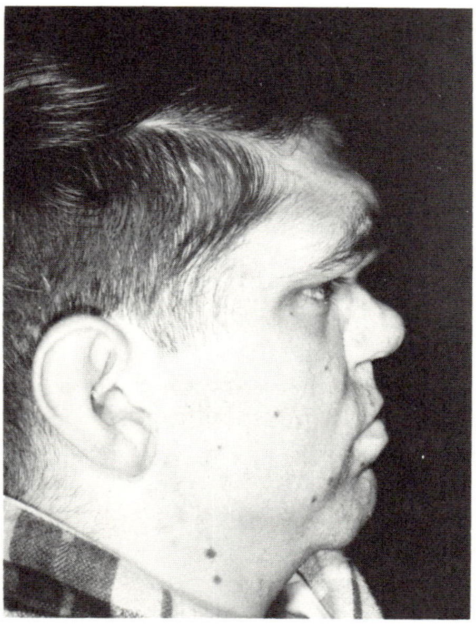

Fig. 7.6. Note marked supraorbital ridge and small chin.

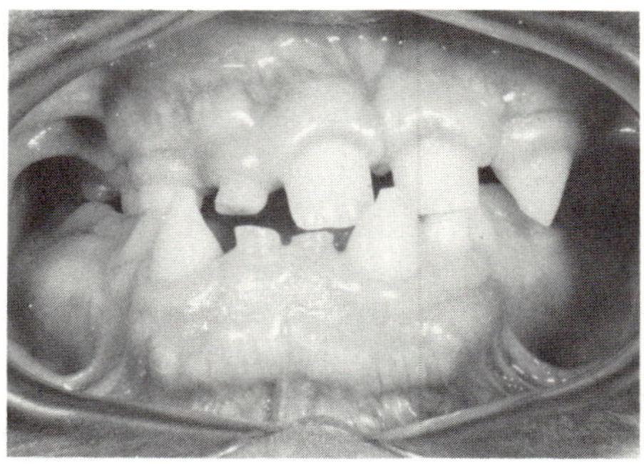

Fig. 7.7. Intraoral view in same patient as Fig. 7.6. showing absence of several permanent teeth with preservation of some deciduous dentition.

Laboratory Aids. None.

References

Gorlin RJ, Cohen MM Jr: Frontometaphyseal dysplasia. A new syndrome. *Am J Dis Child* 118:487–494, 1969.

Gorlin RJ, et al: Genetic craniotubular bone dysplasias and hyperostosis: A critical analysis. *Birth Def* 5(4):79–95, 1969.

Jarvis GA, Jenkins EC: *Syndrome Ident* 3(1):18–19, 1975.

Walker BA: A craniodiaphyseal dysplasia or craniometaphyseal dysplasia. *Birth Def* 5(4):298–300, 1969.

Weiss L, et al: Frontometaphyseal dysplasia—evidence for dominant inheritance. *Birth Def* 11(5):55–56, 1975.

7.5 Gardner Syndrome

This syndrome was first extensively described by Gardner and coworkers in 1953. It is characterized by (1) multiple osteomas, especially of the facies, (2) epidermoid inclusion cysts of the skin which may be present in the face, trunk, and extremities, usually appearing after puberty, (3) polyposis of the large intestine that eventually undergoes malignant transformation, and (4) fibromas and desmoid tumors of the skin or mesentery or both, as well as lipomas or lipofibromas or both. The condition is inherited in an autosomal dominant manner with variable expressivity and marked penetrance.

Facies. Facial asymmetry may be present if the osteomas are of sufficient size (Fig. 7.8). Multiple osteomas also may be found in the calvaria and facial skeleton. The frontal bone is the most frequent site for the osteomas to occur, and they generally precede the appearance of the intestinal polyposis. The osteomas expand and obliterate the paranasal sinuses, especially the sphenoid and ethmoid sinuses. Histologically, the bone shows a mature appearance and a well-developed Haversian system.

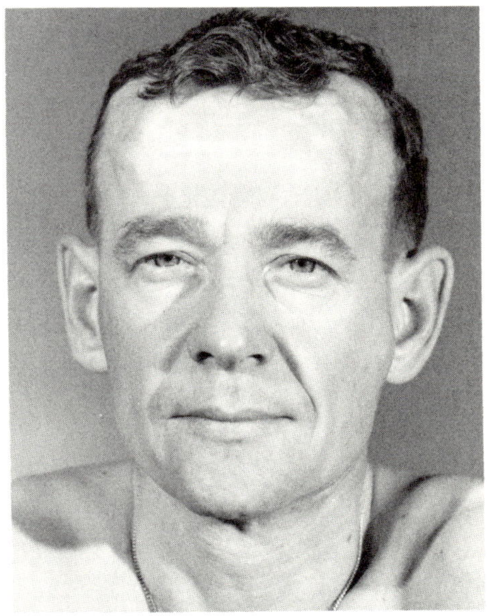

Fig. 7.8. Patient with Gardner syndrome; note protuberant multiple osteomas on the forehead.

Oral Structures. Osteomas are also frequent in the maxilla and mandible (Fig. 7.9). In over half of the reported cases, compound odontomas have been described as part of the syndrome, as well as hypercementosis and unerupted teeth.

Systemic Features. Somatic growth and mental development are within normal limits. The syndrome is characterized by the presence of multiple intestinal polyposis of the colon and rectum with a marked tendency to malignant degeneration. The polyps may be present before puberty. Epidermoid inclusions of the skin may be noted after puberty. In addition, fibromas and desmoid tumors of the skin and mesentery may also be present, as well as lipomas. Long bones also may be the site of osteomas, and when small, these may mimic osteomyelitis.

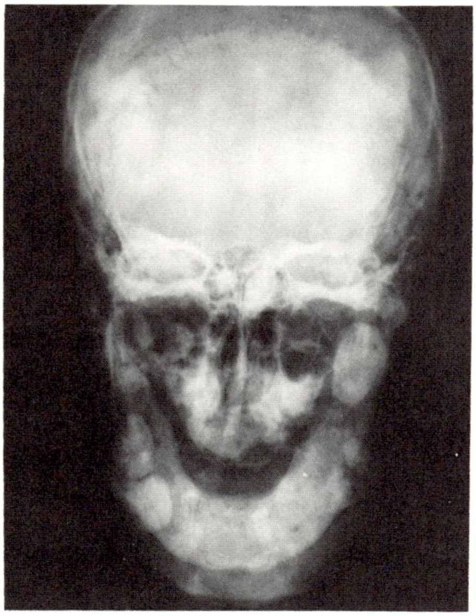

Fig. 7.9. Skull roentgenogram from same patient as Fig. 7.8 showing multiple osteomas of maxilla and especially mandible.

Differential Diagnosis. Intestinal polyposis I, II, IV, juvenile type polyposis coli, and multiple hamartoma syndrome should be included in the differential diagnosis.

Laboratory Aids. Roentgenographic examination of the skeleton and barium contrast survey of the large and small bowel are suggested.

Synonyms. Intestinal polyposis III, osteomatosis-intestinal polyposis syndrome.

References

Gardner EJ, Richards RC: Multiple cutaneous and subcutaneous lesions occurring simultaneously with hereditary polyposis and osteomatosis. *Am J Hum Genet* 5:139–147, 1953.

Gorlin RJ, Chaudhry AP: Multiple osteomas, fibromas, lipomas and fibrosarcomas of the skin and mesentery, epidermoid inclusion cysts of the skin, leiomyomas and multiple intestinal polyposis. *New Engl J Med* 263:1151–1158, 1960.

Leppard B, Bussey HJR: Epidermoid cysts, polyposis, and Gardner's syndrome. *Br J Surg* 62:387–393, 1975.

Pierce ER, et al: Gardner's syndrome: Formal genetics and statistical analysis of a large Canadian kindred. *Clin Genet* 1:65–80, 1970.

Plenk HP, Gardner EJ: Osteomatosis (leontiasia ossea). Hereditary disease of membranous bone formation associated in one family with polyposis of colon. *Radiology* 62:830–840, 1954.

Utsunomiya J, Nakamura T: The occult osteomatous changes in the mandible in patients with familial polyposis coli. *Br J Surg* 62:45–51, 1975.

7.6 Hypertelorism-Hypospadias Syndrome

Opitz and coworkers in 1965 described a syndrome characterized by (1) hypertelorism, (2) hypospadias, and (3) other associated anomalies. The condition is probably inherited in an autosomal dominant manner with incomplete penetrance, variable expressivity, and male sex limitation. Males with the syndrome are severely affected while females have only minor manifestations or are even clinically nonaffected. The condition needs further delineation.

Facies. The face is characterized by marked hypertelorism accompanied by slight antimongoloid or mongoloid obliquity of palpebral fissures (Fig. 7.10). Occasionally strabismus and epicanthal folds may be present. The forehead is generally prominent, and in several instances a widow's peak has been reported. The facial appearance is completed with a frequently brachycephalic, asymmetric cranium with a marked metopic suture. Nevus flammeus of the facial skin is occasionally seen.

Oral Structures. Orodental findings have compromised malocclusion with supernumerary and occasionally fused teeth, micrognathia, and cleft lip-palate.

Systemic Features. Moderate to mild mental retardation is not infrequent. Physical development is within normal limits. Hypospadias is the other constant component of the syndrome. Other findings include cryptorchidism, inguinal hernia, coarctation of the aorta, atrial septal defect, and diastasis recti, among others.

Differential Diagnosis. Isolated hypertelorism and isolated hypospadias as well as the hypospadias-dysphagia syndrome should be included in the differential diagnosis.

Laboratory Aids. None known.

Synonym. Opitz syndrome, BBB syndrome.

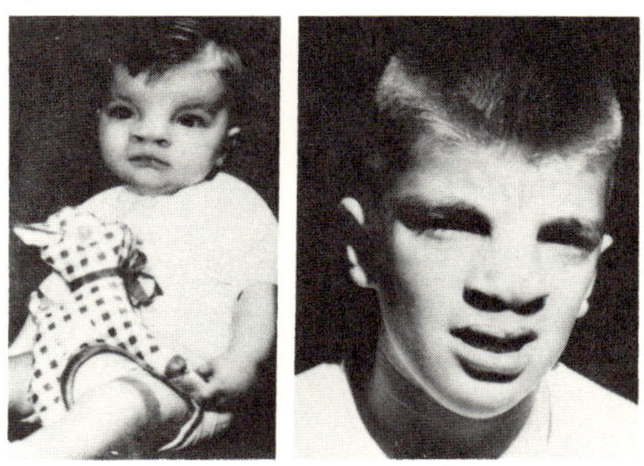

Fig. 7.10. Note marked hypertelorism and broad nasal bridge in the same patient at four months and eleven years old. The child also has hypospadias.

References

Michaelis E, Mortimer W: Association of hypertelorism and hypospadias in the BBB syndrome. *Helv Paediatr Acta* 27:575–581, 1972.

Opitz JM, et al: Hypertelorism and hypospadias: A new recognized hereditary malformation syndrome (Abstr). *J Pediatr* 67:968, 1965.

Opitz JM, et al: The BBB syndrome: Familial telecanthus with associated congenital anomalies. *Birth Def* 5(2): 86–94, 1969.

7.7 Mucopolysaccharidosis IV

MPS IV was independently reported in 1929 by Morquio of Uruguay and Brailsford of England. MPS IV is characterized by (1) the presence of a mucopolysaccharide, keratan sulfate, in the urine of affected individuals, (2) universal platyspondyly with resultant dwarfism, (3) corneal clouding and dental abnormalities, and (4) progressive spinal deformity. It is transmitted in an autosomal recessive manner.

Facies. There is no specific facies. Many patients show a mild ocular hypertelorism and a slightly depressed nasal bridge. The head seems to rest directly on the shoulders, due to shortening of the neck. A mild scaphocephaly also can be present due to premature closure of the sutures.

Oral Structures. Deciduous and permanent teeth present gray crowns with pitted enamel. The enamel is very thin with a tendency to flake off, and the dental cusps are poorly formed (Figs. 7.11–12). The mandibular condyles are flat or concave.

Systemic Features. Intelligence is nearly always normal. After the second year of life, dwarfism becomes prominent. The cervical spine presents marked curvature, producing restricted movement of the neck. Kyphosis with or without scoliosis, universal platyspondyly, genua valga, pes planus, and pectus carinatum are characteristic. Often there is a gibbus-like deformity of the lumbar spine. Radiologic examination may reveal platyspondyly, coxa valga, flared ilia, and dysplasia of the femoral heads. The corneas eventually take on a filmy haze-like opacity.

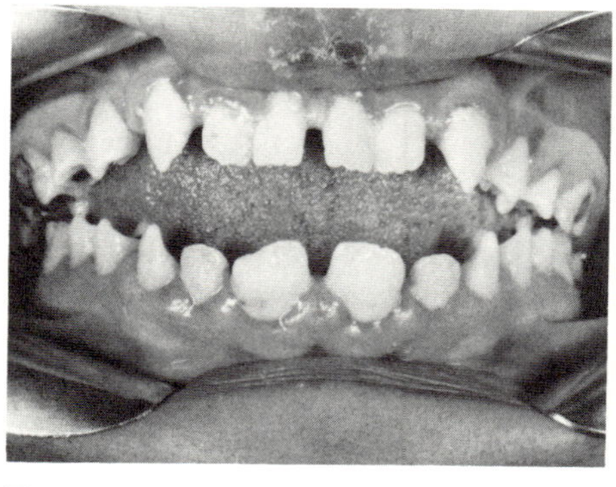

Fig. 7.11. Intraoral view showing marked interdental spaces and pointed cusps in molars and cuspid teeth.

Mild hearing loss usually is noted early in the second decade.

Differential Diagnosis. Aarskog syndrome, Dyggve-Melchior-Clausen syndrome, cartilage-hair hypoplasis, achnodroplasia, pseudoachondroplasia, spondyloepiphyseal dysplasia, spondylometaphyseal dysplasia, diastrophic dwarfism, rickets, and hypophosphatasia should all be considered in making the diagnosis.

Laboratory Aids. Increased excretion of chondroitin 4-sulfate, chondroitin A and C sulfate and keratan sulfate in the urine during childhood, as well as abnormal granules in peripheral neutrophilic granulocytes may be of aid in establishing a diagnosis.

Synonym. Morquio syndrome.

References

Brailsford JF: Chondro-osteo-dystrophy. *Am J Surg* 7:404–409, 1929.

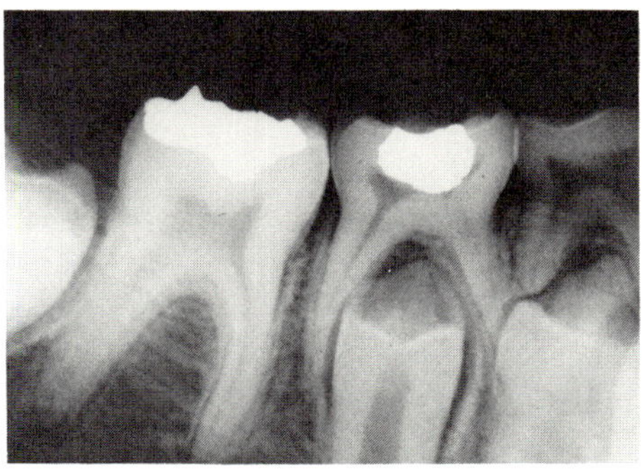

Fig. 7.12. Intraoral radiograph demonstrating thin hypoplastic enamel.

Gardner DG: Dental manifestations of the Morquio syndrome (mucopolysaccharidosis type IV). *Am J Dis Child* 129:1445–1448, 1975.

Garn SM, Hurme VO: Dental defects in three siblings afflicted with Morquio's disease. *Br Dent J* 93:210–212, 1952.

Langer LO, Jr, Carey LS: The roentgenographic features of the KS mucopolysaccharidosis of Morquio (Morquio-Brailsford's disease). *Am J Roentgenol* 97:1–20, 1966.

Morquio L: Sur une forme de dystrophie osseuse familiale. *Arch méd enf* 32:129–140, 1929.

7.8 Multiple Nevoid Basal Cell Carcinoma Syndrome

The syndrome first described by Jarisch in 1894 presents as the major components (1) multiple nevoid basal cell carcinomas, (2) cysts of the jaws, and (3) vertebral and rib anomalies, chiefly splayed and bifid rib. The syndrome is inherited as an autosomal dominant condition with high penetrance and variable expressivity.

Facies. Mild hypertelorism, frontal and biparietal bossing, and mild mandibular prognathism give the face and skull a pagetoid appearance. The facial picture is completed with a broad nasal root. Occasionally strabismus and cataracts are noted. The cutaneous manifestations, ie, nevoid basal cell carcinomas, also occur on the skin of the face (Fig. 7.13).

Oral Structures. The main oral component is numerous cysts of the maxilla and mandible (Fig. 7.14). These cysts are lined by uniformly thick stratified squamous epithelium which generally exhibits a thin layer of parakeratin or orthokeratin. They may be as large as several centimeters in diameter and have a marked tendency to recur after surgical removal. Occasional transformation into ameloblastoma has been reported. The multiple odontogenic keratocysts can appear as early as five to six years of age, interfering with the normal development of the permanent dentition (Fig. 7.15). There is good evidence that the cysts are derived from the overlying oral epithelium.

Systemic Features. Physical development is within normal limits. Mild mental retardation is noted in around 15% of affected individuals. Calcification of the falx cerebri is noted in around 80% of the patients. Medulloblastoma has been reported in several instances, and in some families a sibling of an affected individual has died in early childhood of medulloblastoma. Skeletal anomalies include bifurcation or splaying of one or more ribs, shortened fourth metacarpal, bridging of sella, spina

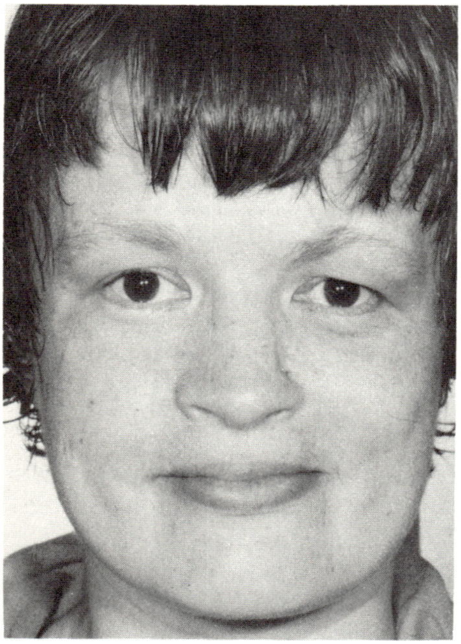

Fig. 7.13. Note multiple pigmented nevi over facial skin. Also note scars under left eye after removal of basal cell carcinoma.

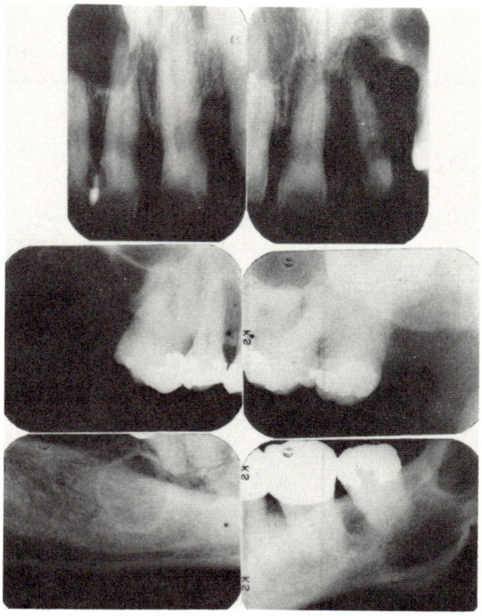

Fig. 7.14. Several intraoral radiographs of a patient with the syndrome showing multiple jaw cysts.

bifida occulta in the cervicothoracic area, and kyphoscoliosis.

The nevoid basal cell carcinomas generally appear in childhood or at puberty, involving the nose, eyelids, cheeks, trunk, arms, and neck. They are flesh-colored to pale brown. Microscopically they cover the wide spectrum of basal cell and adnexal carcinomas. Milia, epithelial inclusion cysts, lipomas, and fibromas are often intermixed with the skin carcinomas. Small pits in the palms and soles are also a component of the syndrome. Various associated eye anomalies have been reported, such as glaucoma, blindness, and coloboma of the choroid and optic nerve. Other less frequent findings include calcified ovarian fibromas, hypogonadism, and lymphatic mesenteric cysts.

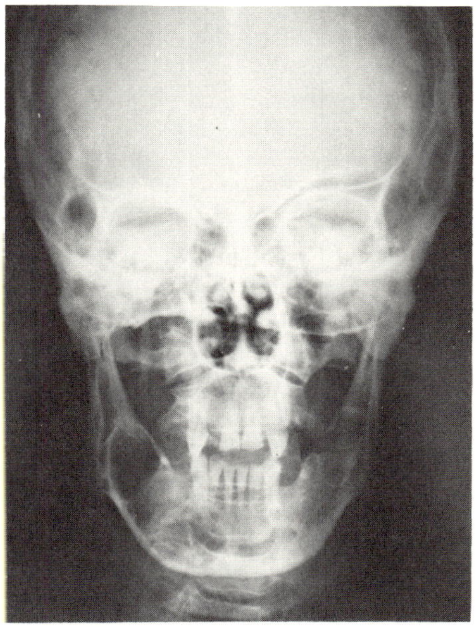

Fig. 7.15. Skull radiograph from another patient also showing multiple intrabony cysts.

Differential Diagnosis. Hypertelorism, dystopia canthorum, and mandibular prognathism are also seen in the Waardenburg syndrome. The multiple lentigines syndrome, multiple cylindromas of the scalp, pseudohyperparathyroidism, epidermal nevus syndrome, and isolated multiple odontogenic keratocysts should be considered in the differential diagnosis.

Laboratory Aids. Biopsy of skin lesions or of the jaw cysts, together with the radiologic findings in the jaws and the chest are conclusive for the diagnosis.

Synonyms. Basal cell nevus syndrome, Gorlin syndrome.

References

Gorlin RJ, Sedano HO: The multiple nevoid basal cell carcinoma syndrome revisited. *Birth Def* 7(8):140–148, 1972.

Kozlowski K, et al: Multiple nevoid basal cell carcinoma syndrome. *Pediatr Radiol* 2:185–190, 1974.

Stoelinga P, et al: Some new findings in the basal cell nevus syndrome. *Oral Surg* 36:686–692, 1973.

Stoelinga P, et al: The origin of keratocysts in the basal cell nevus syndrome. *J Oral Surg* 33:675–684, 1975.

7.9 Osteogenesis Imperfecta

Osteogenesis imperfecta was first described by Ekman in 1788. The syndrome consists of (1) fragile bones, (2) clear or blue sclerae, (3) deafness, (4) loose ligaments, and (5) a dentinogenesis imperfecta-like alteration. The syndrome is inherited as an autosomal dominant condition; however, only about one-third of affected patients will present a familial history of the condition. The remaining two-thirds comprise largely sporadic cases and rarely patients with familial pedigrees that possibly suggest autosomal recessive inheritance. Those having a family history are inclined to have the disease in a milder form and to manifest it later in life (tarda form).

Only about one in three patients presents the complete syndrome. The degree of expressivity is variable. Of patients having blue sclerae, about 60% have the bone disease and possibly only about 30% have otosclerosis. In the congenital type of osteogenesis imperfecta, intrauterine fractures may be so numerous as to be lethal, or the child may survive for only a short time (Fig. 7.16).

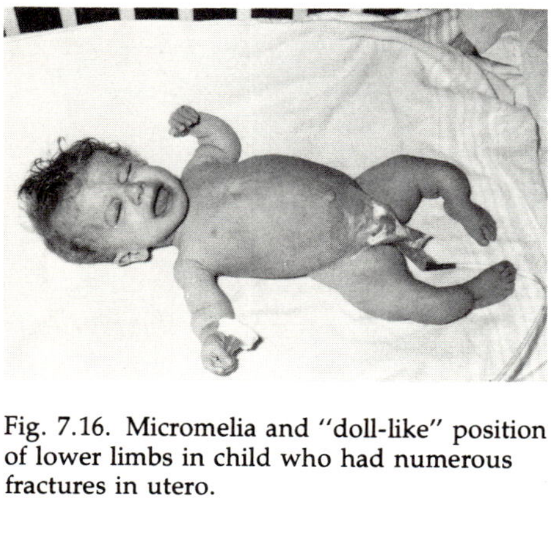

Fig. 7.16. Micromelia and "doll-like" position of lower limbs in child who had numerous fractures in utero.

Facies. The skull is large, especially in the anteroposterior direction. The forehead is broad and bossed, with a temporal bulge and an overhanging occiput. The eyes often present with blue or clear sclerae which may be the only expression of the syndrome. The characteristic scleral appearance has been attributed to thinning of the sclerae with transmittance of choroid pigment, a deficiency of collagen fibers, and variability in collagen fiber aggregation. Additional causes of blue sclerae have included an increase in mucopolysaccharide content and increased translucency due to a thinned fibrous coat.

Oral Structures. The primary teeth are affected in about 80% of patients; the permanent teeth show similar changes in about 35%. The degree of bone involvement appears to have no correlation to the degree of tooth involvement. The crowns of affected teeth are usually vertically smaller than normal. Subsequent to eruption, the dentition may be opalescent or have a translucent appearance. As the patient ages, the teeth darken and the enamel, which is normal, is lost because of the pathology in the underlying dentin. Roentgenographically, the roots of the teeth are thin and shortened and pulp chambers are diminished or absent (Fig. 7.17). Histologic examination of the teeth reveals a reduced degree of scalloping of the dentinoenamel junction. The dentin appears laminated and contains tubules of abnormal size and shape. Biochemical studies indicate diminished calcification manifested by zones of interglobular dentin.

Systemic Features. Mental development is within normal limits. Somatic growth is impeded in patients experiencing numerous fractures and in patients with severe congenital forms. Roentgenographic examination of the skull reveals remarkably thin calvaria and the presence of numerous Wormian bones in the occipital region. The long bones are generally bowed or shortened. Kyphoscoliosis, pectus carinatum and excavatum, and subperiosteal fractures of the shaft and epiphyses may be seen. Twenty-five percent of affected patients have laxity of ligaments with resultant and persistent dislocation of joints. Deafness is frequent and begins in the third decade with progressive hearing loss. The hearing defect may be sensorineural, associated with malformation of the stapes, or involve otosclerosis of the footplate of the stapes. The tympanic membrane is thinned and has a bluish appearance.

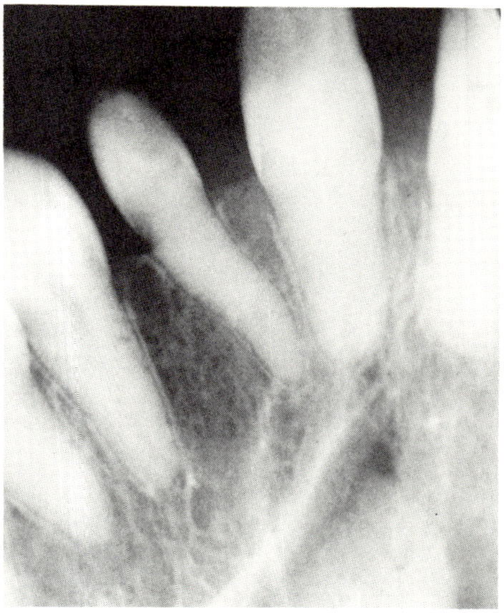

Fig. 7.17. Intraoral radiographs from a patient with osteogenesis imperfecta. Note absent or diminished pulp chambers and small-sized roots.

Differential Diagnosis. Differential diagnosis should include hereditary opalescent dentin, cleidocranial dysplasia, pyknodysostosis, osteoporosis, Ellis-van Creveld syndrome, achondroplasia, and Ehlers-Danlos syndromes.

Laboratory Aids. Increased presence of alpha III type collagen in fibroblast cultures has been described in a small percentage of cases.

Synonym. Brittle bones syndrome.

References

Falvo KA, Bullough PG: Osteogenesis imperfecta—a histometric analysis. *J Bone Joint Surg* 55A:275–286, 1973.

Godfrey JL: A histological study of dentin formation in osteogenesis imperfecta congenita. *J Oral Pathol* 2:85–111, 1973.

Riley FC, et al: Osteogenesis imperfecta: Morphologic and biochemical studies of connective tissue. *Pediatr Res* 7:757–768, 1973.

Witkop CJ Jr, Rao S: Inherited defects in tooth structures. *Birth Def* 7(7):153–184, 1971.

7.10 Pyknodysostosis

The syndrome was first described by Maroteaux and Lamy in 1962. Earlier cases are found in the literature, generally reported either as cleidocranial dysplasia or osteopetrosis. There is good evidence to suggest that Toulouse-Lautrec had this condition. The syndrome consists of (1) dwarfism, (2) increased bone density, (3) partial agenesis of the terminal phalanges of the hands and feet, (4) cranial anomalies, such as persistence of fontanels and failure of closure of cranial sutures, (5) frontal and occipital bossing, and (6) hypoplasia of the angle of the mandible. The condition is inherited in an autosomal recessive manner. The consanguinity rate among the parents of affected individuals is about 35%.

Facies. The face is rather typical, characterized by frontal bulging, a beaked nose and a receding chin. Agenesis of the angle of the mandible, which is a striking feature, and underdeveloped facial bones complete the facial appearance (Figs. 7.18–19).

Oral Structures. Hypoplastic maxillary bones with partial or total absence of the sinuses is a constant finding. Late exfoliation of primary teeth, partial anodontia, and malposition of teeth in the permanent dentition are occasionally seen. Enamel hypoplasia also has been reported in some patients with the syndrome.

Systemic Structures. Adult height is reduced to 134 to 152 cm in most cases. Mental development is normal. Osteopetrosis of all bones is present, but especially of the long bones, spine, and skull base. The increased bone density is responsible for multiple fractures in these patients, but this peculiarity tends to disappear after puberty. The skull is dolichocephalic, due to frontal and occipital bosses. Parietal bulging is also present. Most cranial sutures and fontanels are open, especially the parietooccipital (Fig. 7.20). Wormian bones are commonly observed. The frontal sinuses are consistently absent and the other paranasal sinuses are hypoplastic or absent. The mastoid air cells are often not pneumatized.

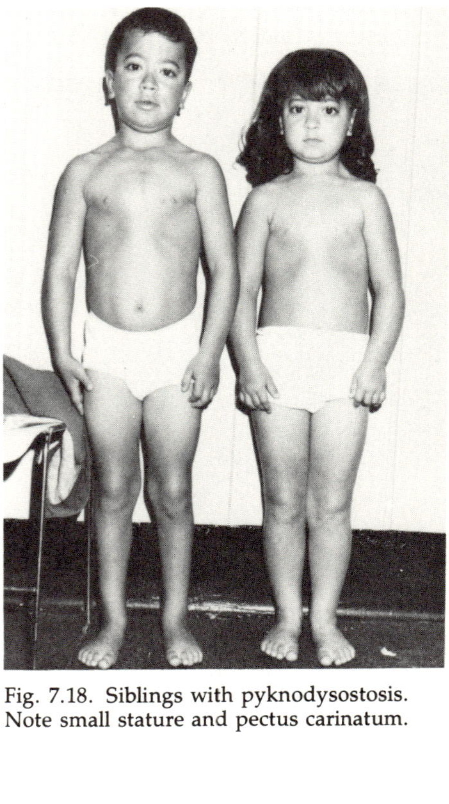

Fig. 7.18. Siblings with pyknodysostosis. Note small stature and pectus carinatum.

The terminal digits of the fingers present an abbreviated appearance. On radiographic examination they are markedly hypoplastic, exhibiting fragmentation of the heads with preservation of the bases, underdevelopment of the unguiculate processes, or narrowing of the ends of otherwise normal terminal phalanges. Dysplastic clavicles with partial aplasia of acromial ends are always present. The skin over the dorsal surfaces of the terminal phalanges of the fingers is generally wrinkled. The nails are flattened and occasionally hypoplastic.

Differential Diagnosis. Acroosteolysis, osteogenesis imperfecta, cleidocranial dysplasia, and osteopetrosis should be included.

Laboratory Aids. None known.

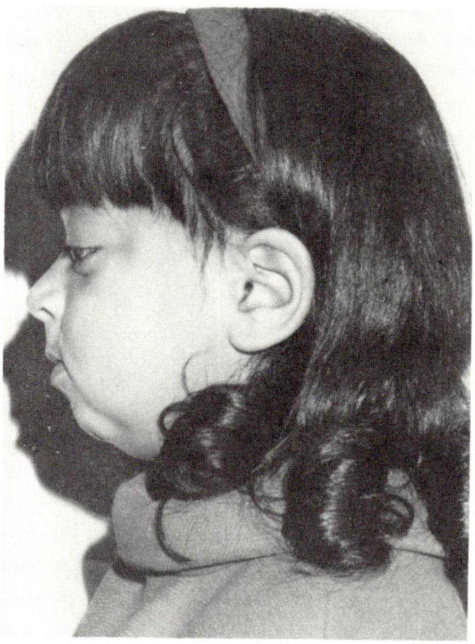

Fig. 7.19. Profile showing beaked nose and receding mandible.

References

Baker RK, et al: Plasma calcitonin in pycnodysostosis. *J Clin Endocrinol Metab* 37:46–55, 1973.

Maroteaux P, Lamy M: La pycnodysostose. *Presse Méd* 70:999–1002, 1962.

Nielsen EL: Pycnodysostosis. *Acta Paediatr Scand* 63:437–442, 1974.

Sedano HO, et al: Pycnodysostosis: Clinical and genetic considerations. *Am J Dis Child* 116:70–77, 1968.

7.11 Rieger Syndrome

Rosano in 1934 and Rieger in 1935 described the syndrome composed of (1) hypodontia (partial anodontia) and (2) hypoplasia of the iridial

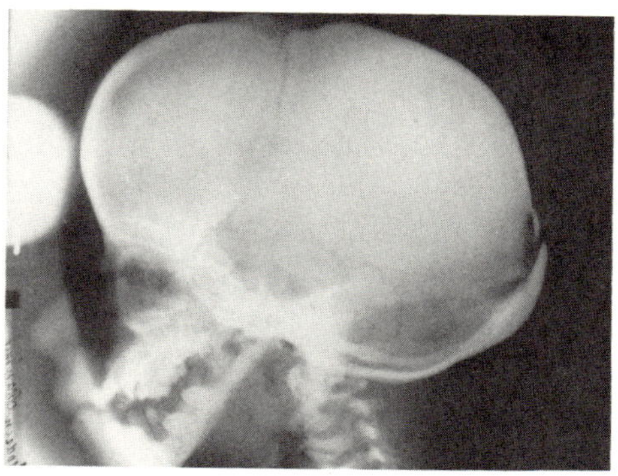

Fig. 7.20. Skull roentgenogram from another patient showing open sutures, closed fontanels, increased bone density, and absence of mandibular angle.

stroma, but the syndrome was probably first noticed by Vossius in 1883. The condition is inherited in an autosomal dominant manner with 95% penetrance and variable expressivity, especially of the dental abnormalities.

Facies. The face is characterized by an apparent mandibular prognathism with a receding upper lip, which gives a sunken appearance to the mouth. In addition the nose is broad, and in over 40% percent of cases there is mild hypertelorism with mild telecanthus.

Oral Structures. Oral manifestations include a relatively underdeveloped premaxilla and marked hypodontia (Fig. 7.21). The maxillary hypoplasia is responsible for the apparent prognathism and the receding upper lip. Severe reduction in the number of teeth has been reported in nearly every case. In less seriously affected patients, the teeth most commonly missing are the maxillary incisors. Enamel hypoplasia, conical crown form, microdontia, and malposition are also associated with the syndrome.

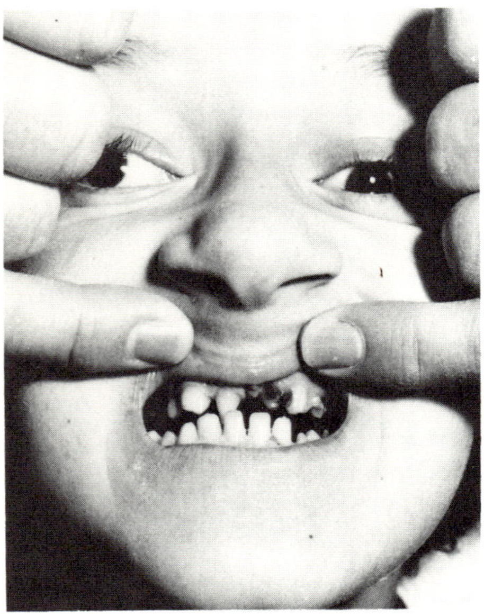

Fig. 7.21. Note strabismus, oligodontia, and conical shaped teeth.

Systemic Features. Physical and mental development are within normal limits. The most frequent ocular findings are hypoplasia and flattening of the anterior surface of the iris and anterior synechiae running from the iris to the cornea across the anterior chamber, producing abnormalities of the iridiocorneal angle. Dyscoria or slit-like pupils result from traction of these synechiae. Other ocular findings include aniridia, optic atrophy, microcornea, and corneal opacity. Pupillary anomalies are present in over 70% of affected individuals, the most frequent finding being ectopic pupil. Secondary juvenile glaucoma is a frequent complication that can cause loss of function and lead to total blindness.

Differential Diagnosis. Incontinentia pigmenti, chondroectodermal dysplasia, and the ectodermal dysplasias should be considered in the differential diagnosis. Gorlin and coworkers (1975) and Sensenbrenner and colleagues (1975) independently described a syndrome composed of Rieger anomaly, severe growth retardation, inguinal hernia, hypermobility of joints, sunken eyes, and delayed teething, inherited in an autosomal recessive manner. This condition should be differentiated from the Rieger syndrome.

Laboratory Aids. None known.

Synonym. Oligodontia and mesodermal dysgenesis of the iris and cornea.

References

Alkemade PPH: *Dysgenesis Mesodermalis of the Iris and the Cornea.* The Netherlands, Van Corcum, 1969.

Feingold M, et al: Rieger's syndrome. *Pediatrics* 44:564–569, 1969.

Gorlin RJ, et al: Rieger anomaly and growth retardation (the S-H-O-R-T syndrome). *Birth Def* 11(2):46–48, 1975.

Langdon JD: Rieger's syndrome. *Oral Surg* 30:788–795, 1970.

Rieger H: Beitrage zur Kenntnis seltener Missbildungen der Iris. *Graefes Arch Ophth* 133:602–635, 1935.

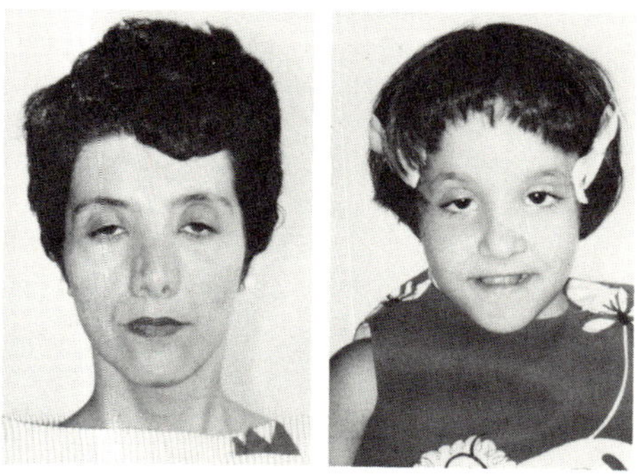

Fig. 7.22. Mother and daughter with the syndrome. Note low-set hairline, ptosis of eyelids, and strabismus. The daughter also has deviated septum.

Rossano R: Absence presque complete du feuillet mésodermique de l'iris dans deux générations. Hypertension oculaire concomitante et polycorie dans un cas. *Bull Soc Ophth* (Paris) 46:8–17, 1934.

Sensenbrenner JA, et al: A low-birthweight syndrome; Rieger syndrome. *Birth Def* 11(2):424–426.

7.12 Saethre-Chotzen Syndrome

The syndrome was first described by Saethre in 1931, followed by Chotzen in 1932. It is characterized by (1) craniosynostosis of variable degree, (2) asymmetric facies, and (3) low-set hairline. The condition is inherited in an autosomal dominant manner with marked penetrance and variable expressivity. Advanced parental age has been reported in isolated cases.

Facies. The typical asymmetric facies is characterized by protruding forehead, large parrot-shaped nose with septum deviation and low frontal hairline (Fig. 7.22). Unilateral or bilateral ptosis of eyelids with mild hypertelorism and strabismus adds to the typical facial appearance. Tear duct anomalies are also a common finding.

Oral Structures. The maxillary bones are almost always mildly hypoplastic, producing a relative prognathism (Fig. 7.23). High-arched palate is an almost constant feature. Clefting of the palate has been reported in several instances.

Systemic Features. Growth and physical development are generally within normal limits, but some patients have been reported to be short. The skull is brachycephalic with marked craniosynostosis. Bilateral parietal bossing, in most cases, is due to early asymmetric involvement of either coronal or sphenobasilar sutures. The early closure of the cranial sutures may cause in some cases an increased intracranial pressure with associated microcephaly, mental retardation of various degrees, and marked visual difficulties due to optic nerve atrophy. Sensorineural deafness has been reported in several patients. Low-set ears with small deformed pinnae are seen in over half of the cases.

The hands are generally small. Clinodactyly of the fifth finger occasionally may be observed. Syndactyly, when present, will manifest as a webbing between the proximal phalanges 2–3 or 2–3–4 in the hands and 2–3 or 4–5 in the feet. Bilateral simian creases are observed in the majority of affected individuals. Hallux valgus is also frequently observed.

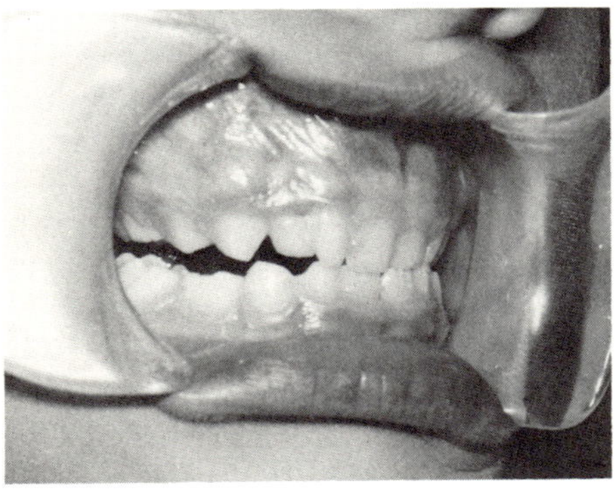

Fig. 7.23. Intraoral view of another patient with the syndrome. Note peg lateral incisors and occlusion type III.

Differential Diagnosis. Acrocephalosyndactyly, OFD I and II, orocraniodigital dysostosis, oculodentoosseous dysplasia, and Crouzon syndrome should be included.

Laboratory Aids. None known.

Synonyms. Acrocephalosyndactyly type III, pseudo-Crouzon syndrome, familial craniosynostosis.

References

Bartsocas CS, et al: Acrocephalosyndactyly type III: Chotzen's syndrome. *J Pediatr* 77:267–272, 1970.

Chotzen F: Eine eigernartige familiäre Entwicklungsstörung. (Akrocephalosyndaktylie, Dysostosis craniofacialis und Hypertelorismus.) *Monatsschr Kinderheilkd* 55:97–121, 1932.

Kreiborg S, et al: The Saethre-Chotzen syndrome. *Teratology* 6:287–294, 1972.

Pantke OA, et al: The Saethre-Chotzen syndrome. *Birth Def* 11(2):190–225, 1975.

Saethre H: Ein Beitrag zum Turmschädelproblem. (Pathogenese, Erblichkeit und Symptomatologie.) *Dtsch Z Nervenheilkd* 117:533–555, 1931.

7.13 Trichodentoosseous Syndrome

The trichodentoosseous syndrome was first described by Robinson and coworkers in 1966. The condition is characterized by (1) taurodont teeth, (2) hypoplastic-hypocalcified enamel, (3) cortical osteosclerosis, (4) tight, curly hair, and (5) thick cornified or splitting nails. The syndrome is inherited in an autosomal dominant manner.

Facies. Affected individuals are dolichocephalic and often demonstrate frontal bossing and a square jaw.

Oral Structures. The teeth are usually taurodont, revealing enlarged and apically placed pulp chambers. The enamel defects are variable; hypoplasia, hypomaturation, and hypocalcification phenotypes have been described in the syndrome. The most frequent enamel change, however, has been enamel hypoplasia (Fig. 7.24). Delayed eruption of the primary teeth with failure of eruption of the secondary dentition has also been described. Radiographically, the mandible is characterized by an obtuse inferior angle and shortened ramus.

Systemic Features. Mental and somatic development are within normal limits. Osteosclerosis of the bone cortex, without cortical thickening, is characteristic but variable, and is present in only half of reported cases. The osseous defect is characterized by a radiographic increase in bone density of both flat and long bones. The base of the skull is the most consistent site of bone involvement. The earliest characteristic of the condition is the development of a full head of tightly curled hair in infancy. This feature may be retained into adulthood, but often is lost and the hair may become straight. Thick, cornified nails or laminated splitting of the nails have been described; however this is the least consistent manifestation of the condition.

Differential Diagnosis. Differential diagnosis should include Vitamin D-resistant rickets (large pulp chamber), Menkes syndrome (hair), and the syndromal association of hypoplastic-hypocalcified enamel, onycholysis and functional hypohidrosis.

Synonyms. Amelogenesis imperfecta, taurodontism, curly hair, and sclerotic bones.

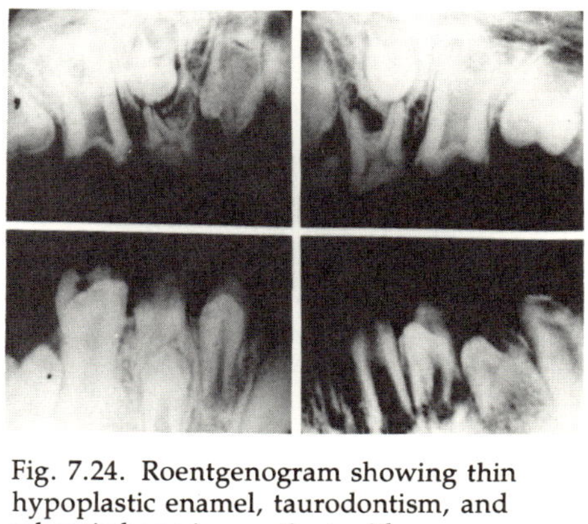

Fig. 7.24. Roentgenogram showing thin hypoplastic enamel, taurodontism, and sclerotic bone in a patient with trichodentoosseous syndrome.

References

Jorgenson RJ, Warson RW: Dental abnormalities in the tricho-dento-osseous syndrome. *Oral Surg* 36:693–700, 1973.

Lichtenstein J, et al: The tricho-dento-osseous (TDO) syndrome. *Am J Hum Genet* 24:569–582, 1972.

Robinson GC, et al: Hereditary enamel hypoplasia; its association with characteristic hair structures, *Pediatrics* 37:498–502, 1966.

Soft Tissue and Teeth

7.14 Chondroectodermal Dysplasia

The syndrome was first described as an entity by Ellis and van Creveld in 1940. Several earlier reports may be found under various designations. Typically the syndrome consists of (1) bilateral manual ulnar polydactyly, (2) chondrodysplasia of long bones, resulting in acromelic dwarfism, (3) hidrotic ectodermal dysplasia affecting principally the nails and teeth, and in half of the cases (4) congenital heart malformations. The syndrome is inherited in an autosomal recessive manner. We have found the consanguinity rate among the parents of affected patients to be 30%. McKusick and coworkers (1964) found 52 cases in 30 families among an Amish isolate.

Facies. The face does not present any striking characteristic. Generally the middle portion of the upper lip presents a slight V-notch, resembling a lip that has undergone cheiloplasty.

Oral Structures. Oral manifestations are quite characteristic and constant, comprising fusion of the anterior portion of the upper lip to the maxillary gingival margin, so that no mucobuccal fold exists anteriorly (Fig. 7.25). This explains the V-notch in the upper lip. The anterior portion of the lower alveolar ridge is often serrated. The two central incisors, either of the primary or secondary dentitions, are generally replaced by an abnormally shaped tooth. Other teeth tend to be somewhat conical in shape, and at times to have hypoplastic enamel. In more than half of the reported cases, teeth are present at birth.

Systemic Features. One-third of the patients are mildly mentally retarded. Dwarfism is due to shortening of the extremities, which progresses distalward (Fig. 7.26). Tubular bones are shortened and thickened with plump diaphyseal ends. Manual polydactyly is almost constant, the extra digit being on the ulnar side. Rarely, extra toes are found. Other skeletal anomalies such as genu valgum, talipes equinovarus and calcaneovalgus, pigeon breast, and curvature of the humerus have occasionally been reported. Congenital heart anomalies of the nature of interseptal defect, cor triloculare, or cor biloculare have been noted in 50% of affected individuals. Usually there is marked koilonychia and hypoplasia of fingernails and toenails. Affected males may show cryptorchidism, epispadias, or hypospadias.

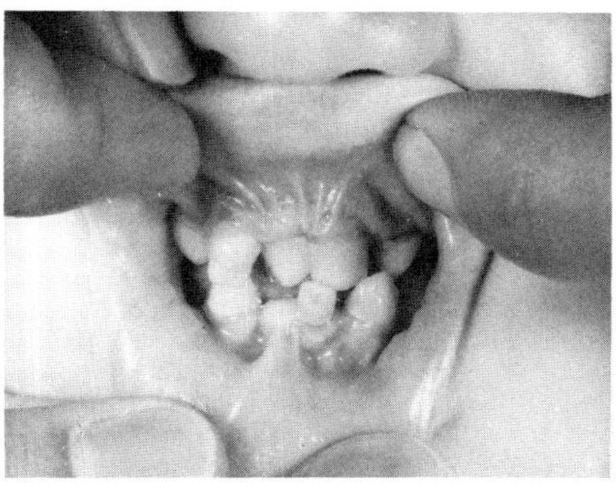

Fig. 7.25. Intraoral photograph showing total absence of superior mucobuccal fold, wide adhesions between lower lip and mandibular gingiva, and malposed abnormal teeth.

Differential Diagnosis. Achondroplasia, asphyxiating thoracic dystrophy, Morquio syndrome, and other chondrodystrophic syndromes should be considered. OFD I and the ectodermal dysplasias also should be included in the differential diagnosis.

Laboratory Aids. None known.

Synonym. Ellis–van Creveld syndrome.

References

Biggerstaff RH, Mazaheri M: Oral manifestations of the Ellis–van Creveld syndrome. *J Am Dent Assoc* 77:1090–1095, 1968.

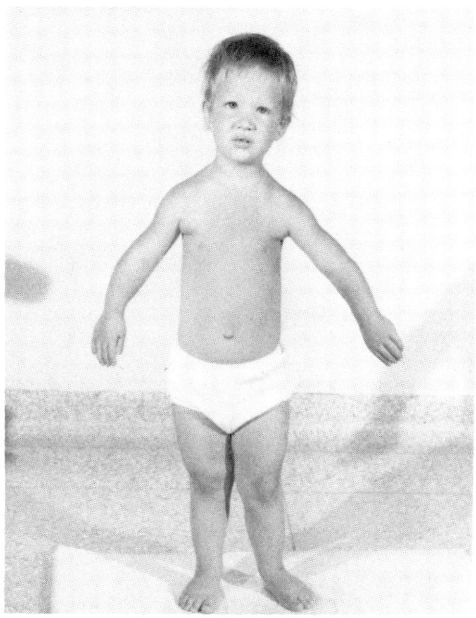

Fig. 7.26. Female, five years old, with the Ellis–van Creveld syndrome. Note apparently long chest due to mesomelia of both upper and lower extremities. Also note mild ocular hypertelorism.

Ellis RWB, van Creveld SA: A syndrome characterized by ectodermal dysplasia, polydactyly, chondro-dysplasia and congenital morbus cordis. *Arch Dis Child* 15:65–84, 1940.

McKusick VA, et al: Dwarfism in the Amish. I. The Ellis–van Creveld syndrome. *Bull Johns Hopkins Hosp* 115:306–336, 1964.

Winter GB, Geddes M: Oral manifestations of chondroectodermal dysplasia (Ellis–van Creveld syndrome). *Br Dent J* 122:103–107, 1967.

7.15 Congenital Hypertrophy of the Gingiva, Altered Eruption of Teeth, and Corneal Dystrophy

Rutherfurd in 1931 described a syndrome consisting of (1) gingival hypertrophy, (2) failure of tooth eruption, and (3) corneal opacities. The condition is inherited in an autosomal dominant manner.

Facies. The intense hypertrophy of the gingiva protrudes the lips, giving a full-mouth appearance.

Oral Structures. The gingival fibromatosis does not reach the immense proportions seen in other gingival fibromatoses. Few teeth may erupt or the complete dentition may remain within the jaws. Occasionally root resorption of the primary teeth may be noted in the unerupted teeth.

Systemic Features. Somatic and mental development are within normal limits. Corneal opacities appear as a result of dense curtain-like structures over the cornea.

Differential Diagnosis. Gingival fibromatosis as a result of Cowden, Cross, Murray, and Zimmermann-Laband syndromes should be considered in the differential diagnosis. In addition, hereditary benign intraepithelial dyskeratosis must be considered in evaluating corneal opacities.

Laboratory Aids. None known.

Synonym. Rutherfurd syndrome.

References

Houston IB, Shotts W: Rutherfurd's syndrome: a familial oculodental disorder. *Acta Paediatr Scand* 55:233–238, 1966.

Rutherfurd ME: Three generations of inherited dental defect. *Br Med J* 2:9–11, 1931.

7.16 Endocrine-Candidosis Syndrome

The syndrome consists of (1) Addison disease, associated with (2) idiopathic hypoparathyroidism and (3) moniliasis. Hypothyroidism, pernicious anemia, juvenile cirrhosis, and ovarian failure also can be present. The condition appears to be inherited in an autosomal recessive manner. Genetic heterogeneity also has been suggested and expressivity is variable.

Facies. The facial skin is dry, scalp hair and eyebrows are sparse, and total alopecia may occasionally ensue. Keratoconjunctivitis, photophobia, and cataracts may also be part of the clinical picture.

Oral Structures. The oral moniliasis involves any or all of the oral mucosa with possible extension into the fauces and larynx (Fig. 7.27). This yeast infection is characterized by thick white plaque-like colonies developing between areas of marked hyperemia. Tongue depapillation as well as angular cheilosis are also observed as part of the infectious process. Later in the course of the disease irregular areas of intraoral pigmentation will be seen directly related to the onset of Addison disease. Enamel hypoplasia and hypocalcification, generally not severe, are observed in the majority of patients (Fig. 7.28). The hypocalcification is characterized by a horizontal linear appearance. Some investigators have noted an increased incidence of dental caries. This finding may be related to the aforementioned areas of hypocalcification. Abnormalities in root formation also have been observed.

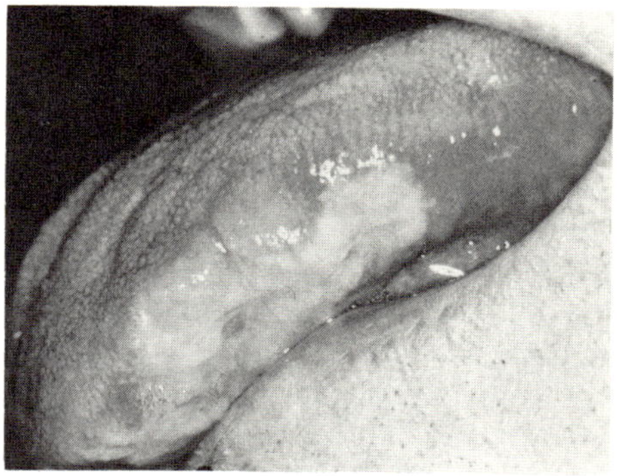

Fig. 7.27. Note extensive monilial granuloma on lateral border of tongue.

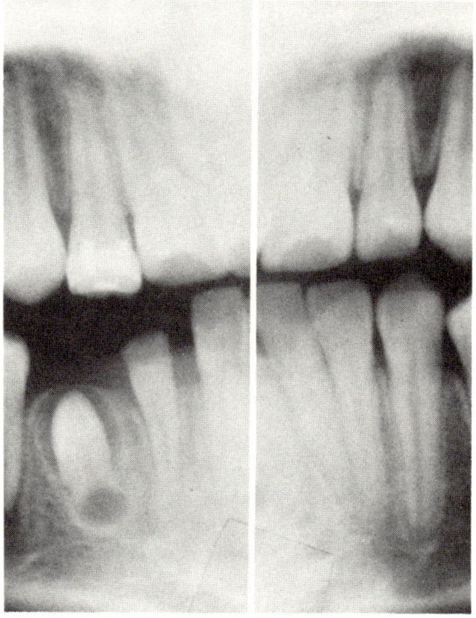

Fig. 7.28. Intraoral radiograph from another patient with the syndrome demonstrating enamel hypoplasia secondary to hypoparathyroidism.

Systemic Features. Somatic and mental development are both within normal limits. All components of the syndrome do not occur simultaneously. The moniliasis is nearly always the first component to appear, generally during the first 6 years of life. It is usually followed by the other components from 3 months to 13 years later. The hypoparathyroidism and hypoadrenal corticalism become manifest most frequently between 9 and 12 years of age, in that order of appearance. The hypoparathyroidism when present is most often associated with tetany.

Other manifestations may include intracranial calcification, epileptiform seizures, abdominal pain and paraesthesias. Fingernails and toenails are frequently affected by candida infections, thus having an irregular brown appearance. Addison disease closely follows the manifestations of hypoparathyroidism and is characterized in the usual way, ie, malaise, hypotension, skin and mucous membrane pigmentation. A high percentage of patients with the syndrome die as a consequence of adrenal crisis.

Differential Diagnosis. Isolated Addison disease, hypoparathyroidism and generalized moniliasis, as well as ectodermal dysplasia and acrodermatitis enteropathica should be included in the differential diagnosis.

Laboratory Aids. Laboratory studies demonstrate low serum sodium and high potassium levels. Adrenal insufficiency can be demonstrated by the injection of ACTH and consequent failure to effect a rise in urinary levels of 17-hydroxycorticosterone and 17-ketosteroids. The serum calcium level is reduced and the serum phosphorus level elevated in the absence of significant disease of the genitourinary and gastrointestinal systems. Furthermore, parathyroid hormone injection results in an increase in the level of serum calcium and in elevated urinary phosphorus excretion.

Synonyms. Addison disease, idiopathic familial juvenile hypoparathyroidism, keratoconjunctivitis, and superficial moniliasis.

References

Greenberg MS, et al: Idiopathic hypoparathyroidism, chronic candidiasis and dental hypoplasia. *Oral Surg* 28:42–53, 1969.

Kirkpatrick CH, et al: Chronic mucocutaneous candidiasis: Model-building in cellular immunity. *Ann Intern Med* 74:955–978, 1971.

Perheentupa J, Hiekkala H: Twenty cases of the syndrome of autoimmune endocrinopathy and candidiasis. *Acta Paediatr Scand* 62:110–111, 1973.

7.17 Epidermolysis Bullosa

Epidermolysis bullosa (EB) has been known since antiquity, but the classic descriptions are those of Hebra and Goldscheiner (in the 1800s). The syndrome occurs in four different clinical forms with several subtypes. The basic classification is as follows: (1) EB simple, autosomal dominant, (2) EB dystrophic, autosomal dominant, (3) EB dystrophic, autosomal recessive, (4) EB lethal, autosomal recessive.

In the simple type, bullae and vesicles in the skin, generally of the extremities, are present at birth or appear during the first months of life. This condition does not interfere with growth and does not result in scarring. Oral manifestations are absent in this type of EB.

The clinical manifestations in the dominant dystrophic type, or Cockayne-Touraine type, generally appear around one year of age in the form of bullae on the ankles, knees, elbows, hands, and feet. Bullae heal with scar formation. The condition becomes less severe with age. The eyes are never affected but there are intraoral bullae and milia.

Infants born with the lethal (Herlitz) form of EB generally die early in infancy. The first manifestations are in the form of blood filled vesicles appearing at the base of the fingernails. The nails are soon shed. Vesiculation and extensive skin involvement soon ensues. Oral manifestations are present in the form of bullae, generally at the junction of the soft and hard palates. Some studies have demonstrated enamel and dentin alteration in both primary and secondary dentitions in an infant with this form of EB.

The most common autosomal recessively inherited dystrophic form of EB will be described in detail.

Facies. The facial skin is often involved in the generalized blister formation characteristic of the syndrome. Microstomia and immobility of the lips are evident, especially in older individuals.

Oral Structures. The oral mucosa is the site of lesions in over 80% of patients. These lesions generally first appear during the nursing period and at the site of feeding pressure. They develop in any area of the oral cavity, the tongue being most frequently affected. Blister formation is followed by rupture, leaving a raw bleeding surface. Healing results in thick fibrous scars which may limit the mobility of lips and tongue. Loss of lingual papillae has been noted as a sequel to recurrent blistering and scarring. Other mucosal manifestations include ecchymosis, leukoplakia-like lesions, and erosions.

Squamous cell carcinoma is known to develop in these patients, especially in the most frequent and severely affected intraoral sites. Enamel hypoplasia is not uncommon (Fig. 7.29). Caries occur with increased frequency, due to the almost impossible task of proper tooth-brushing, and many, if not all, of the teeth are lost on this account. Denture wearing is also difficult for these patients, due to the frequent blister formation at the sites of pressure.

Systemic Features. The bullae are seen on the skin at or shortly after birth, generally at sites of pressure such as feet, elbows, fingers, buttocks, scapulae, occiput, and knees (Fig. 7.30). When the bullae rupture, they leave a raw, painful surface that may become secondarily infected. As the lesions heal, keloid scars form that may produce contraction and pigmentation or depigmentation of various degrees. Fingernails and toenails are dystrophic or absent (Fig. 7.31). Clawhand develops because of scarring (Fig. 7.32). Blisters are also present in the eyes, larynx, and esophagus. Scarring of these sites leads to shrinkage of the conjunctiva, to hoarseness and laryngeal stenosis, and to dysphagia.

Differential Diagnosis. In infants, children, and adolescents, the following conditions should be considered: juvenile dermatitis herpetiformis, viral bullous diseases, pemphigus neonatorum, congenital syphilis, and congenital porphyria, among others. In adults, all the bullae-forming diseases including pemphigus, pem-

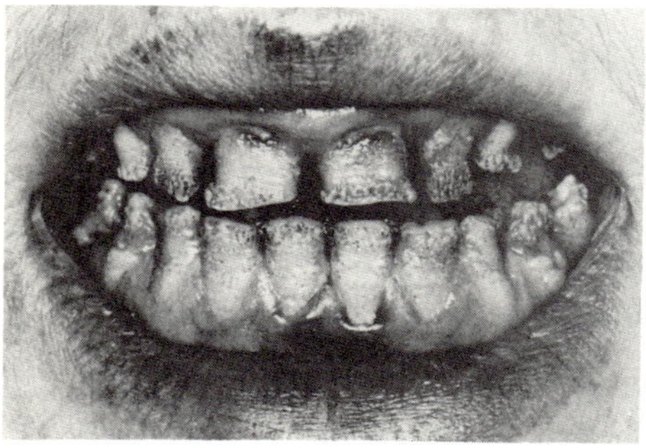

Fig. 7.29. Pitted hypoplastic enamel.

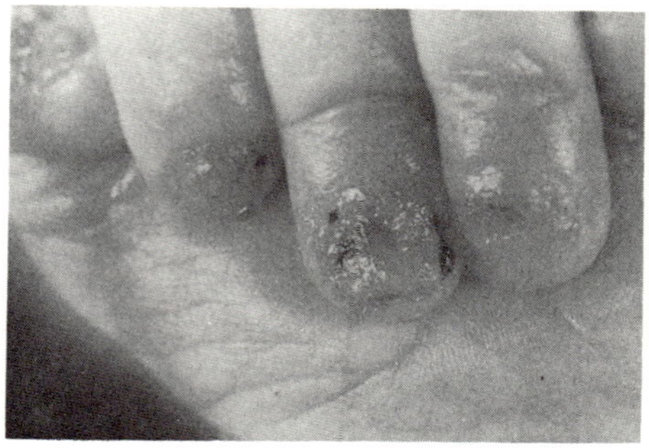

Fig. 7.31. Marked destruction of fingernails in newborn.

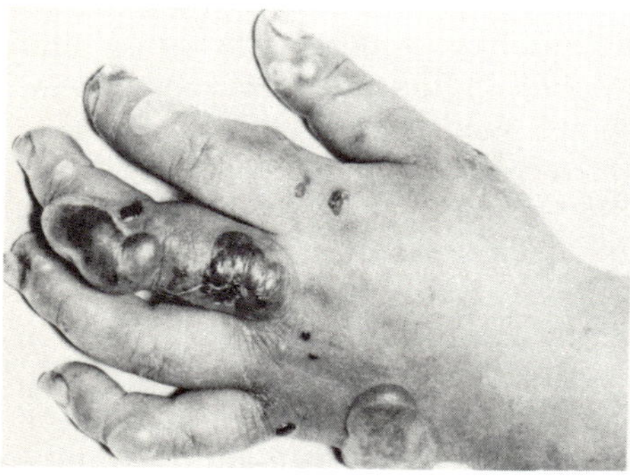

Fig. 7.30. Extensive formation of bullae on hands.

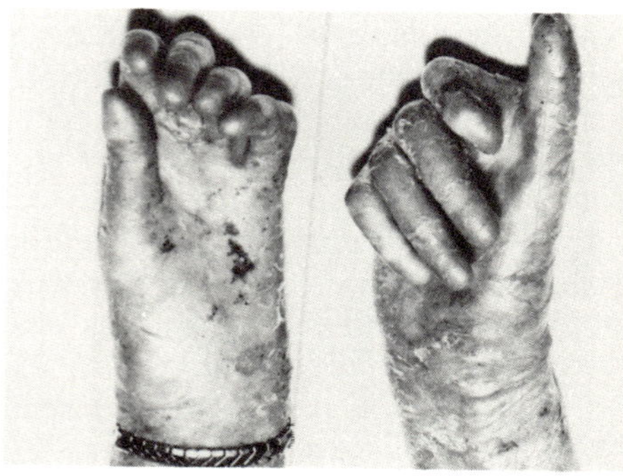

Fig. 7.32. Severe involvement of hands with marked scarring and loss of nails.

phigoid, and erythema multiforme should be included in the differential diagnosis.

Laboratory Aids. Biopsy of affected skin or mucosa will demonstrate either intraepithelial or subepithelial formation of bullae. In the first case, the splitting takes place below the stratum corneum, and this is generally seen in the simple type of EB. Subepithelial bullae are seen in the dystrophic types of the condition. Differential diagnosis, again, should be established with the group of bullous dermatologic diseases.

References

Andreasen JO, et al: Milia formation in oral lesions in epidermolysis bullosa. *Acta Pathol Microbiol Scand* 63:37–41, 1965.

Gedde-Dahl T, Jr: *Epidermolysis Bullosa: A Clinical, Genetic, and Epidemiologic Study*. Baltimore, Johns Hopkins, 1971.

Pearson RW: Epidermolysis bullosa hereditaria letalis. *Arch Dermatol* 109:349–355, 1974.

7.18 Hyalinosis Cutis et Mucosa

The syndrome, first described by Siebenmann in 1908, consists of (1) yellowish nodular hyaline infiltration of skin and mucous membranes and (2) hoarseness. The condition is clearly inherited in an autosomal recessive manner. Familial cases as well as increased consanguinity among the parents of affected patients have been reported frequently.

Facies. Yellow waxy nodules of variable size usually occur on the face. This patchy hyalinization of the skin becomes confluent and fissuring occurs especially around the eyes and lips, giving the face a typical appearance. Rarely, pustular and vesicular lesions may appear. On the margin of the eyelid, bead-like excrescences arise, followed by loss of cilia.

Oral Structures. The mouth is the site of numerous lesions. The majority of the oral tissues, frequently before puberty, become infiltrated with yellowish white, elevated, pea-sized plaques. The lower lip assumes a cobblestone appearance, and radiating fissures appear at the angles of the mouth (Fig. 7.33). Lesions increase in severity with age. The tongue becomes depapillated and macroglossia is evident (Fig. 7.34). The large tongue seems to be bound to the oral floor. Infiltration of the lingual frenum and sublingual areas is also evident. Progression of the lesions on the buccal mucosa will produce total obliteration of the parotid duct opening, with consequent retrograde parotitis. Dysphagia is also seen as a sequel to infiltration of the pharynx. Teeth may fail to develop or may be hypoplastic.

Systemic Features. Mental and physical development are within normal limits. Intracranial calcification, located above the pituitary fossa in the hippocampus, falx cerebri, or temporal lobes, has been found in a considerable number of patients. Epilepsy is seen in about 20% of patients. Discrete or confluent yellowish ivory or waxy nodules of various size are seen on the neck, axillae, and hands early in life. Wartlike hyperkeratotic lesions with a brownish yellow tinge appear on the elbows, knees, and proximal interarticular surfaces of the fingers.

The voice may be hoarse from birth, or may become so at puberty. Early laryngeal involvement is evidenced by the inability to cry, present from birth. Laryngoscopic examination demonstrates plaques and node-like lesions in the epiglottis, in the aryepiglottic folds, and in the interarytenoid region. The vocal cords are thick and nodular with insufficient closure. Dyspnea is a frequent complication and laryngectomy is occasionally performed to clear the airway. Death from severe laryngeal obstruction has occurred occasionally.

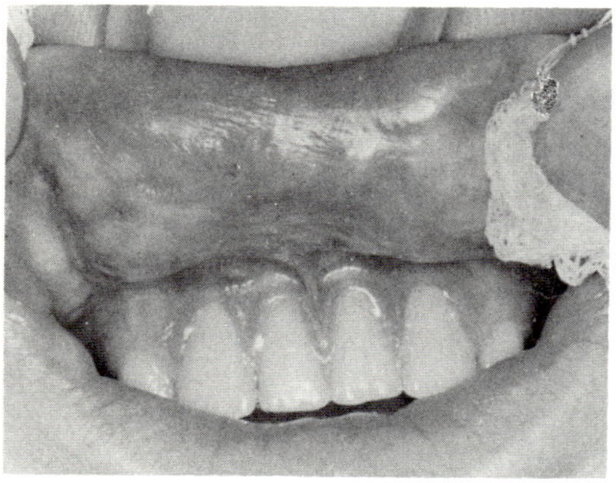

Fig. 7.33. Note cobblestone appearance of lower labial mucosa.

Differential Diagnosis. Primary amyloidosis, pseudoxanthoma elasticum, and adenoma sebaceum should be included among other conditions in the differential diagnosis.

Laboratory Aids. Results of a biopsy are quite specific, and microscopically one notes hyalinosis of the upper layers of the corium or dermis, beginning in the small capillaries or in the sweat glands. The elastic fibers are destroyed. Argyrophilic fibrils appear throughout the dermis. The hyaline material stains intensely with the periodic acid-Schiff (PAS) reaction, and appears to be a glycoprotein with associated free or loosely bound lipid.

Synonyms. Lipoid proteinosis, Urbach-Wiethe syndrome.

References

Gordon H, et al: Lipoid proteinosis. *Birth Def* 7(8):164–177, 1972.

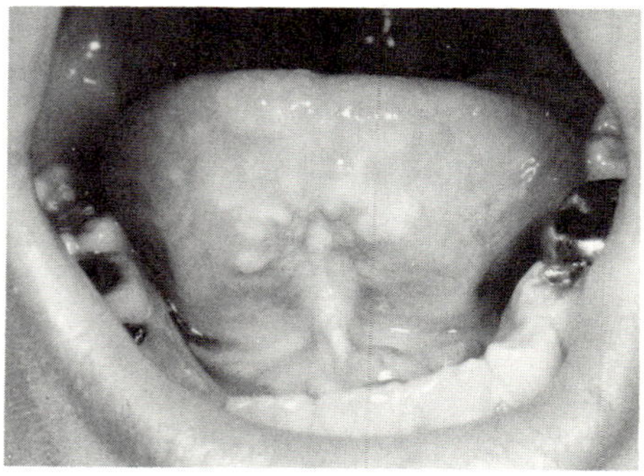

Fig. 7.34. Plaques as seen in the undersurface of the tongue are also present on the lateral borders and dorsum.

Hofer PA, and Öhman J: Laryngeal lesions in Urbach-Wiethe disease. *Acta Pathol Microbiol Scand* 82A:547–558, 1974.

Juberg RC, et al: A case of hyalinosis cutis et mucosae with common ancestors in four remote generations. *J Med Genet* 12:110–112, 1975.

7.19 Hypohidrotic (Anhidrotic) Ectodermal Dysplasia

The syndrome was probably first described by Danz in 1792. Later studies described the major components of the condition as (1) hypodontia, (2) hypotrichosis, and (3) hypohidrosis. Principally affected are structures of ectodermal origin. The syndrome is usually transmitted as an X-linked recessive condition. Therefore, the majority of affected patients are males. However, a great number of females (over 40 cases) have manifested the complete syndrome. The increased parental consanguinity in these cases suggests autosomal recessive inheritance and illustrates the genetic heterogeneity of this syndrome.

Facies. The face is quite characteristic, and affected individuals look enough alike to be mistaken for siblings. The skull resembles an inverted triangle. Marked frontal bossing, depressed nasal bridge (simulating the saddle nose of congenital syphilis), protuberant lips and obliquely inserted ears are the most prominent features (Fig. 7.35). Linear wrinkles are seen about the eyes and mouth.

Oral Structures. The most striking

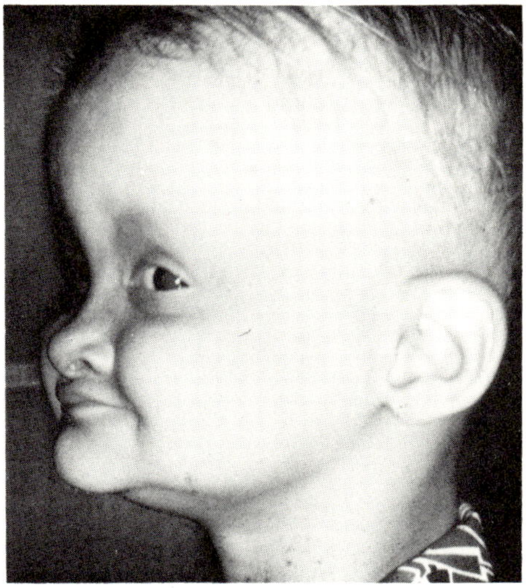

Fig. 7.35. Six-year-old male with the X-linked form of ectodermal dysplasia. Note thin hair, frontal bossing, and depressed nasal bridge.

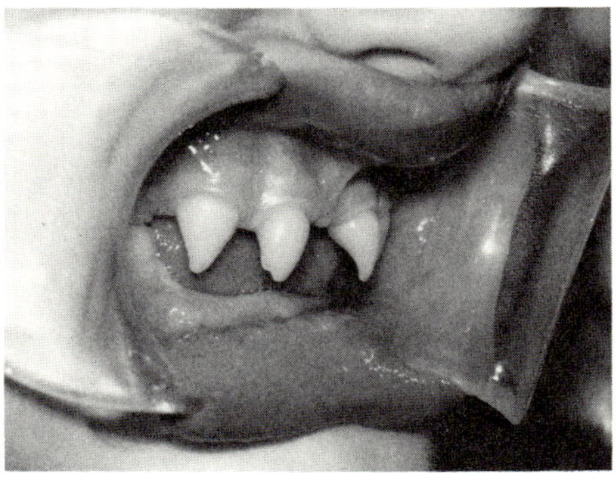

Fig. 7.36. Intraoral view from patient with X-linked form of ED. Teeth are conical; oligodontia is evident.

oral finding is oligodontia, or in some cases, anodontia (Fig. 7.36). The few teeth that may be present, generally incisors and canines, have a conical crown form. The alveolar process will not develop in the absence of teeth, resulting in loss of vertical dimension, with consequent protruding lips.

Systemic Structures. Physical and mental development are within normal limits. Hypohidrotic ectodermal dysplasia may not be clinically manifested until the second year of life, and because the physical features are not so apparent, the child may have a "fever of unknown origin." The inability to sweat, due to marked aplasia of the eccrine sweat glands, results in intolerance to heat, with severe hyperpyrexia. The skin is soft and thin, presenting severe dryness, due to diminished numbers of sebaceous glands, but eczema is uncommon. Small hyperkeratotic plaques are frequently noted on the palms and soles.

At birth, the body is devoid of lanugo hair; after puberty, the beard is generally normal, but axillary and pubic hair is scant. The scalp hair is generally blond, fine, stiff, and short. The eyelashes and especially the eyebrows are often entirely missing. The fingernails and toenails are usually normal or slightly spoon-shaped.

Differential Diagnosis. Dominant hidrotic forms of ectodermal dysplasia are different syndromes from the one considered here. Progeria and congenital syphilis should be included in the differential diagnosis. Table 7.1 lists all the disorders published to date that present involvement of structures derived from ectoderm.

Laboratory Aids. The ability to sweat is easily demonstrated by employing the starch-iodine test. Other methods are available, such as agar plates with silver nitrate and potassium chromate, and O-phthalaldialdehyde in xylene. Sweat pore counts using dental rubber base can also be performed.

Synonym. Christ-Siemens-Touraine syndrome.

References

Crump JA, Danks DM: Hypohidrotic ectodermal dysplasia. *J Pediatr* 78:466–473, 1971.

Gorlin RJ, et al: Hypohidrotic ectodermal dysplasia in females: A critical analysis and argument for genetic heterogeneity. *Z Kinderheilkd* 108:1–11, 1970.

Witkop CJ, Jr, et al: Hypoplastic enamel, onycholysis and hypohidrosis inherited as an autosomal dominant trait. A review of ectodermal dysplasia syndromes. *Oral Surg* 39:71–86, 1975.

7.20 Mucolipidosis II

Mucolipidosis II was originally described as a distinct entity by DeMars and Leroy in 1967 as characterized by (1) short stature, (2) psychomotor retardation, (3) Hurler-like facies, (4) gingival enlargement, and (5) death from heart failure early in life. The condition is another example of genetic heterogeneity, with the majority of the cases inherited in an autosomal recessive manner. The fibroblasts of ML-II contain numerous granular inclusions in their cytoplasm, which are believed to be altered lysosomes. At present there is no convincing evidence that storage of either a specific mucopolysaccharide or lipid exists. Both culture medium of ML II cells grown in vitro and the serum of affected patients have shown an increased activity of several acid hydrolases, suggesting lisosomal leakage. However, some investigators have interpreted these data to indicate that ML II cells contain improperly processed enzyme molecules, which lack specificity for uptake into lysosomes. To date the basic defect remains unknown.

Facies. The facies is typified by inapparent supraorbital ridges and full cheeks covered with fine telangiectasias (Fig. 7.37). The lips are protuberant and the eyelids are puffy. The orbits are small and there is some exophthalmus present. Tortous veins have been noted about the temporal region and around the orbits. A significant nasal discharge may be present, but to a lesser degree than in MPS I-H. Clinically the corneas appear clear.

Oral Structures. The gingiva are greatly enlarged and may completely cover the teeth or prevent their eruption. Macroglossia may result in a chronically open mouth. The enamel is hypocalcified and the storage material may be noted about the unerupted teeth, especially the first molars.

Systemic Features. Severe shortness of stature is characteristic. Psychomotor retardation is present and severe. Muscular hypotonia and inguinal hernia may be the first characteristics noted after birth. Hepatomegaly is minimal and splenomegaly is usually not evident. Joint mobility is reduced. The hands, fingers, neck, and thoracic cavity are all shortened. The spine often reveals

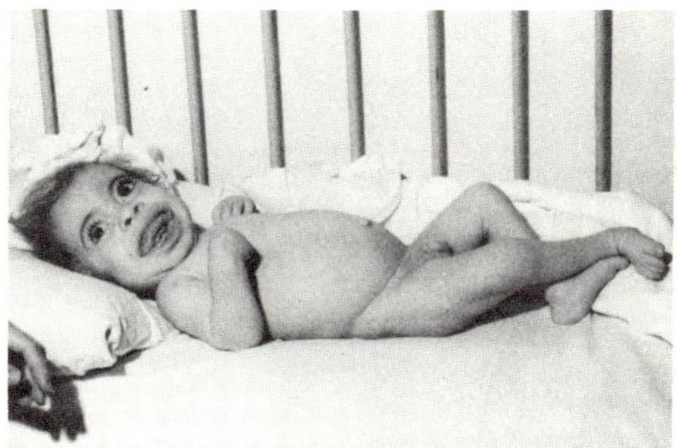

Fig. 7.37. Infant with I-cell disease. Note Hurleroid features.

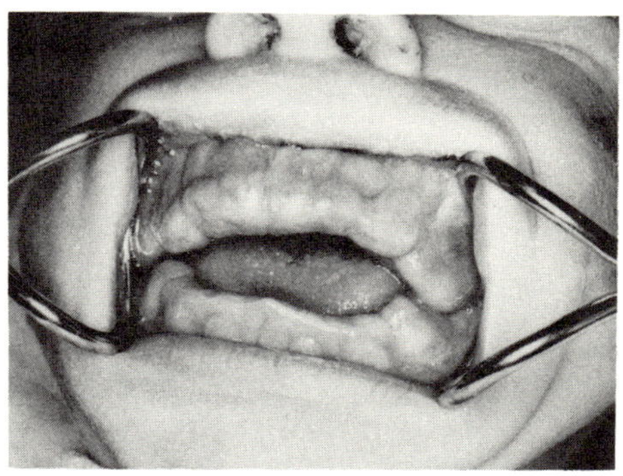

Fig. 7.38. Intraoral view of same patient showing prominent thickening of gingival mucosa and anterior open bite.

TABLE 7.1 *Ectodermal structures affected in various forms of ectodermal dysplasia**

CONDITION	HAIR	DENTITION
Hypohidrotic ectodermal dysplasia, X-linked	Hypotrichosis	Missing and conical teeth
Hypohidrotic ectodermal dysplasia, autosomal recessive	Hypotrichosis	Missing and conical teeth
Pachyonychia congenita Type II (Jackson and Lawler)	Dry hair, occasionally alopecia	Natal teeth
Epidermolysis bullosa dystrophica; several genetic types	Hypotrichosis in some patients	General hypoplasia or pitting of enamel; severity related to genetic type; eruption retarded in some patients
Focal dermal hypoplasia	Sparse hair in focal areas of scalp, pubis	Small malformed teeth, hypoplastic enamel, notching of incisors, extra incisors
Dyskeratosis congenita	Loss of cilia secondary to chronic blepharitis and ectropion	Teeth infrequently malformed
Odontotrichomelic hypohidrotic dysplasia	Hypotrichosis	Small, conical and missing teeth
Hypohidrotic ectodermal dysplasia with cleft lip/ palate and ocular, genital, and digital anomalies	Stiff, sparse, "steel wool," sparse eyebrows and lashes, no axillary or pubic hair	Missing teeth; short, square incisors and canines; hypoplastic enamel
Ectodermal dysplasia, cleft lip and palate, popliteal pterygia	Hypotrichosis	Small and conical teeth
Xeroderma, talipes and enamel defect-XTE syndrome	Dry, slow growing, no lashes on lower lids, scanty follicles in body skin	Yellow enamel (probably hypomaturation of enamel)
Coffin-Siris syndrome	Hypotrichosis of scalp hair; hypertrichosis of eyebrows and forehead	Small teeth
Rothmund-Thomson syndrome	Sparse to alopecia	Anomalous cusps and ridge pattern
Tooth and nail syndrome	Fine hair in a few patients; sparse to absent eyebrows	Missing and conical teeth
Tricho-dento-osseous syndrome	Tight curly hair	Taurodontism; hypoplastic enamel
Incontinentia pigmenti	Alopecia (pseudopelade) in 20 to 25%	Missing, small, conical, and impacted teeth
Palmoplantar keratosis, hypodontia, hypotrichosis and cysts of eyelids	Male type alopecia of scalp, little body hair	Missing teeth
Premolar aplasia, hyperhidrosis and canities premature (Böök syndrome)	White hair	Missing premolars

NAILS	SWEAT	INHERITANCE PATTERN
Infrequently spoon-shaped	Decreased number of sweat glands	X-linked recessive
Spoon-shaped	Decreased number of sweat glands	Autosomal recessive
Congenital to infantile onset of extremely thick subungual hyperkeratosis	Palmar and plantar hyperhidrosis	Autosomal dominant
Moderate to marked dystrophy, depending on genetic type	Palmar hyperhidrosis may be present in some cases	Autosomal recessive and dominant forms (genetic heterogeneity)
Dystrophic, thin nails, spoon-shaped or absent in about 50 per cent of patients	Dyshidrosis, hypo- or hyperhidrosis, mostly palmoplantar	Possibly X-linked dominant, lethal in the male
Dystrophic with onset late childhood or at puberty; short atrophic nails	Palmoplantar hyperhidrosis with palmar keratosis	X-linked and autosomal recessive forms (genetic heterogeneity)
Possibly hypoplastic	Hyporesponsiveness to pilocarpine	Possibly autosomal recessive
Small, dysplastic, with soft-tissue tufting	Reduced sweat on iontophoresis; no skin appendages on biopsy; fewer sweat glands; reduced response to pilocarpine and heat; hyperthermia	Possibly autosomal dominant
Dysplastic	Hypohidrosis	Possibly autosomal recessive
Small malformed toenails	Reduced number of sweat glands	Probably autosomal recessive, possibly homozygous autosomal dominant
Absent to hypoplastic fifth fingernails and toenails; other nails hypoplastic	No	Not an inherited disorder
Dystrophic in about one-fourth of patients	No	Autosomal recessive
Slow nail growth in children; small and frequently spoon-shaped; toenails most severely involved; adult fingernails may appear normal	No	Autosomal dominant
Thick, split	No	Autosomal dominant
Rarely dystrophic	No	X-linked dominant, lethal in the male
Fragility	No	Possibly autosomal recessive
No	Palmoplantar hyperhidrosis	Autosomal dominant

No: Not affected

Ectrodactyly, ectodermal dysplasia, and cleft lip/palate (EEC syndrome)	Sparse and fine; cilia absent	Small and conical teeth
Pachyonychia congenita, Type I (Jadassohn-Lewandowski)	Dry hair; infrequent alopecia	No
Freire-Maia syndrome	Partial alopecia with follicular hyperkeratosis of scalp	No
Hypoplastic enamel, onycholysis and hypohidrosis	No	Hypoplastic-hypocalcified enamel
Monilethrix and anodontia	Monilethrix	Conical and missing teeth in few cases
Gorlin-Chaudhry-Moss syndrome	Hypertrichosis	Missing; bell-shaped roots; reduced pulp chambers
Oculomandibulodyscephaly (Hallermann-Streiff syndrome)	Hypotrichosis	Conical, missing natal and supernumerary teeth; hypoplastic enamel
Tricho-rhino-phalangeal syndrome	Thin, slow-growing hair	Supernumerary incisors
Oculodento-osseous dysplasia	Dry, short hair in some cases	Hypoplastic enamel
Hypertrichosis lanuginosa	Facial and body hypertrichosis	Missing teeth
Orofacial digital syndrome I	Alopecia and dryness	Missing mandibular lateral incisors
Ungual type ectodermal dysplasia (hidrotic ED)	Alopecia, lanugo, or fine, short, dry, straight hair	No
Palmoplantar hyperkeratosis and alopecia	Alopecia to hypotrichosis of scalp; alopecia of brows and lashes	No
Curly hair-ankyloblepharon-nail dysplasia syndrome (CHANDS)	Curly	No
Focal facial dermal dysplasia	Focal hairless pigmented temporal forehead and chin lesions; may have absent or double row of eyelashes	No
Ectodermal dysplasia and deafness	No	Missing and conical teeth
Chondroectodermal dysplasia (Ellis-van Creveld syndrome)	No	Missing, conical, and natal teeth
Ectodermal dysplasia, deafness and ocular anomalies (Marshall syndrome)	No	Missing, small, and conical teeth
Palmoplantar hyperkeratosis with reticular pigmentation	No	Teeth infrequently involved with yellow flecks in enamel
Onycholysis	No	No
Onychodystrophy and deafness	No	No
Otodental syndrome	No	Globodontia, large globe-shaped teeth, cuspids through molars affected

*Modified from Witkop CJ, Jr., et al., Hypoplastic enamel, onycholysis, and hypohidrosis inherited as an autosomal dominant trait. A review of ectodermal dysplasia syndromes. *Oral Surg.* 39:711–86, 1975.

No	Hypohidrosis (starch test negative)	Autosomal dominant
Congenital to infantile onset of extremely thick subungual hyperkeratosis	Palmar and plantar hyperhidrosis	Autosomal dominant
Severe onychogryposis	Hypohidrosis unresponsive to pilocarpine	Inheritance pattern if any is unknown
Onycholysis	Hypofunction of sweat glands	Autosomal dominant
No	No	Possibly autosomal dominant
No	No	Autosomal recessive
No	No	Not an inherited disorder
No	No	Autosomal recessive and dominant forms (genetic heterogeneity)
No	No	Autosomal dominant
No	No	Possibly autosomal dominant
No	No	Autosomal dominant, lethal in the male
Children—convex nails with onycholysis of outer third; adults—longitudinal striations, convex ends, and thick horny subungual keratosis	No	Autosomal dominant
Small dystrophic with onycholysis	No	Autosomal dominant
Small dysplastic	No	Autosomal recessive
No	Absent sweat glands in focal lesions	Autosomal dominant
Small dystrophic with furrows	Sweat chloride possibly elevated	Autosomal dominant
Hypoplastic spoon-shaped and wrinkled nails	No	Autosomal recessive
No	Mild hypohidrosis	Autosomal dominant
No	Palmoplantar hypohidrosis with keratosis	Autosomal dominant
Onycholysis with scleronychia	No	Autosomal dominant
Slow-growing, small dystrophic nails	No	Autosomal recessive
No	No	Autosomal dominant

No: Not affected

a kyphosis in the thoracolumbar region. The lower limbs appear hypotrophic and are usually immobile. The calvaria reveal only minor involvement as compared to the "dysostosis multiplex" of MPS I-H.

Differential Diagnosis. MPS I-H and Gm_1 gangliosidosis should be considered in establishing a diagnosis.

Laboratory Aids. Serum liposomal hydrolases are usually increased. Cultured fibroblasts contain an abundance of coarse cytoplasmic inclusions with a characteristic inclusion-free perinuclear zone. Peripheral lymphocytes contain large cytoplasmic inclusions.

Synonym. I-cell disease.

References

DeMars RI, Leroy JG: The remarkable cells cultured from a human with Hurler's syndrome. *In Vitro* 2:107–118, 1967.

Galili D, et al: Massive gingival hyperplasia preceding dental eruption in I-cell disease. *Oral Surg* 37:533–539, 1974.

Leroy JG, et al: I-cell disease: A clinical picture. *J Pediatr* 73:360–365, 1971.

Leroy JG, et al: I-cell disease: Biochemical studies. *Pediatr Res* 6:752–757, 1972.

Weissmann U, et al: Mucolipidosis II (I-cell disease). A clinical and biochemical study. *Acta Paediatr Scand* 63:9–16, 1974.

7.21 Mucopolysaccharidosis III

Meyer and collaborators (1958) first described and identified MPS III. The condition is characterized by (1) severe mental retardation, (2) neurologic degeneration, (3) excessive heparan sulfate excretion in the urine, and (4) mild Hurler-like clinical appearance. The condition exists in two forms. MPS III-A is a deficiency of heparan sulfate-n-sulfatase and MPS III-B is deficiency of n-acetyl-α-D-glucosaminidase. The two conditions are not allelic mutations, so phenotypic expression of either condition requires a homozygous state. Defective degradation and storage of heparan sulfate by either deficient heparan sulfate-n-sulfatase (MPS III-A) or n-acetyl-α-D-glucosaminidase (MPS III-B) accounts for MPS III.

Facies. Although there is no characteristic facies for young children, older children may resemble patients affected with Hurler syndrome. However, the degree of facial involvement is never as distinct as that seen in MPS I-H. The nasal bridge may be sunken in the vast majority of cases. The hair is coarse and triangular in cross section (Fig. 7.39). Corneal clouding is not a feature of the condition.

Oral Structures. Generalized obliteration of pulp chambers and canals by irregular secondary dentin has recently been reported. Macroglossia occurs late in the disorder.

Systemic Features. Height is normal or slightly reduced. Intelligence and motor skills diminish with time. Joint mobility is usually slightly restricted at the elbows and knees. The posterior calvaria are usually thickened and the mastoid bones often appear sclerotic. Hypoplasia of the supra-acetabular portions of the ilia and oval-shaped vertebral bodies are the most common skeletal anomalies. Hepatomegaly is noted in a large percentage of cases.

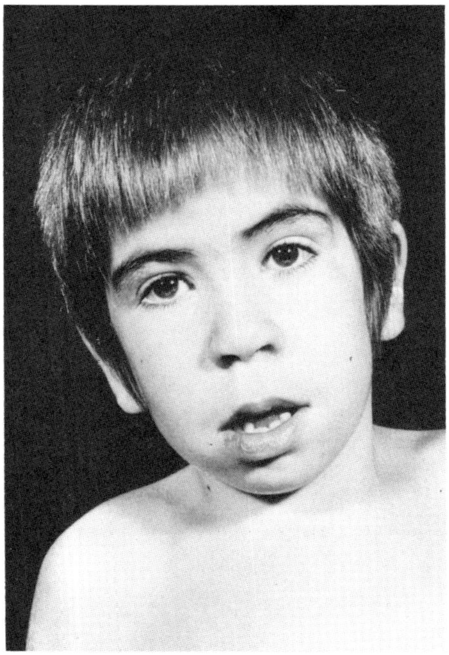

Fig. 7.39. Note coarse, thick features and abundant scalp hair in a patient with MPS III, Sanfilippo syndrome.

Differential Diagnosis. MPS II and MPS I-H should be included in the differential diagnosis.

Laboratory Aids. Metachromasia of coarse granules in peripheral lymphocytes, plasma cells and reticulohistiocytes, excessive urinary excretion of heparan sulfate, accumulation of S^{35}-labeled AMPS in fibroblasts and diminished or absent n-acetyl-α-D-glucosaminidase in tests may all be useful in attaining a diagnosis for MPS III-B.

Synonym. Sanfilippo syndrome.

References

Danks DM et al: The Sanfilippo syndrome: clinical, biochemical, radiological, haematological, and pathological features of nine cases. *Aust Paediatr J* 8:174–186, 1972.

Farriaux JP et al: Etude comparative des aspects cliniques, radiologiques, biochemiques et genetiques de la maladie de Sanfilippo de type A et type B. *Helv Paediatr Acta* 29:349–370, 1974.

Meyer K, et al: Excretion of sulfated mucopolysaccharides in gargoylism (Hurler's syndrome). *Proc Soc Exp Biol Med* 87:275–279, 1958.

Sanfilippo SJ et al: Mental retardation associated with acid mucopolysaccharidiuria (heparitin sulfate type). *J Pediatr* 63:837–838, 1963.

7.22 Mucopolysaccharidosis VI

Maroteaux and Lamy (1963) were first to describe MPS VI in a patient with an MPS I-H phenotype but with normal intelligence. The condition has an autosomal recessive mode of inheritance. A mild and a severe form of the condition have been recognized and may represent allelic mutations. A deficiency of arylsulfatase B appears to be the basis of the condition. Clinical and biochemical findings are caused by intracellular accumulation of AMPS. Dermatan sulfate is the most prominent AMPS stored.

Facies. The facies closely resembles that of MPS I-H. The forehead is prominent, the nasal bridge depressed, the cheeks full and the lips large. In addition, there is a significant hypertelorism, large cranium, relatively broad jaws, corneal opacities, and prominent eyebrows and scalp hair.

Oral Structures. The teeth are widely spaced as a result of macroglossia. The permanent mandibular molars are usually delayed in eruption and may have an angulated position in the mandible. The unerupted molar may be surrounded by radiolucent areas which probably represent accumulations of dermatan sulfate in the tooth follicles.

Systemic Features. The stature is diminished; however, intelligence may be within normal limits. The chest reveals a prominent sternum. Claw-like hand deformities or multiple contractures of the joints are noted after the first year of life. Hepatomegaly and splenomegaly are common findings. Cardiac anomalies may include valvular incompetence and narrowing of coronary arteries. Conductive and sensorineural hearing loss and impaired vision are also frequent.

Differential Diagnosis. MPS I-H and MPS II (severe type) should be considered in establishing the diagnosis.

Laboratory Aids. Granulocytes, monocytes, and lymphocytes reveal an accumulation of dense coarse inclusions. Dermatan sulfate is excreted in abundance in the urine; however, this diminishes with age. Cultured fibroblasts show abnormally high amounts of S^{35}-labeled MPS accumulation.

Synonym. Maroteaux-Lamy disease.

References

Barton RW, Neufeld EF: A distinct biochemical deficit in the Maroteaux-Lamy syndrome (mucopolysaccharidosis VI). *J Pediatr* 80:114–116, 1972.

Maroteaux M, et al: Une nouvelle dysostose avec élimination urinaire de chondroitin-sulfate B. *Presse Méd* 71:1849–1852, 1963.

Spranger J, et al: Mucopolysaccharidosis VI (Maroteaux-Lamy disease). *Helv Paediatr Acta* 25:337–362, 1970.

Stumpf DA, et al: Mucopolysaccharidosis type VI (Maroteaux-Lamy syndrome). *Am J Dis Child* 126:747–755, 1973.

Soft Tissue and Jaw Bones

7.23 Craniocarpotarsal Dysplasia

This syndrome was originally described by Freeman and Sheldon in 1938. Burian in 1963 coined the term "whistling face syndrome." The condition is most probably inherited in an autosomal dominant manner.

Facies. The characteristic facies presents deeply sunken eyes and true ocular hypertelorism. Convergent strabismus is common, as well as a mild degree of blepharophimosis and ptosis of the eyelids. Antimongoloid obliquity of the palpebral fissures is due to hypoplasia of the malar bones (Fig. 7.40). The small nose reveals narrow nostrils and a long philtrum. The nasal alae are often bent, thus simulating nostril colobomas. Near the nasal tip, the alae are of normal thickness, but they thin out backward and insert close to the columella. The nasolabial folds are seen only near the sides of the nose. The central parts of the cheeks bulge excessively during whistling, suggesting a muscle deficiency.

Oral Structures. Microstomia is almost always present; the intercommissural (interangular) distance is about two-thirds that of a normal child of the same age. The lips are held as if the patient were whistling. The palate is highly arched and the mandible generally is hypoplastic and retrognathic. A fibrous band, demarcated by two paramedian grooves extending from the middle of the lower lip to the chin, is a constant finding. This scar-like structure often presents an H or V shape. Biopsy of the buccinator muscles reveals replacement of muscle bundles by fibrous connective tissue.

Systemic Features. Height is generally below the third percentile. Flexion contractures of the fingers have been present in all patients, and the thumbs are generally involved at the metacarpophalangeal joint. Ulnar deviation of fingers, without bone anomalies, and talipes equinovarus, generally bilateral, are constant features. Less frequently associated anomalies include kyphoscoliosis, mild pectus excavatum, mild pterygium colli, asymmetric pinnae, and spina bifida occulta.

Differential Diagnosis. Arthrogryposis multiplex congenita may be included in the differential diagnosis; however, there is usually little confusion with other conditions.

Laboratory Aids. None known.

Synonyms. Whistling face syndrome, Freeman-Sheldon syndrome.

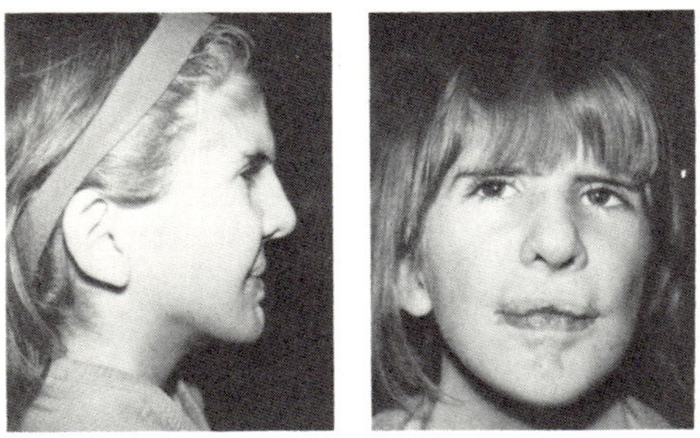

Fig. 7.40. Note flat middle face and characteristic H-shaped cutaneous defect of chin.

References

Burian F: The "whistling face" characteristic in a compound cranio-facio-corporal syndrome. *Brit J Plast Surg* 16:140–163, 1963.

Cervenka J, et al: Cranio-carpo-tarsal dysplasia or whistling face syndrome. *Arch Otolaryng* 91:183–187, 1970.

Freeman EA, Sheldon JH: Cranio-carpotarsal dysplasia—an undescribed congenital malformation. *Arch Dis Child* 13:277–283, 1938.

Rinsky LA, Bleck EE: Freeman-Sheldon ("whistling face") syndrome. *J Bone Joint Surg* 58A:148–150, 1976.

Sauk JJ, et al: Electromyography of oral-facial musculature in cranio-carpotarsal dysplasia. *Clin Genet* 6:132–137, 1974.

7.24 Cryptophthalmos Syndrome

The syndrome consists of (1) extension of the skin of the forehead to completely cover one or both eyes, (2) total or partial soft tissue syndactyly of fingers or toes or both, (3) coloboma of the alae nasi, (4) abnormal hairline, and (5) various urogenital abnormalities. The syndrome, which was first described by Zehender and Manz in 1873, is inherited in an autosomal recessive manner.

Facies. The frontal hairline is low and extends bilaterally over the temple area, ending in the skin of the supraorbital region with a typical "arrowhead" configuration. Total or partial absence of eyebrows is a constant finding. Unilateral or bilateral colobomas of the nostrils are commonly seen. The facial appearance is accentuated by small, low-set pinnae. Frequently the upper skin of the helix is continuous with that of the scalp (Fig. 7.41).

The most striking facial finding is the cryptophthalmus, which is bilateral in almost 60% of patients. The ocular globes are not missing and they can be palpated under the covering skin. Occasionally, strong light will induce skin reflexes due to contraction of the orbicularis muscles. Lid coloboma, microphthalmia, or epibulbar dermoid can affect the uncovered eye in the unilateral cases.

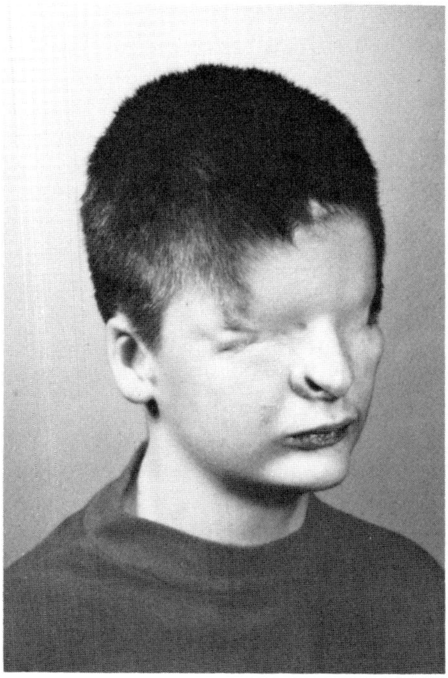

Fig. 7.41. Extension of skin of forehead over eyes, coloboma of nasal alae, bizarre hairline, and unusual form of pinnae with attachment to scalp.

Total or partial obstruction of the conjunctival sac can also be present. Levator palpebrae and orbicularis muscles are normal, but the lens may be absent, hypoplastic or calcified, and generally displaced. The cornea is differentiated from the sclera.

Oral Structures. Cleft lip or palate or both and ankyloglossia have been noted in several cases, as well as atresia or hypoplasia of the larynx.

Systemic Features. Physical development is within normal limits. Mental development may be slow as a consequence of ocular, auditory, oral, and laryngeal involvement. Meningoencephalocele has been noted in about 10% of the cases. The external auditory meatuses are narrower than normal. Air conduction loss and abnormal ossicles have also been seen. Syndactyly of hands and feet has been present in about 40% of the patients. Umbilical hernia occurs in about 20% and a vast array of urogenital abnormalities have been observed, including cryptorchidism, hypospadias, male and female pseudohermaphroditism, chordee, micropenis, and agenesis of a kidney.

Differential Diagnosis. The face is so characteristic as to be quite distinctive; nevertheless, anophthalmia and frontonasal dysplasia should be included in the differential diagnosis.

Laboratory Aids. None known.

References

Azevedo ES, et al: Cryptophthalmos in two families from Bahia, Brazil. *J Med Genet* 10:389–392, 1973.

Dinno ND, et al: The cryptophthalmos-syndactyly syndrome. *Clin Pediatr* 13:219–224, 1974.

Waring JO, Shields JA: Partial unilateral cryptophthalmos with syndactyly, brachydactyly, and renal anomalies. *Am J Ophthalmol* 79:437–440, 1975.

7.25 Generalized Gm_1 Gangliosidosis

Landing and coworkers (1964) first recognized Gm_1 gangliosidosis. The condition is characterized by ML II or MPS I-H phenotype with (1) progressive mental retardation and (2) death before the age of two years. Autosomal recessive inheritance has been established. Absence of β-galactosidase activity with resultant intracellular accumulation of Gm_1 ganglioside and keratan sulfate are responsible for the clinical and biochemical manifestations of the condition.

Facies. Full cheeks, puffy eyes, prominent philtrum, and depressed nasal bridge all may appear at birth. Cherry-red macular spots are common, while corneal opacities are rare.

Oral Structures. Enlargement of alveolar processes and macroglossia are common oral findings.

Systemic Features. Early kyphoscoliosis and radiologic evidence of an early dyostosis multiplex more severe than that in MPS I-H typifies generalized gangliosidosis. Psychomotor retardation is a prominent finding. The inability to swallow, tonic-clonic seizures, and blindness occur after the first year of life and are evidence of cerebral degeneration. Hepatosplenomegaly is present in most cases.

The hands are short and exhibit flexion contractures of the joints. The ribs are wide and the vertebral bodies short, with hook-shaped deformities in the thoracolumbar region. The ilia are hypoplastic and periosteal cloaking may be present on the shafts of the long bones in infants. The short tubular bones are thickened with proximal pointing of the metacarpals.

Differential Diagnosis. Tay-Sachs disease, ML II, metachromatic leukodystrophy, Sandhoff disease, infantile Neimann-Pick disease, Faber lipogranulomatosis, Goldberg syndrome, and MPS I-H should all be considered in the differential diagnosis.

Laboratory Aids. Acid β-galactosidase is diminished in leukocytes, cultured fibroblasts, blood, and urine. Lymphocytes and bone marrow histiocytes reveal numerous fine vacuoles.

Synonym. GM_1 gangliosidosis, type I.

References

Landing BH et al: Familial neurovisceral lipidosis. *Am J Dis Child* 108:503–522, 1964.

O'Brien JS: Generalized gangliosidosis. *J Pediatr* 75:167–186, 1969.

O'Brien JS: Gm_1 gangliosidosis. in Stanford, JB, et al, *The Metabolic Basis of Inherited Disease,* 3rd Ed. St Louis, McGraw-Hill, 1972.

7.26 Gingival Fibromatosis, Hypopigmentation, Microphthalmia, Oligophrenia, and Athetosis

Cross, McKusick, and Breen first described the syndrome complex in 1967. The syndrome is characterized by (1) hypopigmentation, (2) microphthalmia, (3) oligophrenia, and (4) athetoid movements and spasticity. The condition appears to have autosomal recessive inheritance.

Facies. The facies is athetoid. Microphthalmia and protuberant lips, probably secondary to gingival enlargement, are present. The corneas are cloudy and highly vascularized, and often there is a coarse, jerky nystagmus. The scalp hair is hypopigmented, as is the skin.

Oral Structures. The gingiva is hyperplastic, as are the alveolar processes. The palate is highly arched and there is palatal constriction of the maxillary arch in the region of the premolars.

Systemic Features. Somatic growth is within normal limits. Mental development is severely retarded. By the age of three months, patients reveal oligophrenia with spasticity and athetoid movements.

Differential Diagnosis. Tyrosinase positive and tyrosinase negative albinism should be included in the differential diagnosis, as well as the syndromes of gingival fibromatosis and the mucopolysaccharidoses and mucolipoidoses.

Laboratory Aids. Hair bulb test for tyrosinase is weakly positive.

Synonym. Cross Syndrome.

References

Cross HE, et al: A new oculocerebral syndrome with hypopigmentation. *J Pediatr* 70:3, 1967.

7.27 Mucopolysaccharidosis II

Hunter (1917) first described the syndrome in two brothers. Presently, two forms of the condition are recognized: (1) a mild form, in which the affected individual's life expectancy is extended into adulthood; and (2) a severe form, in which there is a rapid deterioration of psychomotor systems and the development of physical deformities. The syndrome is inherited in an X-linked manner with mild and severe forms of the condition representing allelic mutation. The incidence of the syndrome is approximately 0.66 per 100,000 births. A deficiency of sulfoiduronate sulfatase with defective degradation of AMPS is believed to be responsible for the condition.

Facies. The head is grossly enlarged. The neck is short (Fig. 7.42). The general character of the facies is similar to that of MPS I-H but is less striking in the mild form of the condition.

Oral Structures. Macroglossia occurs after five years of age with resultant wide spacing of teeth (Fig. 7.43). Bony alterations of the jaws and skull in the severe form of Hunter syndrome resemble those of Hurler syndrome.

Systemic Features. Intelligence may be only slightly impaired in the mild form of the condition but may be severely retarded after age 3 in the severe form. Affected patients are usually shorter than normal, especially after age 3. Muscle reflexes become progressively hyperactive as muscle tone increases. The physical habitus reveals a short neck, broad chest, and protruding abdomen with

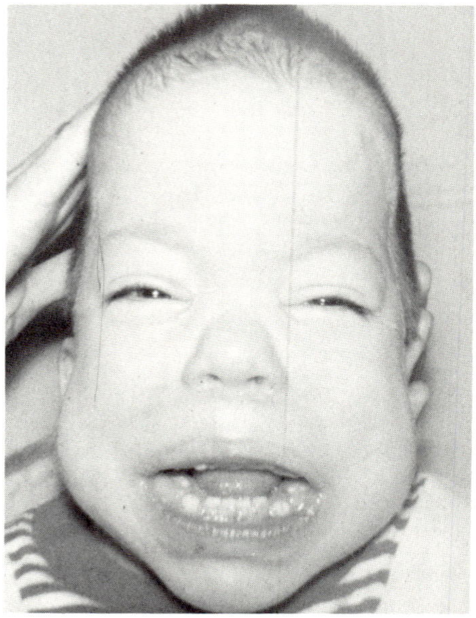

Fig. 7.42. Severe MPS II (type B): note coarse scalp hair, coarse facies, open mouth, and depressed nasal bridge.

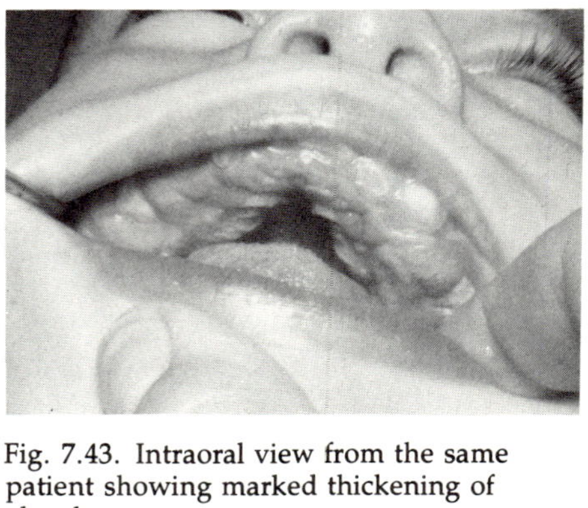

Fig. 7.43. Intraoral view from the same patient showing marked thickening of alveolar processes.

umbilical hernia. Hepatosplenomegaly and cardiovascular pathology are usual. Thoracolumbar kyphosis may be present. The joints reveal diminished mobility, and clawing deformation of the hands is common. Other common manifestations are deafness (15%) and hard, irregular, nontender papules of the skin.

Differential Diagnosis. The differential diagnosis should include other MPSs and MLs.

Laboratory Aids. Tests for excretion of equal amounts of urinary heparan sulfate and dermatan sulfate, accumulation of S^{35}-labeled AMPS in fibroblasts, lymphocyte metachromasia, and Alder-Reilly granules in peripheral granulocytes are useful; however, demonstration of deficient sulfoiduronate sulfatase activity is desirable.

Synonym. Hunter syndrome.

References

Bach G, et al: The defect in the Hunter syndrome: Deficiency of sulfoiduronate sulfatase. *Proc Nat Acad Sci* 70:2134–2138, 1973.

Hunter C: A rare disease in two brothers. *Proc Roy Soc Med* 10:104–115, 1917.

Leroy JG, Crocker AC: Clinical definition of the Hurler-Hunter phenotypes. *Am J Dis Child* 112:518–530, 1966.

7.28 Myotonic Dystrophy

Myotonic dystrophy was first described in 1909 by Steinert, Batten, and Gibb. The condition is characterized by (1) myotonia, (2) progressive muscle wasting, (3) hypogonadism, (4) cataracts, and (5) progressive deterioration. The disorder is inherited in an autosomal dominant manner with complete penetrance; however, there is great variation in clinical expression. Genetic heterogeneity has been suggested on the basis of differences in the time of onset. One form of the condition has an onset in infancy and rarely occurs after age 30. Another form of the condition has an initial onset between the ages of 20 and 60, while a third form occurs between age 4 and 25. Prenatal detection is feasible since the gene for myotonic dystrophy is closely linked to that of the secretor locus. The basic defect associated with myotonic dystrophy originates within muscles, and is believed to result from disturbances in the ability of the sarcoplasmic reticulum to bind and release calcium in addition to disturbances in the energetics in muscle fibers.

Facies. The facies is narrow, expressionless, and mask-like as a result of progressive atrophy and weakness of facial muscles and the muscles of mastication (Fig. 7.44). Severe involvement of the sternocleidomastoid muscles may result in an exaggerated curvature of the neck.

Oral Structures. Lingual myotonia resulting in indistinct speech may be the initial presenting sign of the disorder. Retention of saliva in the oral cavity and a high incidence of dental caries have been reported. Less consistent findings include malocclusion, high-arched palate, micrognathia, and prognathism.

Systemic Features. Mental deficiency is common and mental deterioration may occur with progression of the disease. Muscle wasting and weakness are usually progressive and result in increased debility. Death usually results from cardiac failure, pneumonia, or recurrent illness. However, the latter does not occur until the fifth or sixth decade of life. Involvement of the extremities is usually progressive, first affecting proximal musculature, extending distally, resulting in gait disturbances and pseudohypertrophy. Ptosis of the eyelids is common. Opacities in the thin zone of the lens cortex occur in the early stages of the disease. Mature cataracts, present in 85% of the patients, usually do not appear until later in the course of the disease. Other ophthalmologic findings have included ophthalmoplegia, keratitis sicca, blepharitis, corneal dystrophy, microphthalmia, enophthalmos, choroidal coloboma, epiphoria, pigmentary defects of the macula and retina, and optic atrophy.

Atrophic skin and calcifying epitheliomas of Malherbe have been described, as well as partial alopecia

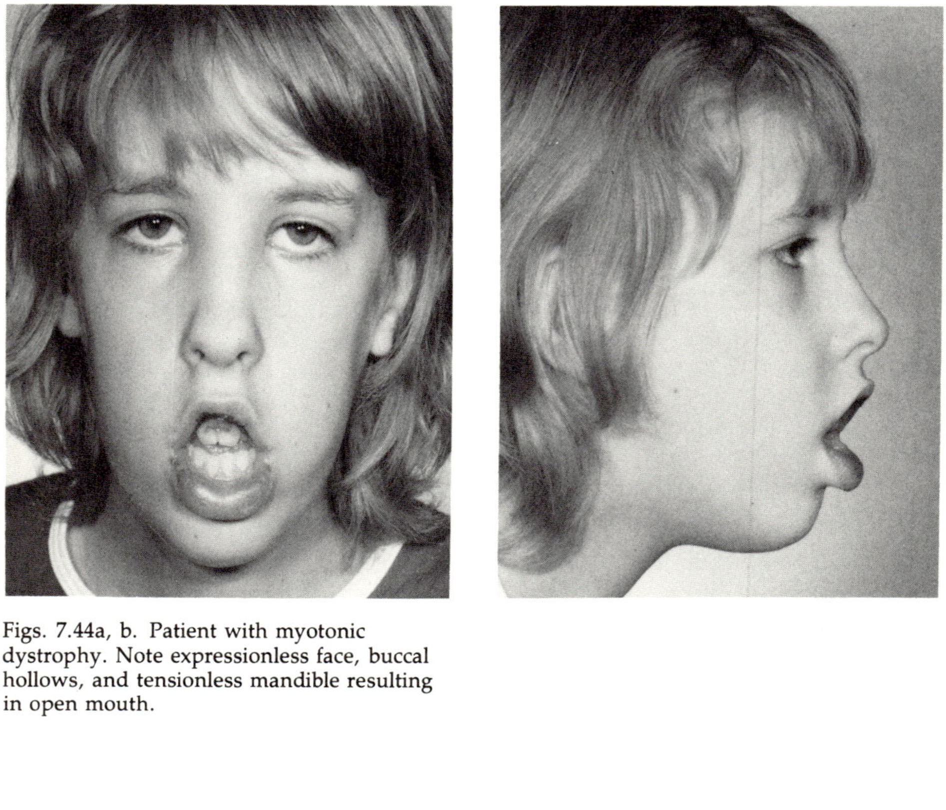

Figs. 7.44a, b. Patient with myotonic dystrophy. Note expressionless face, buccal hollows, and tensionless mandible resulting in open mouth.

of the frontal and parietal scalp in males. Cardiologic manifestations have commonly included conduction defects and arrhythmias. Weakening of the thoracic musculature and inability of the esophagus to clear often result in respiratory distress, pulmonary infections, and chronic pulmonary disease. Reduced amplitude of peristaltic contractions, esophageal and gastric retention, cholelithiasis, reduced small intestinal mobility, steatorrhea, diarrhea and constipation have all been associated with increased frequency in myotonic dystrophy. Testicular atrophy and cryptorchidism have been reported in males, while females may manifest amenorrhea, dysmenorrhea, and ovarian cysts. Diabetes mellitus, hypothyroidism, and thyroid adenoma have been reported occasionally. Skeletal changes have included hyperostosis frontalis interna, small sella turcica, large paranasal sinuses, ocular hypotelorism, pectus excavatum, kyphoscoliosis, neonatal thin ribs, and talipes equinovarus.

Differential Diagnosis. Myotonia may also be associated with Kok syndrome, Gamstorp-Wohlfart syndrome, generalized myotonia, paramyotonia congenita of Eulenburg, and myotonia congenita (Thomsen syndrome).

Laboratory Aids. Muscle biopsy, slit lamp examination for "myotonic dust," abnormal electromyographic studies, serum immunoglobulin determination of IgG and IgM, and insulin secretion studies may be of aid in establishing the diagnosis.

Synonym. Steinert syndrome.

References

Bundey S: Detection of heterozygotes for myotonic dystrophy. *Clin Genet* 5:107–109, 1974.

Kuiper DH: Gastric bezoar in a patient with myotonic dystrophy: A review of the gastrointestinal complications of myotonic dystrophy. *Am J Dig Dis* 16:529–534, 1971.

Pruzanski W: Myotonic dystrophy—a multisystem disease: Report of 67 cases and a review of the literature. *Psychiatr Neurol* (Basel) 149:302–322, 1965.

Radu H, et al: Quantitative study of the myotonic state. *Europ Neurol* 4:100–107, 1970.

7.29 Trichorhino-phalangeal Syndrome

Giedion in 1966 described a syndrome comprising (1) cone-shaped epiphyses, (2) sparse, fine hair, (3) a somewhat pear-shaped nose, and (4) growth retardation. The trichorhinophalangeal syndrome is genetically heterogeneous. Autosomal dominant and recessive forms are known to occur. They are differentiated by pedigree studies, since the clinical manifestations are identical for both inherited forms.

Facies. The facial appearance is often overlooked. The nose is rather broad and pear-shaped, and the philtrum appears to be overly long (Fig. 7.45). The medial part of the eyebrows is broad, but the lateral portion is narrow and thin. The scalp hair is sparse from the time of birth. Its texture is fine and its growth is slow. The hair is especially sparse in the frontotemporal areas, somewhat simulating male pattern baldness.

Oral Structures. An enlarged and prominent philtrum gives the facies a more or less typical appearance. In addition, mild micrognathia may be present.

Systemic Features. Height is between the third and tenth percentiles. Bone age is often several years behind chronologic age. Mental development is within normal limits. The fingers become progressively deformed from age six, but these alterations tend to level off at puberty. Characteristically there is swelling of the middle phalangeal joints with axial deviation of the fingers distal to this point (Fig. 7.46). Roentgenographically, the middle phalanges of the second, third, and fourth fingers are the sites of cone-shaped epiphyses. One or more metacarpals are commonly shortened, usually the fourth or fifth. Multiple cone-shaped epiphyses are also noted in the toes.

Pes planus is also a frequent finding. Scoliosis or lordosis has been described by several investigators. The scapulae are often winged. The pubic and axillary hair is scant. The nails are thin. Increased susceptibility to upper respiratory tract infections has also been observed.

Differential Diagnosis. All other forms of peripheral dysostosis, as well as hypohidrotic ectodermal dysplasia and the Langer-Giedion syndrome, should be considered.

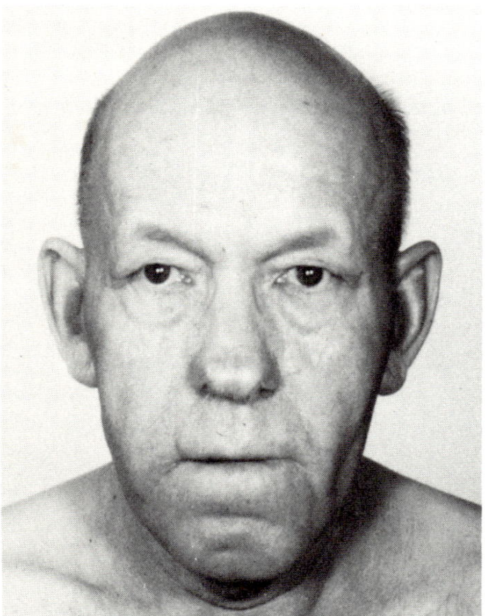

Fig. 7.45. Adult patient with the TRP syndrome showing somewhat pear-shaped nose and long philtrum.

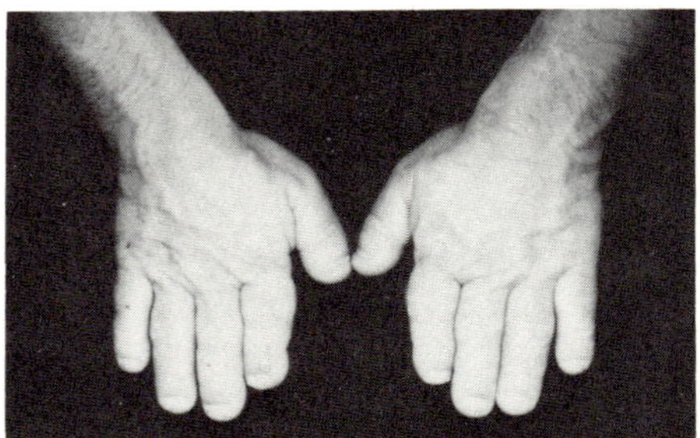

Fig. 7.46. Abbreviated thumbs and swollen middle phalangeal joints with axial deviations of the fingers distal to this point.

Laboratory Aids. None known.

References

Beals RK: Tricho-rhino-phalangeal dysplasia. *J Bone Joint Surg* 55A:821–826, 1973.

Giedion A: Das tricho-rhino-phalangeale Syndrom. *Helv Paediatr Acta* 21:475–482, 1966.

Giedion A: Cone-shaped epiphyses of the hands and their diagnostic value: The tricho-rhino-phalangeal syndrome. *Ann Radiol* 10:322–329, 1967.

Giedion A, et al: Autosomal dominant transmission of the tricho-rhino-phalangeal syndrome. *Helv Paediatr Acta* 28:249–259, 1973.

Gorlin RJ, et al: Tricho-rhino-phalangeal syndrome. *Am J Dis Child* 118:595–599, 1969.

7.30 Tuberous Sclerosis

Tuberous sclerosis, first described by Bourneville (1880) and by Pringle (1890), is one of the neurocutaneous syndromes. Its more important characteristics are (1) epilepsy, (2) mental deficiency, and (3) fibroangiomas. The components of the triad may appear in any order. Some patients manifest signs at birth, but in the majority of cases the seizures and skin changes first appear in the two- to six-year-old. Most patients die before the third decade of life, but some may survive into middle age. Pneumonia, cachexia, status epilepticus, or acute heart failure have all been reported as contributing causes of death. The syndrome is found in less than 1% of persons institutionalized for epilepsy and mental retardation and in about 1 in 300,000–500,000 of the general population. It is inherited in an autosomal dominant manner.

Facies. Characteristic of the syndrome are the numerous fibroangiomas distributed over the face (Fig. 7.47). The skull often exhibits thickened calvaria with an irregular outer table and exostoses on the inner table of the frontal bone.

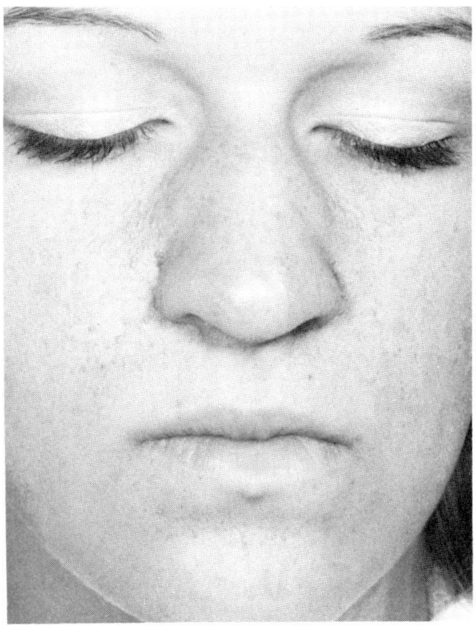

Fig. 7.47. Rounded seed-like masses formed by hyperplastic connective and vascular tissues over the facial skin.

Oral Structures. In 10% of patients, the oral mucosa may be the site of fibrous growths, which may be found on the gingiva, lip, buccal mucosa, dorsum of tongue, palate, or uvula (Fig. 7.48). The tongue of affected patients has been found to be long and narrow as a consequence of thickening of the alveolar process, and of hyperostosis. Retarded eruption of teeth and hypoplastic pitted changes in the enamel have been reported but not consistently.

Systemic Features. Somatic growth is within normal limits. However, about 50% of affected patients are mentally retarded. The cerebral cortex and ependymal lining of the ventricles may show proliferation of glial elements and ganglion cells in addition to intracranial calcifications. Throughout the skull, areas of increased radiopacity can be noted, especially in the parietal bones. Affected patients may have petit mal, Jacksonian, or grand mal epilepsy. When present the severity of

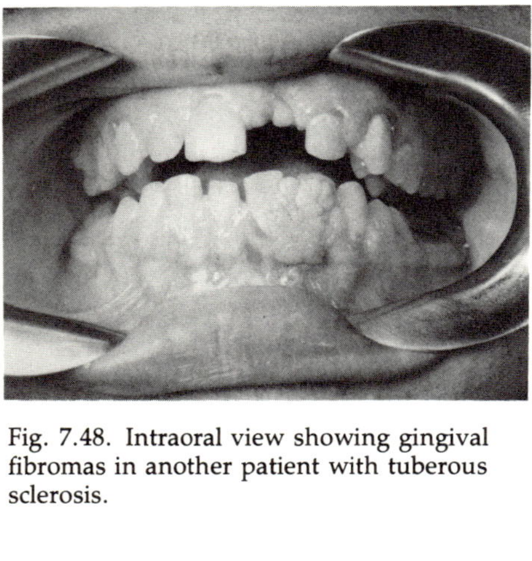

Fig. 7.48. Intraoral view showing gingival fibromas in another patient with tuberous sclerosis.

epilepsy increases with age. Glial cell, nerve cell, and vascular tissue proliferation of the retina occurs in 20% of affected patients.

The skin lesions may consist of small, reddish, flat or rounded seedlike masses composed of hyperplastic connective and vascular tissues. These lesions are usually noted over the nose, cheeks, nasolabial furrows, and chin. The onset of puberty seems to cause an increase in their number. Soft polypoid fibromatous tumors may sometimes be noted on the dorsal trunk or scalp. Occasionally similar lesions may occur beneath the nail beds (subungual fibromas). Flat, round plaques may also be noted in the lumbar area. Especially helpful in diagnosis of the condition in the infant with epilepsy is the presence on the trunk of ovoid areas of depigmentation resembling the leaf of a mountain ash.

About two-thirds of patients have cyst-like areas in the phalanges and irregular periosteal new-bone formation along the shafts of the metacarpals and metatarsals. Approximately 80% of patients have (mixed type) renal tumors. Rarely is there a malignant change. Rhabdomyomas of the heart and cystic defects ("honeycomb") of the lungs, as well as hepatic and pancreatic hamartomas, are not uncommon.

Differential Diagnosis. Differential diagnosis should include multiple trichoepitheliomas, multiple syringocystadenomas, and colloid milia in the presence of skin pathology. Radiologic differential diagnosis should include Stürge-Weber syndrome, Hippel-Lindau syndrome, calcifying subdural hematoma, Paget's disease of bone, melorheostosis, periostitis, toxoplasmosis, and cysticerosis.

Laboratory Aids. Biopsy of fibroangiomas, pneumoencephalographic studies, and Wood's light identification of ovoid areas of depigmentation on the trunk of infants with epilepsy are useful in the diagnosis of this condition.

Synonym. Bourneville-Pringle syndrome.

References

Anderson D, Tannen RL: Tuberous sclerosis and chronic renal failure. Potential confusion with polycystic kidney disease. *Am J Med* 47:163–168, 1969.

Bjornberg A: Adenoma sebaceum. Review, case reports and discussion of eugenic aspects. *Acta Dermatovener* 41:213–223, 1961.

Fitzpatrick TB, et al: White leaf-shaped macules. *Arch Derm* 98:1–6, 1968.

Nevin NC, Pearce WG: Diagnostic and genetical aspects of tuberous sclerosis. *J Med Genet* 5:273–280, 1968.

Soft Tissue, Jaw Bones, and Teeth

7.31 Coffin-Lowry Syndrome

In 1966 Coffin and collaborators first described a syndrome characterized by (1) retarded mental and physical development, (2) peculiar facies, and (3) spinal, digital, and other osteocartilaginous anomalies. All severely affected patients reported to date have been males. Milder clinical manifestations have been described in female relatives of affected individuals. This would suggest X-linked inheritance.

Facies. The facies is characterized by prominent frontal bossing, hypertelorism, and antimongoloid obliquity of palpebral fissures (Fig. 7.49). Thick nasal septum, convergent strabismus, and epicanthal folds are common features. The supraorbital ridges are thick and markedly protruded. The ears are low set.

Oral Structures. The maxilla and zygoma are hypoplastic, and consequently the upper lip is thin with a long philtrum and a pouting lower lip. The mandible is prognathic, and a wide open angle has been noted. High-arched palate with crowding of teeth and malocclusion are constant findings. Also constant are oligodontia, especially of mandibular incisors, and a deep midline furrow of the entire dorsal lingual surface (Fig. 7.50).

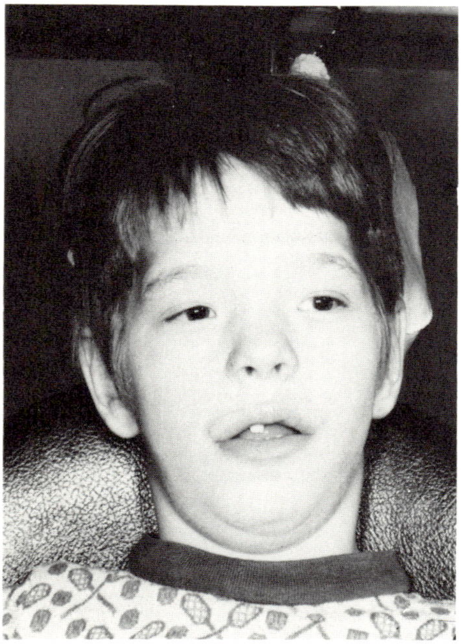

Fig. 7.49. Note hypertelorism, short upturned nostrils, and thick lower lip.

Systemic Features. All patients are small in stature, within the third percentile and more than two standard deviations from the mean. Bone age is delayed. Patients have a slow gait and a striking posture with bent knees and stooped back. Mental retardation is marked; IQ values of 20–25 have been reported. Affected individuals are nonaggressive, with a pleasant and cooperative attitude. Microcephaly and thick calvaria have been present in all reported males.

The hands are unusually soft and with ulnar deviation. The fingers have a cone-shaped configuration with a broad base and narrow tip,

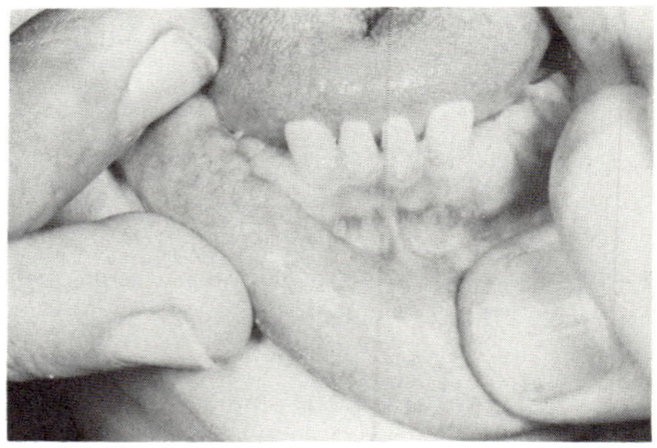

Fig. 7.50. Intraoral view demonstrating oligodontia and abnormally shaped teeth.

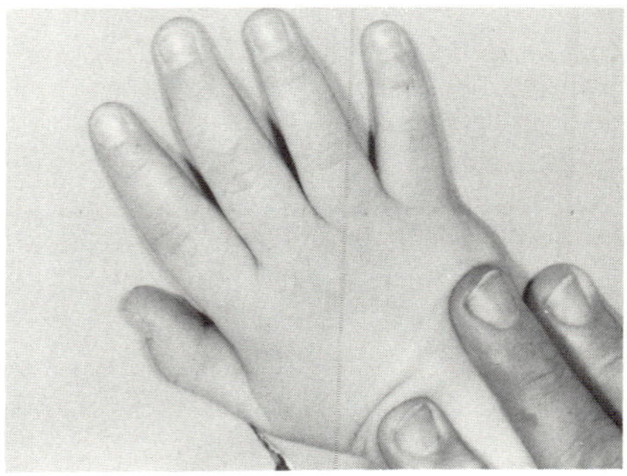

Fig. 7.51. Hand of the same patient as in Fig. 7.50 showing fingers with a thick base and narrow tips.

giving the hands a peculiar appearance (Fig. 7.51). Tufting of terminal phalanges of fingers with constriction of the adjacent shaft, resulting in a drumstick appearance, has been described in every case. There are extra ossification centers at the base of each metacarpal. Pectus carinatum as well as limited extension of elbows have been reported in all cases. Other major findings have been anterior notch defect in lumbar vertebrae, kyphosis, scoliosis, and lordosis.

Differential Diagnosis. Juvenile cerebral gigantism and the mucopolysaccharidoses should be included in the differential diagnosis.

Laboratory Aids. None are known, but skin biopsy in several cases has demonstrated a greatly reduced number of elastic fibers.

Synonym. Mental retardation with osteocartilaginous anomalies.

References

Coffin GS, et al: Mental retardation with osteocartilaginous anomalies. *Am J Dis Child* 112:205–213, 1966.

Lowry B, et al: A new dominant gene mental retardation syndrome. *Am J Dis Child* 121:491–500, 1971.

Martinelli B, Campailla E: Contributo alla conoscenza della sindrome di Coffin, Siris, Wegienka, *Giorn Psich Neuropat* 97:449–458, 1969.

Temtamy SA, et al: The Coffin-Lowry syndrome: An inherited faciodigital mental retardation syndrome. *Pediatrics* 86:724–731, 1975.

7.32 Dubowitz Syndrome

Dubowitz (1965) described a syndrome characterized by (1) short stature, (2) microcephaly, (3) mental retardation, (4) eczema, and (5) characteristic facies. The condition is inherited in an autosomal recessive manner.

Facies. The facies is characterized by a high forehead with flat supraorbital ridges (Fig. 7.52). The nasal bridge is high, accentuating the small nasal tip and alae. True ocular hypertelorism and dystopia canthorum, together with ptosis of the eyelids, gives the facies a "sad-clown" appearance. Other facial findings include slight antimongoloid or mongoloid obliquity of palpebral fissures, blepharophimosis, and micrognathia. The facial appearance is completed by microcephaly, flared and low-set ears, eczema, and sparse scalp hair and eyebrows.

Oral Structures. In addition to micrognathia, delayed eruption of teeth, bifid uvula, high-arched palate, and submucous cleft may be found.

Systemic Features. Mental retardation is generally present to a mild degree. Some patients with normal intelligence have been reported. Growth retardation with primordial dwarfism is present in every case. Eczema of the skin is also present in the extremities, especially during infancy. Other associated anomalies have included chronic rhinorrhea, high-pitched voice, hypospadias, cryptorchidism, and pilonidal dimples.

Differential Diagnosis. The Bloom syndrome and the fetal alcohol syndrome should be differentiated.

Laboratory Aids. None known. There is a single report of associated normochromic, microcytic, or slightly hypochromic anemia.

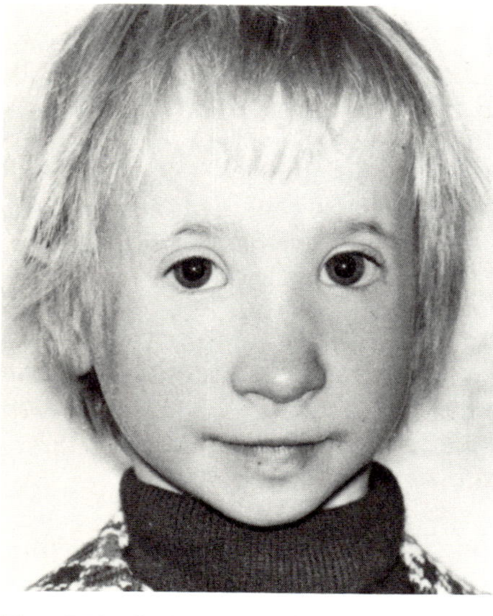

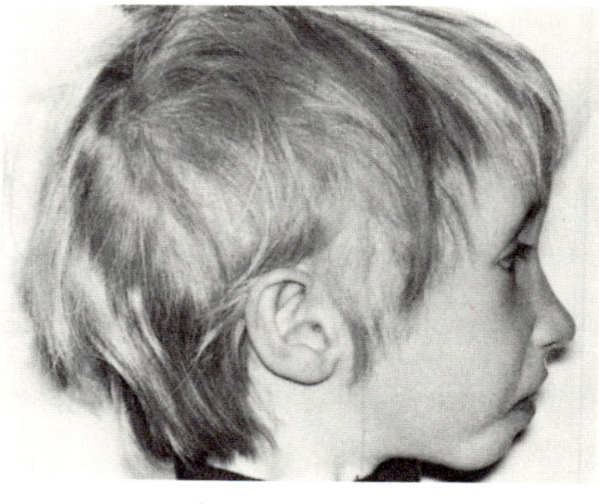

Figs. 7.52a, b. Note high forehead, hypertelorism, depressed nasal bridge, and small retrognathic mandible.

References

Dubowitz V: Familial low birthweight dwarfism with an unusual facies and a skin eruption. *J Med Genet* 2:12–17, 1965.

Grosse FR, et al: The Dubowitz syndrome. *Z Kinderheilkd* 110:175–187, 1971.

Opitz J, et al: The Dubowitz syndrome: Further observations. *Z Kinderheilkd* 116:1–12, 1973.

7.33 Ehlers-Danlos Syndromes

Ehlers (1901) described a syndrome consisting of (1) hyperelastic skin, (2) skin hemorrhages, and (3) loose-jointedness. Later, Danlos (1908) added (4) cutaneous pseudotumors to the syndrome. Presently, Ehlers-Danlos syndromes may be divided into seven types based on genetic and clinical findings and on pathogenesis. E-D type I is the most severe classic form of the condition and is inherited in an autosomal dominant manner, but the basic defect remains unknown. E-D type II, which is the classic mild form, is also inherited in an autosomal dominant manner. E-D type III represents the benign form of the syndrome, manifested as hypermobility and inherited in an autosomal dominant manner.

E-D type IV (Sack type) is the ecchymotic or arterial form, inherited in an autosomal recessive mode with a deficiency of type 3 collagen as the basic defect. E-D type V represents the X-linked form of the condition and has as its basic defect a deficiency of lysyl oxidase. E-D type VI is an autosomal recessive condition, in which lack of lysyl hydroxylase is the basic defect. E-D type VII is inherited in an autosomal recessive manner and results from a deficiency of procollagen peptidase.

Facies. The facies in the different syndromal types is not characteristic (Fig. 7.53). The ears may project outward and downward and stretch on physical pressure, except in E-D type IV. Bilateral epicanthal folds with an apparent broad nasal root are also frequent findings.

Oral Structures. The oral mucosa appears normal; however, it is very fragile and easily bruised. There is no evidence of abnormal healing or excessive scar formation, but tissue approximation after suturing is usually poor. The gingivae and periodontium are both susceptible to injury and destructive disease at an early age. Severe bleeding has been reported subsequent to tooth extraction. The teeth of patients with Ehlers-Danlos syndrome are smaller than normal and have deformed roots and large pulp stones in the coronal pulp chambers. The bicuspid and molar teeth may present high cusps and deep occlusal fissures. Hypoplastic enamel, irregularities of the amelodentinal and cementodentinal junctions, and formation of pathologic dentin have all been reported. Recurrent subluxation of the temporomandibular joint and the ability of patients to touch the tip of the nose with the tip of the tongue

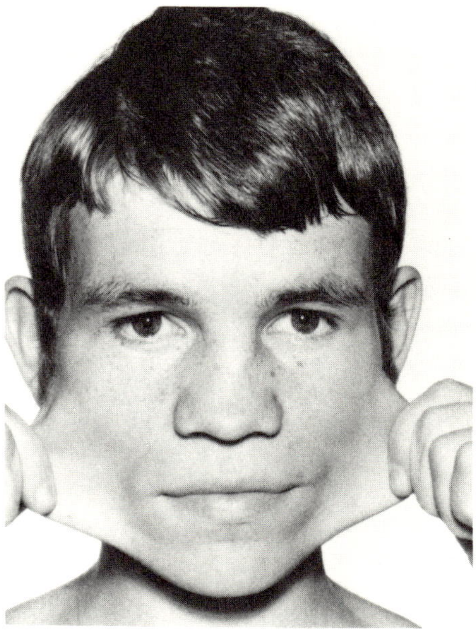

Fig. 7.53. Hyperelastic facial skin assumes normal shape after release.

(Gorlin sign) have both been reported (Fig. 7.54).

Systemic Features. Mental development is usually within normal limits. Joint hyperextensibility is perhaps the most outstanding feature of some forms of the syndrome (types I, II, III, VI, and VII) (Fig. 7.55). E-D types IV and V usually only manifest hypermobility of the digits. Habitual dislocation of the joints, pes planus, and genu recurvatum are commonly seen. Scoliosis and kyphoscoliosis are not severe when present, except in E-D type VI, where severe scoliosis may be prominent. Osteoarthritic changes probably due to recurrent dislocation involve the weight-bearing joints of the majority of affected adults.

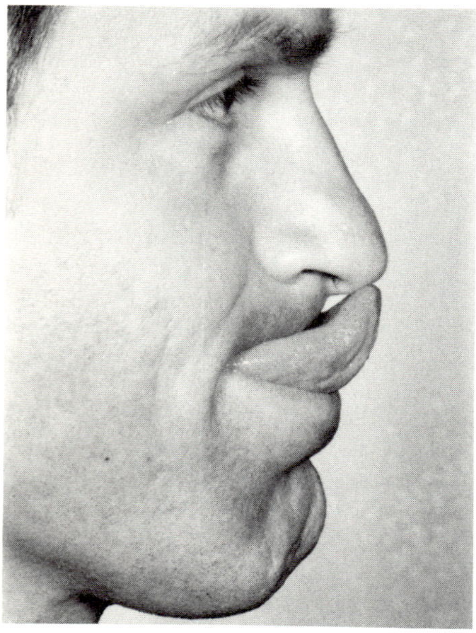

Fig. 7.54. The ability to touch the nose with the tip of the tongue is present in 50% of patients with the syndrome, in contrast to only 10% of nonaffected individuals.

Talipes has been noted in 5% of patients. The ulnar styloid process may be elongated. Inguinal or umbilical hernia has been found in 10–20% of affected patients.

The skin, especially over the joints, is hyperelastic and velvety in texture except in the ecchymotic type in which the skin is especially translucent and elastosis perforans is frequent. Skin fragility is usually responsible for gaping wounds and easy bruising with marked subcutaneous bleeding (E-D types III and V usually show minimal bruising and skin fragility). Healing of the skin may result in papyraceous scars. Molluscoid pseudotumors at the heels and other major joints are also common. Calcified subcutaneous spheroids may be found over bony prominences of the forearms and shins in about one-third of cases. Myopia and strabismus have been reported with increased frequency. Blue sclerae have been noted in only about 10% of reported cases. Less common opthalmologic findings have included microcornea, retinal detachment, keratoconus, and angioid streaks.

Gastrointestinal complications have included intestinal diverticula, diaphragmatic eventration, hiatus

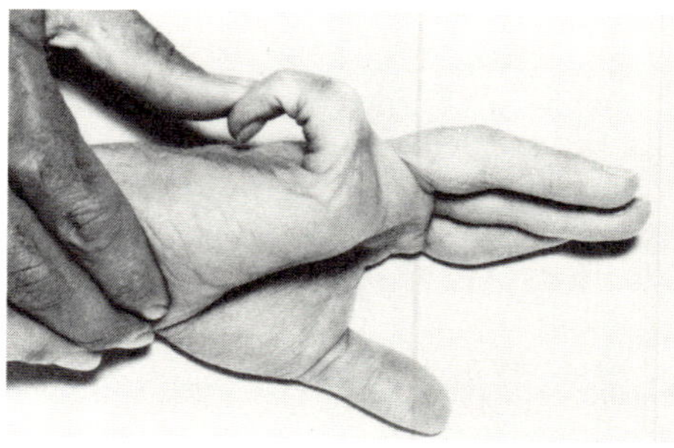

Fig. 7.55. Marked joint hypermobility.

hernia, and rectal prolapse during infancy. Massive gastrointestinal hemorrhage has been noted in the ecchymotic form of the syndrome. E-D type IV may also manifest spontaneous rupture of arteries or aortic dissection or both. Pulmonary arterial stenosis and multiple arterial lesions have been described. Varicose veins are common in E-D types I and V. Acrocyanosis also has been reported with increased frequency.

Differential Diagnosis. Familial generalized articular hypermobility, as well as Marfan syndrome and several other connective tissue disorders should be included.

Laboratory Aids. The degree of joint mobility may be measured by the Ellis-Bundick method and elasticity of skin by the method of Graham and Beighton.

Synonyms. Cutaneous fragility, hyperelasticity and articular hyperlaxity, cutis hyperelastica.

References

Barabas AP: Vascular complications in the Ehlers-Danlos syndrome with special reference to the "arterial type" or Sack's syndrome. *J Cardiovas Surg* 13:160–167, 1972.

Beighton PH: X-linked recessive inheritance in the Ehlers-Danlos syndrome. *Brit Med J* 2:409–411, 1968.

Beighton PH, et al: Variants of the Ehlers-Danlos syndrome. Clinical, biochemical, hematological and chromosomal features of 100 patients. *Ann Rheum Dis* 28:228–245, 1969.

Graham R, Beighton PH: Physical properties of the skin in the Ehlers-Danlos syndrome. *Ann Rheum Dis* 28:246–251, 1969.

Krane SM, et al: Lysyl-protocollagen hydroxylase deficiency in fibroblasts from siblings with hydroxylysine-deficient collagen. *Proc Nat Acad Sci* 69:2899–2903, 1972.

Lichtenstein JR, et al: Defect in conversion of procollagen to collagen in a form of Ehlers-Danlos syndrome. *Science* 182:298–299, 1973.

7.34 Fetal Face Syndrome

Described initially by Robinow and coworkers in 1969, the syndrome consists of (1) characteristic facies, (2) forearm brachymelia, and (3) hypoplastic genitalia. The syndrome is probably inherited in both autosomal dominant and recessive manners.

Facies. The facies resembles that of a fetus of about 8 weeks, with large neurocranium, marked frontal bossing, ocular hypertelorism, S-shaped lower eyelids, short nose with anteverted nostrils, and the so-called fish-mouth configuration (Fig. 7.56).

Oral Structures. Oral manifestations include triangular mouth with downturned angles, teeth malpositioned after eruption with consequent crowding and malocclusion, gingival hypertrophy, and macroglossia. Occasional reports include cleft lip, cleft palate, cleft tongue, and cleft lower lip.

Systemic Features. Mental development has been within normal limits in the majority of patients. Sporadic cases associated with mental retardation have been reported. Growth is within normal limits at birth and during the neonatal period, but by the third year of life falls below the third percentile. Adults remain shorter than normal.

Forearm brachymelia is a constant feature, with excessive ratios between upper and lower arm. Hemivertebrae and minor anomalies of the radius, ulna, metacarpals, and phalanges, as well as brachydactyly and clinodactyly of the fifth fingers have been noted. The penis is markedly hypoplastic at birth, but the degree of hypoplasia diminishes with age. The scrotum and testicles are normal. Affected females present hypoplastic clitoris and labia minora.

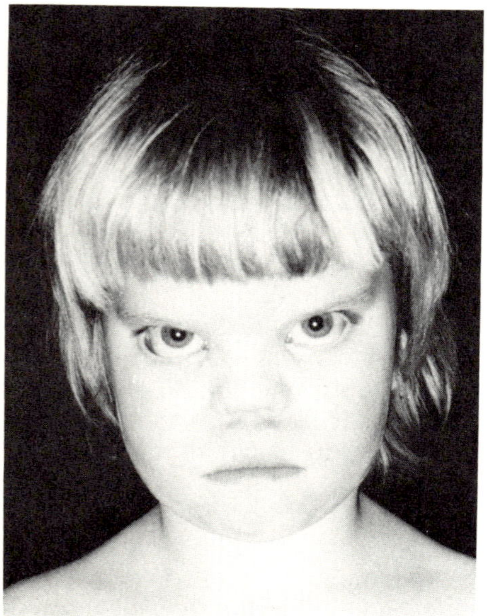

Fig. 7.56. Note ocular hypertelorism, bulging forehead, bizarre lower eyelids, and short upturned nose.

Differential Diagnosis. Achondroplasia, acrodysostosis, and Aarskog syndrome should be included in the differential diagnosis. Mild cases of frontonasal dysplasia should also be considered.

Laboratory Aids. None known.

Synonym. Robinow syndrome.

References

Kelly TE, et al: The Robinow syndrome. *Am J Dis Child* 129:383–386, 1975.

Robinow M, et al: A newly recognized dwarfing syndrome. *Am J Dis Child* 117:645–651, 1969.

7.35 Focal Dermal Hypoplasia Syndrome

The syndrome originally described by Goltz and coworkers in 1962 consists of (1) atrophy and linear pigmentation of the skin, (2) localized superficial fatty deposits in the skin, (3) multiple papillomas of mucous membranes or periorificial skin, and (4) anomalies of the extremities, including syndactyly, oligodactyly, and adactyly. The syndrome appears to be transmitted in an X-linked dominant manner with variable clinical expressivity. The condition is lethal in the male.

Facies. The face is asymmetrical with pointed chin and notching of the alae nasi. The eyes are sunken and may present several abnormalities, including iris coloboma and strabismus. The eyebrows and scalp hair are sparse. The facial picture is completed by asymmetric ears and skin and lip anomalies as described below.

Oral Structures. Cleft lip-palate has been described in several cases. The most striking oral component is the presence of multiple frambesiform papillomas of the lips (Fig. 7.57). The buccal mucosa is less commonly affected with similar lesions. Dental abnormalities include hypodontia, microdontia, and hypoplasia of enamel.

Systemic Features. Physical growth is often retarded. Mental retardation of varying degree is frequent, as is microcephaly. Streaky hypopigmentation, atrophy, telangiectasia, and papillomas of the skin or mucosae of the oral, anal, and genital regions, as well as of the skin of the axillary, inguinal, and periumbilical areas are also a constant finding (Fig. 7.58). Hypotrichosis and "paper-thin" nails have been associated with the syndrome. Reddish yellow nodules of subcutaneous fat can be seen throughout the thin dermis. Bilateral syndactyly of variable degree, polydactyly, absence or hypoplasia of a digit or hand bone, clinodactyly, scoliosis, spina bifida, and hypoplasia of the right clavicle are fre-

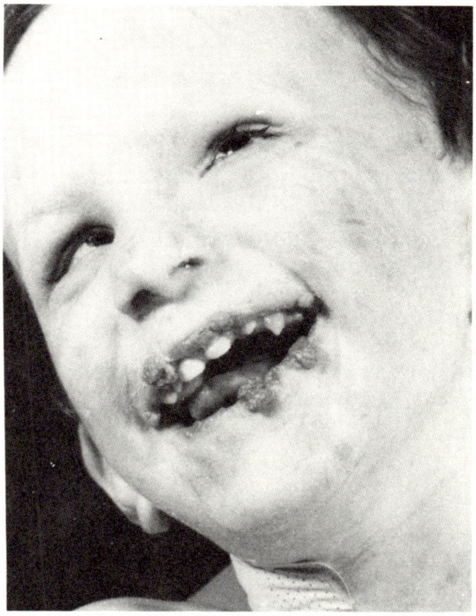

Fig. 7.57. Note multiple frambesiform lesions of both lips, focal dermal defect on the facial skin, and strabismus.

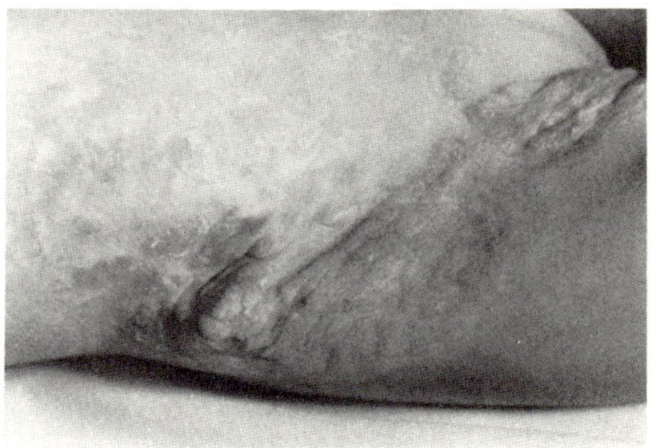

Fig. 7.58. Skin of the hip and thigh in patient. Note multiple sacular growths.

quent findings. Umbilical or inguinal hernia or both, joint hypermobility, strabismus, coloboma of the iris or choroid or both, and microphthalmia have also been noted.

Differential Diagnosis. Poikiloderma congenita, epidermal nevus syndrome, and incontinentia pigmenti should be included in the differential diagnosis.

Laboratory Aids. Biopsy of the skin from affected areas will demonstrate normal subcutaneous fat beneath the epithelium.

Synonym. Goltz-Gorlin syndrome.

References

Ginsburg LD, et al: Focal dermal hypoplasia syndrome. *Am J Roentgenol* 110:561–571, 1970.

Goltz RJ, et al: Focal dermal hypoplasia syndrome. *Arch Dermatol* 86:708–714, 1962.

Goltz RW, et al: Focal dermal hypoplasia syndrome. *Arch Dermatol* 101:1–11, 1970.

Zergollern L, et al: Focal dermal hypoplasia. *Dermatologia* 148:240–246, 1974.

7.36 Hyperkeratosis Palmoplantaris and Periodontoclasia in Childhood

The syndrome first described by Papillon and Lefèvre in 1924 consists of (1) hyperkeratosis of the palms and soles and (2) premature destruction of the periodontal ligament of both deciduous and permanent dentitions, with subsequent loss of teeth. The condition is inherited in an autosomal recessive manner.

Facies. No characteristic facial features or findings are known to be associated with the syndrome.

Oral Structures. After normal eruption of the deciduous teeth, and concurrent with the initial appearance of the palmar and plantar hyperkeratosis, the gingiva becomes red, swollen, and boggy, and bleeds easily (Figs. 7.59–60). Severe halitosis is noted. When the last primary molars complete eruption, destruction of the periodontal ligament begins, leading to the formation of deep periodontal pockets which exude pus upon pressure. Roentgenograms show a marked destruction of the supporting alveolar bone. The complete dentition becomes mobile, and by 4 to 5 years old all the teeth are shed in approximately the same sequence in which they erupted. After the primary teeth are lost, gingival inflammation subsides and the oral cavity resumes its normal appearance, the patient being completely edentulous. The process is repeated in essentially the same manner, but with more marked symptoms, after eruption of the permanent dentition has begun. The patient generally becomes totally edentulous by the 16th year, with only the third molars exempt from exfoliation. When all permanent teeth are lost, the gingiva resumes its normal appearance and dentures are tolerated well.

Systemic Structures. Physical and mental development are within normal limits. Occasionally, ectopic calcification of the tentorium and choroid has been noted. Hyperkeratosis palmoplantaris, usually of the diffuse type, generally precedes periodontal involvement of the primary dentition. The palms usually present a well-demarcated, red, scaly hyperkeratosis extending to the margins and over the thenar eminences (Fig. 7.61). The soles are involved to a greater degree, the process frequently spilling over the edges and onto the Achilles tendon. Occasionally, tibial tuberosities, external malleoli, and dorsum of finger and toe joints present hyperkeratotic plaques. The degree of hyperkeratosis increases in severity coincidentally with the acute periodontal manifestations. Fetid hyperhidrosis, especially of the feet, is frequent.

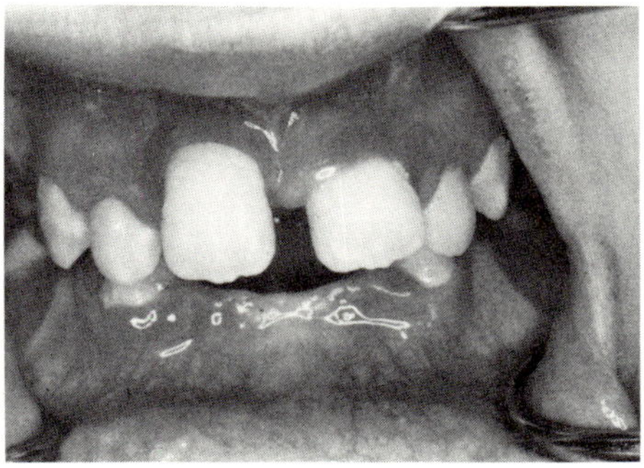

Fig. 7.59. Intraoral view showing marked gingival inflammation. Note that mandibular incisors are absent due to premature exfoliation.

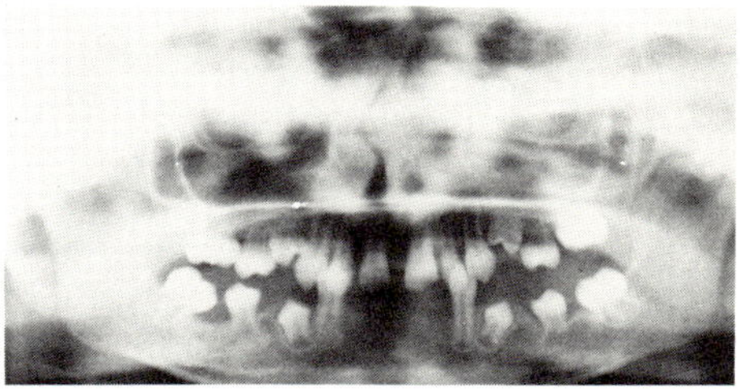

Fig. 7.60. Panoramic radiograph from the patient in Fig. 7.59 showing similar dental findings.

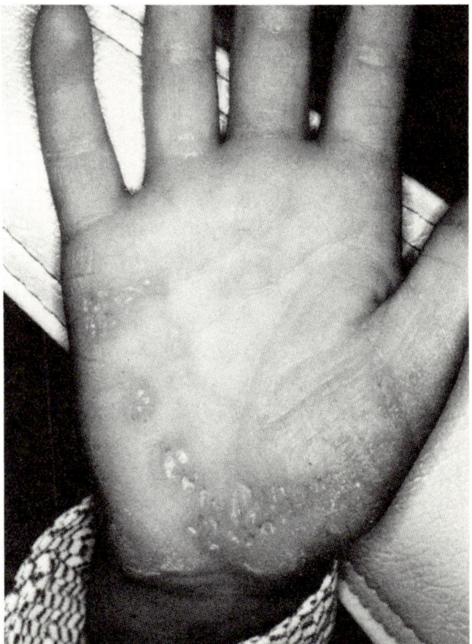

Fig. 7.61. Note palmar hyperkeratosis. Similar lesions were present in both soles.

Palmoplantar hyperkeratosis persists throughout life.

Differential Diagnosis. All other forms of keratosis palmoplantaris, pachyonychia congenita, and a host of conditions associated with premature loss of teeth in childhood should be considered.

Laboratory Aids. None known.

Synonym. Papillon-Lefèvre syndrome.

References

Giansanti GS, et al: Palmar-plantar hyperkeratosis and concomitant periodontal destruction. (Papillon-Lefèvre syndrome). *Oral Surg* 36:40–48, 1973.

Gorlin RJ, et al: The syndrome of palmar-plantar hyperkeratosis and premature periodontal destruction of the teeth. *J Pediatr* 65:895–908, 1964.

Papillon –, Lefèvre P: Deux cas de kératodermie palmaire et plantaire symétrique familiale (maladie de Méléda) chez le frère et la soeur. Coexistance dans le deux cas d'altérations dentaires graves. *Bull Soc Fr Dermatol Syphilgr* 31:82–84, 1924.

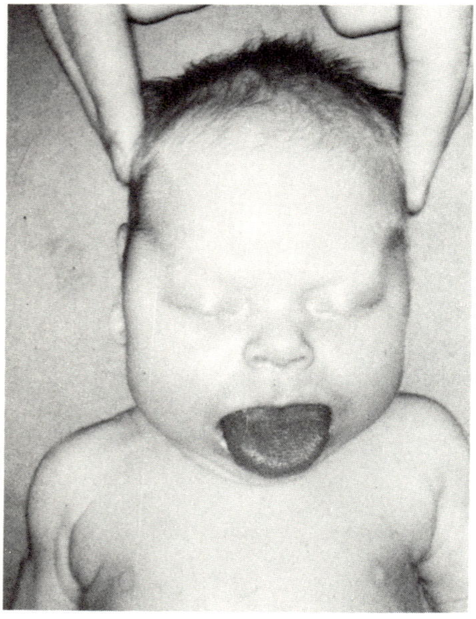

Fig. 7.62. Newborn with impressive macroglossia. The infant also had omphalocele.

7.37 Macroglossia-Omphalocele-Visceromegaly Syndrome

The syndrome originally was reported by Beckwith in 1963 and consists of (1) macroglossia, (2) omphalocele or umbilical hernia, (3) postnatal gigantism, (4) visceromegaly, and (5) linear indentations of the ear lobe. Evidence suggests that the syndrome is most probably inherited in an autosomal dominant mode with incomplete penetrance and variable expressivity. The majority of cases represent isolated examples.

Facies. The facies is characterized primarily by open mouth due to macroglossia (Fig. 7.62). Microcephaly has also been reported. Recently, linear indentations of the ear lobes have been included as a significant feature of the syndrome in one-third of reported cases.

Oral Structures. Macroglossia is the most constant feature of the complex, being present in 90% of cases. Biopsy of the tongue has shown that the muscle cells are within normal limits in size and number. Hypoplasia of the middle third of the face and class III malocclusion together with anterior open bite and retroclined mandibular incisors are also frequent oral manifestations.

Systemic Features. Gigantism at birth is present in less than half the cases. Growth may even be subnormal for a few months, but in most cases somatic gigantism eventually results, and height and weight are often above the ninetieth percentile. Advanced bone age is invariably present, and occasionally there may be widening of the metaphyses and cortical thickening of long bones. Mild to moderate retardation may occasionally be a feature of the syndrome, probably resulting from undetected hypoglycemic episodes in infancy. Polycythemia seems to be a constant feature and posterior eventration of the diaphragm and glabellar nevus flammeus are frequently associated with the syndrome. Such lesions tend to become less prominent during the first year of life.

Hemihypertrophy has also been noted. Visceromegaly has been described in about half of the patients, hepatomegaly and nephromegaly being most frequent with cardiomegaly occurring less often. Pancreatomegaly has been noted at autopsy. Either omphalocele or umbilical hernia has been reported in about 90% of cases. Some patients have diastasis recti.

Differential Diagnosis. Differential diagnosis should include neonatal hypoglycemia, isolated macroglossia, and isolated omphalocele. Also the facies should be differentiated from that seen in Hurler and Hunter syndromes and congenital cretinism.

Laboratory Aids. Beckwith estimated that symptomatic hypoglycemia may be a feature in one-third to one-half of affected patients. Hyperlipemia and hypercholesterolemia have also been noted, as well as hypocalcemia, adrenal cortical carcinoma, nephroblastoma, and gonadoblastoma.

Synonyms. Beckwith-Wiedemann syndrome, EMG syndrome.

References

Beckwith JB: Macroglossia, omphalocele, adrenal cytomegaly, gigantism, and hyperplastic visceromegaly. *Birth Def* 5(2): 188–196, 1969.

Cohen MM Jr: Macroglossia, omphalocele, visceromegaly, cytomegaly of the adrenal cortex and neonatal hypoglycemia. *Birth Def* 7(7):226–232, 1971.

Filippi G, McKusick VA: The Beckwith-Wiedemann syndrome (the exomphalos-macroglossia-gigantism syndrome): Report of two cases and review of the literature. *Medicine* 49:279–298, 1970.

Thorburn MJ, et al: Exomphalos-macroglossia-gigantism syndrome in Jamaican infants. *Am J Dis Child* 119:316–321, 1970.

7.38 Mucopolysaccharidosis I-H

Hurler in 1919 was the first to describe the syndrome. The most characteristic features include (1) retarded growth after infancy, (2) corneal clouding, (3) characteristic physical and craniofacial anomalies, (4) severe mental retardation, (5) urinary excretions of increased acid mucopolysaccharides (AMPS) and (6) intracellular storage of AMPS. Mucopolysaccharidosis I-H occurs with a frequency of about 1 in 100,000 births and has autosomal recessive inheritance. The etiology of the syndrome is due to absence of α-iduronidase and resultant accumulation of undegraded AMPS in affected cells and tissues.

Facies. The head is enlarged, with bulging of the frontal bones (Fig. 7.63). Scaphocephaly may result from hyperostosis and premature closure of sagittal and metopic sutures. Radiographically the skull reveals a depressed sphenoidal plane and a J-shaped sella. The orbital roofs are thickened and dense and the orbits are shallow. The nose usually reveals a broad tip, wide anteverted nostrils and depressed nasal bridge. In addition to corneal clouding, the eyes reveal an increased interpupillary distance and prominent lower eyelids. The cheeks, nasolabial folds, and ear lobes all appear thickened. A chronic nasal discharge is usually present.

Oral Structures. The mouth is generally open. The lips are thickened, flattening the philtrum and elongating the upper lip. The tongue usually protrudes from the chronically open mouth. The alveolar ridges are usually hyperplastic and the teeth are widely spaced (Fig. 7.64). The enlarged tongue results in an anterior open-bite. Tooth eruption is delayed in half of the affected patients. Usually, the mandibular second primary molars and permanent molars are positioned distoangularly. Localized bone destruction resembling "dentigerous cysts" is very common in the mandibular molar by age 3 (Fig. 7.65). We believe that these bone lesions represent hyperplastic dental follicles engorged by dermatan sulfate. The mandible is characteristically short and broad with short and narrow rami. The condyles are

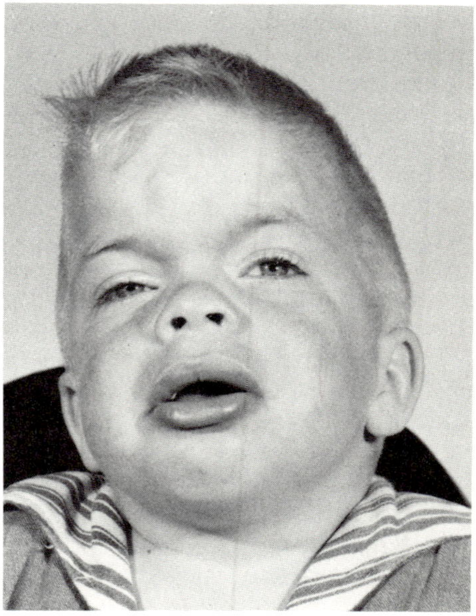

Fig. 7.63. Note chronically open mouth and coarse facial features.

often limited in movement and modified, presenting a cup-shaped excavation or an inclined flat surface. A cleft may exist at the mandibular notch or the notch may be irregular.

Systemic Features. Although somatic growth may be above the 87th percentile in the first year of life, by age 3 affected children are usually below the 3rd percentile. There is a short neck, pectus carinatum and excavatum, and a kyphosis or gibbus in the lumbodorsal region. Radiologically, bone trabeculation is coarse. The ribs are wide and the vertebrae are dysplastic, revealing a hook-shaped morphology with biconcave end plates of the lower thoracic and upper lumbar vertebral bodies. The iliac wings are flared and the basilar portions of the ilia are hypoplastic. Diaphyseal widening and deformed epiphyses are noted in the long tubular bones. Hands reveal a claw deformity.

Hepatic and splenic enlargement, laxity of the abdomen, shortened spine and deformed chest result in a protruding abdomen. Inguinal and umbilical hernias are common. Cardiomegaly secondary to AMPS deposition is usual. The skin is coarse, dry, pale, and covered by fine lanugo hair.

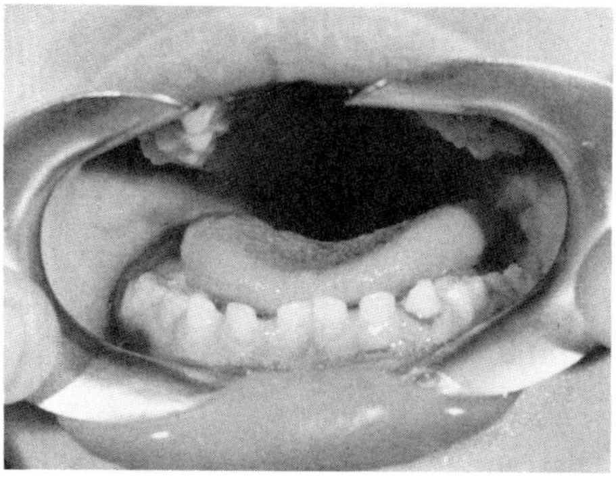

Fig. 7.64. Intraoral view of same patient as Fig. 7.63 showing widely spaced teeth and macroglossia.

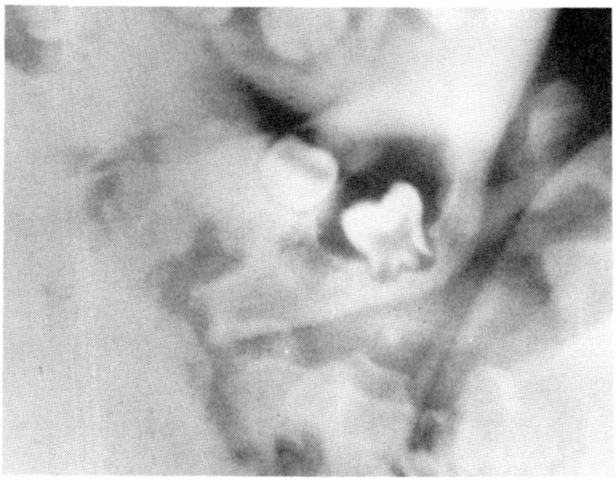

Fig. 7.65. Panoramic radiograph demonstrating dentigerous cyst-like bone destruction around the germ of a permanent molar.

Differential Diagnosis. Differential diagnosis should include other mucopolysaccharidoses and mucolipoidoses.

Laboratory Aids. Excretion of excess urinary dermatan sulfate and heparan sulfate; histochemical evidence of AMPS in peripheral leukocytes in bone marrow and in cultured fibroblasts; gross albumin turbidity; toluidine blue spot test; and demonstration of diminished or absent α-iduronidase activity are all useful in establishing the diagnosis.

Synonym. Hurler syndrome.

References

Bach G, et al: The defect in the Hurler and Scheie syndrome: Deficiency of α-L-iduronidase. *Proc Nat Acad Sci* 69:2048–2051, 1972.

Gardner DG: The oral manifestations of Hurler's syndrome. *Oral Surg* 32:46–57, 1971.

Hurler G: Über einen Typ multipler Abartungen, vorwiegend am Skelettsystem. *Ztschr Kinderheilkd* 24:220–234, 1919.

Leroy JG, Crocker AC: Clinical definition of Hurler-Hunter phenotypes. *Am J Dis Child* 112:518–530, 1966.

Worth HM: Hurler's syndrome: A study of radiologic appearances in the jaws. *Oral Surg* 22:21–35, 1966.

7.39 Orofacialdigital Syndrome I

The syndrome of (1) multiple hyperplastic frenula, (2) cleft tongue, (3) dystopia canthorum, (4) hypoplasia of nasal alar cartilages, (5) median cleft of upper lip, (6) asymmetric cleft palate, (7) various digital malformations, and (8) mild mental retardation was first defined by Papillon-Leage and Psaume in 1954. Similar cases had been reported earlier under various names. The syndrome is inherited in a X-linked dominant manner, limited to females and lethal in males.

Facies. The facies is characterized by frontal bossing, hypoplasia of alar cartilages, and broad nasal root. Lateral displacement of the inner canthi and resultant hypertelorism are also noted. The upper lip is short, presenting a pseudocleft in the midline (Fig. 7.66). Milia of the face and ears are common but they disappear before age 3. Dryness or alopecia of the scalp or both is present in about 65% of affected individuals.

Oral Structures. Oral manifestations include a thick hyperplastic upper frenum which produces partial obliteration of the anterior fold. The frenum also extends through the upper lip beyond the vermilion border producing a small midline cleft.

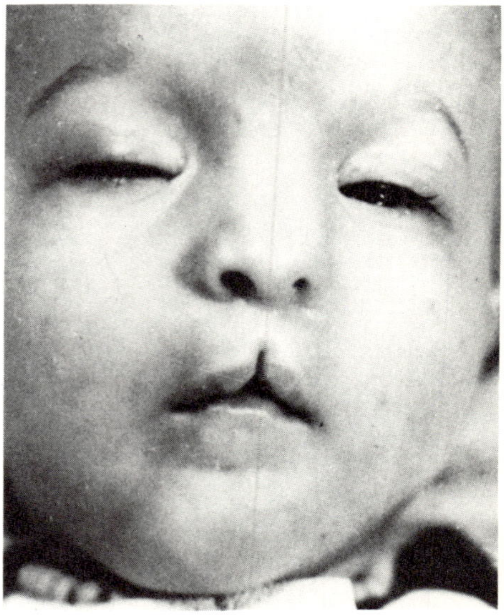

Fig. 7.66. Note lack of flare of the nasal alae and pseudocleft in midline of upper lip.

Lateral clefts of the palate are produced by bilateral grooves arising from the maxillary buccal frenula. The palate is then divided into an anterior segment and two posterior processes (Fig. 7.67). The soft palate can also be the site of asymmetric clefting. The lower mucobuccal fold is traversed by thick fibrous bands, especially in the region of the lower lateral incisors, which produce clefting of the alveolar process and, by extension, bi-, tri-, or tetra-furcation of the tongue (Fig. 7.68).

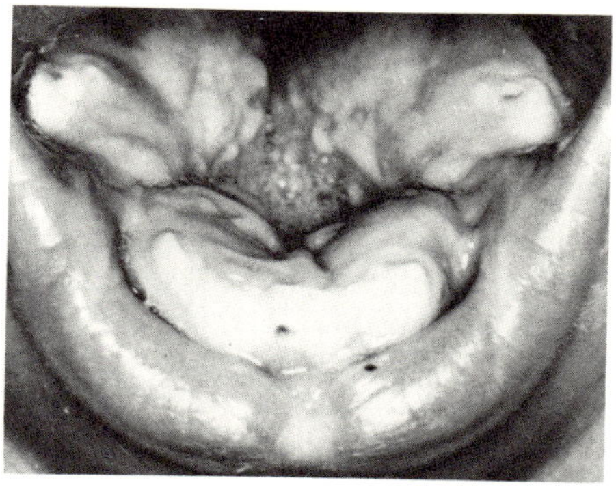

Fig. 7.67. Intraoral view in another patient showing division of the maxilla into an anterior portion containing incisors and canine teeth, and two posterior segments.

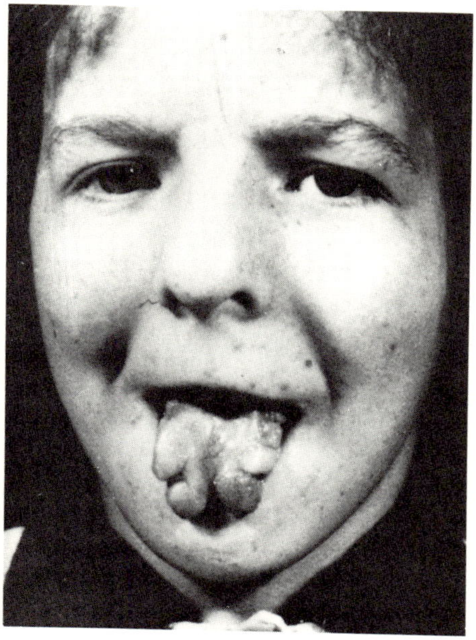

Fig. 7.68. Tetrafurcation of the tongue in a third patient with the OFD I syndrome.

About 50% of patients will present a small, whitish hamartoma at the midline of the ventral surface of the tongue. This mass is formed by fibrous connective tissue, salivary gland tissue, striated muscle fibers, and occasionally cartilage. One-third of the patients present ankyloglossia. Malposition of maxillary canine teeth, supernumerary canines and premolars, and infraocclusion are common. Aplasia of mandibular lateral incisors is noted in 60% of reported cases. The mandible has been described as small or hypoplastic with a short ramus. The cranial base angle, nasion-sella-basion, is increased.

Systemic Features. Somatic growth is within normal limits. One-third to one-half of the patients are mildly mentally retarded. Several digital malformations are associated with the syndrome, such as clinodactyly, syndactyly, brachydactyly, and polydactyly, in decreasing order of frequency. Toe malformations are less common and include unilateral hallucal polysyndactyly, syndactyly, and brachydactyly. Roentgenograms of hands and feet show the short tubular bones to be shorter and thicker than normal with some degree of osteoporosis.

Differential Diagnosis. OFD-II, Mohr-Rimoin syndrome, which is inherited in an autosomal recessive manner, and Ellis-van Creveld syndrome should be included in the differential diagnosis.

Laboratory Aids. None known.

Synonyms. OFD-I syndrome, dysplasia linguofacialis.

References

Gorlin RJ: The oral-facial-digital (OFD) syndrome. *Cutis* 4:1345–1349, 1968.

Gorlin RJ, Psaume J: Orodigitofacial dysostosis—a new syndrome. *J Pediatr* 61:520–530, 1962.

Lauterstein A, Pruzansky S: Tooth anomalies in the oral-facial-digital syndrome. *Teratology* 2:137–146, 1969.

Papillon-Leage (Mme), Psaume J: Une malformation hereditaire de la muquesuse buccale et freins anormaux. *Rev Stomatol (Paris)* 55:209–227, 1954.

Ruess AL, et al: The oral-facial-digital syndrome: A multiple congenital condition of females with associated chromosomal abnormalities. *Pediatrics* 29:985–995, 1962.

7.40 Orofacialdigital Syndrome II

Mohr in 1941 and Claussen in 1946 delineated a syndrome consisting of (1) lobed tongue, (2) manual polydactyly, and (3) bilateral polysyndactyly of the halluces. The syndrome is inherited in an autosomal recessive manner.

Facies. A midline cleft of the upper lip is observed frequently but may be absent (Fig. 7.69).

Oral Structures. The most constant feature of the syndrome is cleft tongue. Generalized ankyloglossia has been reported in a few instances, in addition to cleft palate and bifid uvula. Multiple frenula are frequently present but to a lesser extent than is observed in OFD-I syndrome. A number of patients have been reported with fatty hamartomas of the dorsum of the tongue.

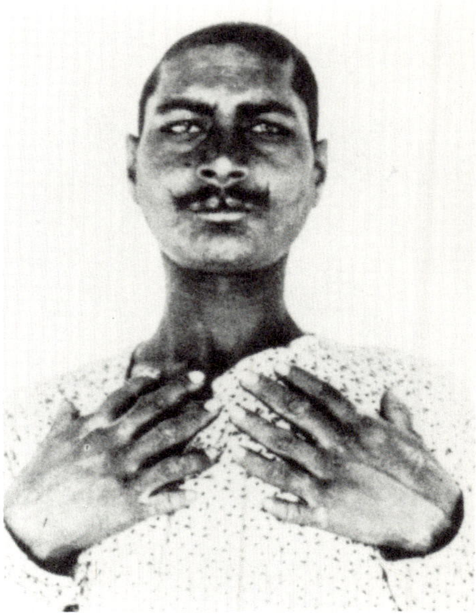

Fig. 7.69. Note pseudocleft of midline of upper lip and bimanual hexadactyly.

Systemic Features. Retarded mental development has been reported in addition to other neurologic abnormalities including microcephaly, choroid coloboma, muscular hypotonia, and conduction deafness. Skeletal abnormalities are limited to the hands and feet. Bilateral manual ulnar hexadactyly and bilateral polysyndactyly of the halluces are both characteristic, although bimanual hexadactyly is not a requirement for establishing the diagnosis. Other findings have included increased susceptibility to respiratory infection, tachypnea, cryptorchidism, and inguinal hernia.

Differential Diagnosis. Premaxillary variant of holoprosencephaly, frontonasal dysplasia, and OFD-I syndrome should be included in the differential diagnosis.

Laboratory Aids. None known.

Synonyms. Mohr syndrome, OFD II syndrome.

References

Claussen O: Et arveligt syndrom omfattende tungemissdannelse og polydaktyli. *Nord Med* 30:1147–1151, 1946.

Goldstein E, Medina JL: Mohr syndrome or oral-facial-digital II: Report of two cases. *J Am Dent Assoc* 89:337–382, 1974.

Gustavson KH, et al: Syndrome characterized by lingual malformation, polydactyly, tachypnea and psychomotor retardation (Mohr syndrome). *Clin Genet* 2:261–266, 1971.

Mohr OL: A hereditary sublethal syndrome in man. *Nor Vidensk Akad Oslo I Mat Naturv Klasse* 14:3–18, 1941.

Pfeiffer RA, et al: Das Syndrom von Mohr und Claussen. *Klin Pediätr* 185:224–229, 1973.

Miscellaneous

7.41 Jaw-Winking and Winking-Jaw Syndromes

Marcus Gunn in 1883 first described the jaw-winking syndrome as consisting of (1) unilateral congenital eyelid ptosis and (2) exaggerated elevation of the ptotic lid on moving the lower jaw to the contralateral side. The syndrome is most likely inherited in an autosomal dominant manner. The lid winking in conjunction with jaw movement can be best explained by an aberrant innervation of the levator palpebrae superioris muscle from the motor branch of the trigeminal nerve, with a possible supranuclear, or at least combined supranuclear-nuclear, involvement. Several cases have been reported in which the syndrome has diminished or disappeared at approximately 25 years of age. There is no sex predilection.

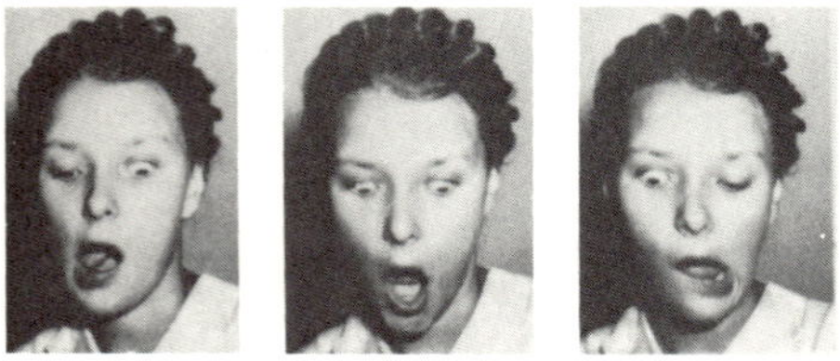

Fig. 7.70. Exaggerated eye-opening in patient with jaw-winking syndrome. Left lid opened when jaw was opened to the right and vice versa. Both eyes showed exaggerated lid opening when jaw was opened wide without deviation.

Facies. Ptosis of one eyelid, most prevalent on the left side, is congenitally present in approximately 90% of affected individuals (Fig. 7.70). The lid can not be raised to any significant degree. Some patients present bilateral ptosis and occasionally others have the syndrome without ptosis. Rarely, paresis of the extraorbital eye muscles can be present, but pupillary and corneal reflexes are normal.

Oral Structures. In about 40% of patients the syndrome is produced

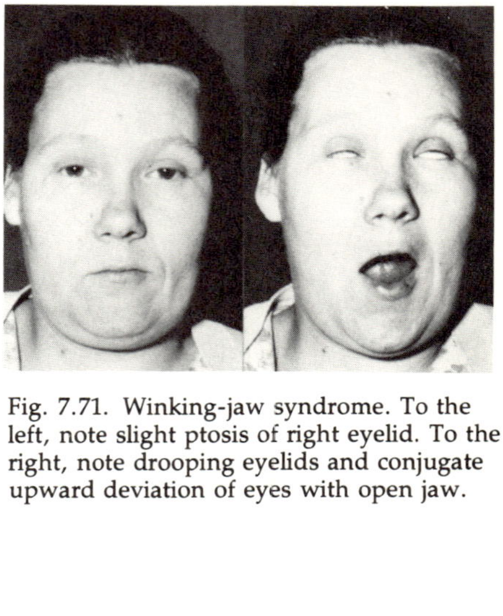

Fig. 7.71. Winking-jaw syndrome. To the left, note slight ptosis of right eyelid. To the right, note drooping eyelids and conjugate upward deviation of eyes with open jaw.

both upon depressing the mandible and upon moving it to the side opposite the affected eye. Another 40% need only to depress the mandible. The remaining 20% have the condition triggered by various stimuli, such as movement of the lips in whistling, clenching the teeth, puffing out the cheeks, protrusion of the tongue, swallowing, or rarely, closing the other eye.

Systemic Features. None seem to be affected in this syndrome.

Differential Diagnosis. The winking-jaw syndrome is manifest as a brisk movement of the mandible to the contralateral side when the cornea is touched (Fig. 7.71). Both these syndromes are considered to be release phenomena, probably due to a supranuclear lesion that reunites the orbicularis oculi and external pterygoid muscles.

Laboratory Aids. None known.

Synonyms. Marcus Gunn syndrome, inverse Marcus Gunn syndrome.

References

Feric-Seiwerth F, et al: Marcus-Gunn Syndrome. *Klin Monatsbl Augenheilkd* 154:519–524, 1969.

Jancar J: Inverse jaw-winking with exaggerated Bell's phenomenon. *Ophthalmologica* 151:548–554, 1966.

Kirkham TH: Familial Marcus Gunn phenomenon. *Br J Ophthalmol* 53:282–283, 1969.

Glossary of Dental Terms

Alveolus	Cavity within alveolar bone that contains the roots of the teeth.
Angular cheilosis	*See* cheilosis.
Ankyloglossia	Tongue-tie due to anterior attachment or hyperplasia of lingual frenulum.
Anodontia	Total developmental absence of teeth.
Attrition	Physiological wear of the hard dental tissues, especially the enamel.
Bite, open	Similar to malocclusion, type III.
Cheilitis	Inflammation of the lip(s).
Cheiloplasty	Generally refers to surgical repair of cleft lip.
Cheilosis, angular	Cracking of labial commissures, generally secondarily infected with Candida albicans.
Cryptodontia	Multiple intrabony retention of teeth.
Cyst, dentigerous	A developmental cyst associated with an impacted tooth, the tooth crown being in the cyst cavity.
Cyst, radicular	An inflammatory cyst attached to the periapical portion of the tooth root.
Dentigerous cyst	*See* cyst.
Dentin, interglobular	The dentin that calcifies in a globular pattern. Normally seen in the root and occasionally the crown.
Dentin, mantle	The layer of dentin that is formed first. In a fully developed tooth, the layer of dentin immediately below the enamel.
Halitosis	Bad breath.
Horns, pulp	*See* pulp.
Interglobular dentin	*See* dentin.
Macroglossia	Large tongue.
Mantle dentin	*See* dentin.
Microdontia	Small teeth.
Micrognathia	Small mandible.
Odontoma	Hamartomatous lesion characterized by formation of either small denticles or haphazardly arranged hard and soft dental tissues.
Oligodontia	Marked developmental suppression of teeth formation.
Peg lateral	Maxillary lateral incisor with peg crown form.
Prognathism	Generally refers to protruding mandible. Relative prognathism used for cases in which the mandible is normal and the maxilla is hypoplastic.
Pulp horns	Extension of the dental pulp into the cusp areas.
Pulp stones	Deposits of amorphous calcification within the dental pulp.
Radicular cyst	*See* cyst.
Retrognathia	Receded mandible due to small size.

Syngnathia	Fused mouth due to fibrous or bony adhesions between maxilla and mandible.
Taurodontism	Molars, less often premolars, are generally square with large pulp chambers and pyramidal roots.
Vertical dimension	The normal distance between maxilla and mandible attained by holding the mandible in a relaxed position with the lips closed.
Xerostomia	Dry mouth.

Photo Credits

Fig. 1.5 W. G. Young, Minneapolis, MN.
Fig. 1.6 From Gorlin & Goldman, eds., *Thomas's Oral Pathology*, ed. 6, 1970, C. V. Mosby Co., St. Louis, MO, U.S.A.
Fig. 1.15 W. G. Young, Minneapolis, MN.
Fig. 1.22 R. Bevis, Minneapolis, MN.
Fig. 1.23 R. Bevis, Minneapolis, MN.
Figs. 1.24–Fig. 1.29 J. Brand, Minneapolis, MN.
Figs. 2.4–2.5 C. J. Witkop, Jr., Minneapolis, MN.
Fig. 2.1 D. Waite, Minneapolis, MN.
Fig. 2.3 I. Schübel, Munich, Germany
Figs. 2.6–2.8 C. J. Witkop, Jr., Minneapolis, MN.
Fig. 2.11 C. J. Witkop, Jr., Minneapolis, MN.
Figs. 3.2–3.4 From Goodman and Gorlin, *Atlas of the Face in Genetic Disorders*, ed. 2, 1977, The C. V. Mosby Co., St. Louis, MO, U.S.A.
Figs. 3.5–3.6 From Gorlin and Sedano, *Modern Medicine* ©, 1971 by Harcourt Brace Jovanovich, Inc.
Figs. 3.7–3.8 From Hudson, C. D. & Witkop, C. J., Jr.: Autosomal dominant hypodontia with nail dysgenesis, & Oral Surg. Oral Med. Oral Pathol. *39:* 409–423, 1975.
Fig. 3.9 From Gorlin & Sedano, *Modern Medicine,* © 1971 by Harcourt Brace Jovanovich, Inc.
Fig. 3.12 From Archard, H. O. and Witkop, C. J., Jr., Hereditary hypophosphatemia (vitamin D-resistant rickets) presenting primary dental manifestations, Oral Surg. Oral Med. Oral Pathol. *22:* 184–193, 1966.
Fig. 3.13 C. J. Witkop, Jr., Minneapolis, MN.
Fig. 3.14 From Witkop, C. J., Jr., *Scweiz Monatschr. Zahnheilkd.* 82: 917, 1972
Figs. 3.22–3.23 From Witkop, C. J., Jr., et al.: Globodontia in the otodental syndrome, Oral Surg. Oral Med. Oral Pathol. *41:* 472–483, 1976
Fig. 3.25 R. Bruckner, Portland, Oregon
Fig. 3.28 J. M. Moragas, Barcelona, Spain, through W. Reed, Burbank, CA.
Fig. 3.29 J. M. Moragas, Barcelona, Spain, through W. Reed, Burbank, California, from Gorlin & Sedano *Modern Medicine,* © 1973 by Harcourt Brace Jovanovich, Inc.
Fig. 4.1 From Gorlin & Sedano, *Modern Medicine,* © 1970 by Harcourt Brace Jovanovich, Inc.
Fig. 4.2 From J. Keutel et al., *Z. Kinderheilkd.* 101: 165–180, 1967.
Fig. 4.4 P. Weary, Charlottesville, VA.
Fig. 4.9 From Gorlin & Sedano, *Modern Medicine,* © 1971 by Harcourt Brace Jovanovich, Inc.
Figs. 4.10 & 4.11 From Goodman and Gorlin, *Atlas of the Face in Genetic Disorders,* ed. 2, 1977, the C. V. Mosby Co., St. Louis, MO., U.S.A.
Figs. 4.15–4.16 From Gorlin & Sedano, *Modern Medicine,* © 1968 by Harcourt Brace Jovanovich, Inc.
Fig. 4.17 P. F. LaBand, San Francisco, CA.
Fig. 4.18 C. J. Witkop, Jr., Minneapolis, MN.
Fig. 4.19 G. B. Winter, London, England.
Figs. 4.21–4.22 From E. Drescher et al., *J. Pediatr. Surg.* 2: 427, 1967.
Figs. 4.23–4.24 C. J. Witkop, Jr., Minneapolis, MN.
Fig. 4.25 From Gorlin & Sedano, *Modern Medicine,* © 1968 by Harcourt Brace Jovanovich, Inc.
Fig. 4.27 C. J. Witkop, Jr., Minneapolis, MN.
Fig. 4.30 W. B. Reed, Burbank, CA., from Gorlin & Sedano, *Modern Medicine,* © 1972 by Harcourt Brace Jovanovich, Inc.
Fig. 4.31 From Homans, John, *A Textbook of Surgery,* 6th ed., 1945. Courtesy Charles C. Thomas, Publisher, Springfield, IL.
Figs. 4.35–4.36 From Goodman and Gorlin, *Atlas of the Face n Genetic Disorders,* ed. 2, 1977, The C. V. Mosby Co., St. Louis, MO, U.S.A.
Fig. 4.38 D. Rimoin, Los Angeles, California.
Fig. 4.39 From Pietruschka, G. et al., **Klin. Mbl. Augenheil k** 54: 525, 1969.
Fig. 4.43 From Gorlin & Sedano, *Modern Medicine,* © 1969 by Harcourt Brace Jovanovich, Inc.
Figs. 4.46–4.47 From Eddy, D. D. and Farber, E. M., *Arch. Dermatol.* 86: 729. Copyright 1962, American Medical Association.
Fig. 4.48 W. B. Reed, Burbank, CA, from Gorlin & Sedano, *Modern Medicine,* © 1970 by Harcourt Brace Jovanovich, Inc.
Fig. 4.49 C. J. Witkop, Jr., Minneapolis, MN.
Fig. 4.50 C. Lopez, Guatemala City, Guatemala.
Figs. 4.51–4.52 From Gorlin & Sedano, *Modern Medicine,* © by Harcourt Brace Jovanovich, Inc.
Fig. 4.53 M. M. Cohen, Jr., Seattle, WA.
Figs. 5.4–5.5 J. E. Jan, Vancouver, Canada.
Figs. 5.6–5.8 From Gorlin & Sedano, *Modern Medicine,* © 1972 by Harcourt Brace Jovanovich, Inc.
Fig. 5.9 From Gorlin & Sedano, *Modern Medicine,* © 1971 by Harcourt Brace Jovanovich, Inc.
Fig. 5.13 From Gorlin & Sedano, *Modern Medicine,* © 1968 by Harcourt Brace Jovanovich, Inc.
Fig. 5.14 From Millard, D. R., Jr. et al., *Amer. J. Surg.* 113: 615, 1967.
Fig. 5.15 From Macpherson, R. I., *J. Canad. Assoc. Radiol.* 25: 22, 1974.
Fig. 5.16 From Gorlin & Sedano, *Modern Medicine,* © 1972 by Harcourt Brace Jovanovich, Inc.
Figs. 5.20–5.21 from Wilner, H. I. and Finby, N., *J.A.M.A.* 187: 490. Copyright 1964, American Medical Association.
Figs. 5.25–5.26 From Schumacher, H. P., *Z. Kinderheilk.* 105: 88, 1969.
Fig. 5.27 From Gorlin & Sedano, *Modern Medicine,* © 1972 by Harcourt Brace Jovanovich, Inc.
Fig. 6.3 From Gorlin & Sedano, *Modern Medicine,* © 1972 by Harcourt Brace Jovanovich, Inc.
Fig. 6.10 R. A. Rüdiger, Hamburg, Germany.
Fig. 6.11 From Gorlin & Sedano, *Modern Medicine,* © 1972 by Harcourt Brace Jovanovich, Inc.
Fig. 6.12 N. Fitch, Montreal, Canada.
Fig. 6.13 From Gorlin & Sedano, *Modern Medicine,* © 1973 by Harcourt Brace Jovanovich, Inc.
Fig. 7.2 From Gorlin & Sedano, *Modern Medicine,* © 1968 by Harcourt Brace Jovanovich, Inc.
Fig. 7.3 From Forland, M., *Amer. J. Med.* 33: 792, 1962.
Fig. 7.4 From Gorlin & Sedano, *Modern Medicine,* © 1968 by Harcourt Brace Jovanovich, Inc.
Fig. 7.5 R. Noonan, Louisville, KY, from Gorlin & Sedano, *Modern Medicine,* © 1971 by Harcourt Brace Jovanovich, Inc.
Figs. 7.6–7.7 From Gorlin , R. J. and Cohen, M. M., Jr., *Amer. J. Dis. Child.* 118: 487, 1969.
Fig. 7.10 From Opitz, J. M. et al., The BBB Syndrome: Familial telecanthus with associated congenital abnormalities. In Bergsma D. (ed.): Part II. "Mallamation Syndromes." White Plains: The National Foundation–March of Dimes BD:OAS V(2) 86–94, 1969.
Fig. 7.15 From Gorlin & Pindborg, *Syndromes of the Head and Neck,* Copyright 1964 by. Used with permission of McGraw-Hill Book Company.
Figs. 7.18–7.19 Weisskopf, Louisville, KY.
Fig. 7.20 From Shuler, S. E., *Arch. Dis. Child.* 38: 629, 1963.
Fig. 7.21 From Frandsen, E., *Acta Ophthalmol. (Kbh)* 41: 757, 1963.
Figs. 7.22–7.23 From Gorlin & Sedano, *Modern Medicine,* © 1972 by Harcourt Brace Jovanovich, Inc.
Fig. 7.24 From Crawford, J. L., *J. Dent. Child.* 37: 171, 1970.
Fig. 7.26 From Gorlin & Sedano, *Modern Medicine,* © 1968 by Harcourt Brace Jovanovich, Inc.
Fig. 7.28 C. J. Witkop, Jr., Minneapolis, MN.
Fig. 7.29 From Rodermund, O. E., *Dermatol. Wochenschr.* 153: 350, 1967.
Fig. 7.30 A. Lodin, Stockholm, Sweden.
Fig. 7.32 From Winstock, D., *Br. J. Dermatol.* 74: 431, 1962.
Fig. 7.35 From Gorlin & Sedano, *Modern Medicine,* © 1969 by Harcourt Brace Jovanovich, Inc.
Figs. 7.37–7.38 From Galili, D. et al., Massive gingival hyperplasia preceding dental eruption in I-cell disease, Oral Surg. Oral Med. Oral Pathol. *37:* 533–539, 1974.
Fig. 7.39 From Harper, P. S. et al., *J. Med. Genet.* 11: 123, 1974.
Fig. 7.41 C. H. Ide and P. B. Wollschlaeger, Columbia, MO, from Gorlin & Sedano, *Modern Medicine,* © 1969 by Harcourt Brace Jovanovich, Inc.
Figs. 7.42–7.43 C. J. Witkop, Jr., Minneapolis, MN.
Figs. 7.45–7.46 From Gorlin & Sedano, *Modern Medicine,* © 1972 by Harcourt Brace Jovanovich, Inc.
Fig. 7.48 From Gorlin & Sedano, *Modern Medicine,* © 1970 by Harcourt Brace Jovanovich, Inc.
Fig. 7.52 A & B From Grosse, R. et al., *Z. Kinderheilk.* 110: 1757, 1971.
Figs. 7.53 & 7.55 From P. E. Beighton, *The Ehlers-Danlos Syndrome,* William Heinemann Med. Books Ltd., London, England, 1972
Fig. 7.56 M. Robinow, Yellow Springs, OH.
Fig. 7.57 R. Goltz, Minneapolis, MN, from Goodman-Gorlin, *Atlas of the Face in Genetic Disorders,* ed. 2, 1977, The C. V. Mosby Co., St. Louis, MO, U.S.A.
Fig. 7.58 L. D. Ginsburg, Long Beach, CA.
Fig. 7.65 From Worth, H. M.: Hurler's syndrome A Study of radiologic appearances in the jaws, Oral Surg, Oral Med, Oral Pathol. *22:* 21–35, 1966.
Fig. 7.65 From Worth, H. M.: Hurler's syndrome A Study of radiologic appearances in the jaws, Oral Surg, Oral Med. Oral Pathol. *22:* 21–35, 1966.
Fig. 7.67 From Gorlin, R. J. and Psaume, J., *J. Pediat.* 61: 520, 1962.
Fig. 7.69 From Thurston, E. O., *Lancet* 2: 996, 1909.
Fig. 7.70 From Kanter, D., *Klin. Monatsbl. Augenheilk.* 126: 50, 1955.
Fig. 7.71 From Jancar, J., *Ophthalmologica (Basel)* 151: 548, 1966.

INDEX